Katherine L. Applegate, Ph.D.
Duke University Medical Center
Durham, NC 27710

GROUP PSYCHOTHERAPY
FOR PSYCHOLOGICAL TRAUMA

Group Psychotherapy for Psychological Trauma

ROBERT H. KLEIN
VICTOR L. SCHERMER

Editors

Foreword by K. Roy MacKenzie

THE GUILFORD PRESS
New York   London

© 2000 The Guilford Press
A Division of Guilford Publications, Inc.
72 Spring Street, New York, NY 10012
www.guilford.com

Printed in the United States of America

This book is printed on acid-free paper.

Last digit is print number: 9 8 7 6 5 4 3 2 1

Library of Congress Cataloging-in-Publication Data

Group psychotherapy for psychological trauma / Robert H. Klein, Victor L.
     Schermer, editors.
       p. cm.
  Includes bibliographical references and index.
  ISBN 1-57230-557-6 (hc : alk. paper)
     1. Post-traumatic stress disorder—Treatment. 2. Group psychotherapy.
  3. Psychic trauma—Treatment. I. Klein, Robert H. II. Schermer, Victor L.
  RC552.P67 G76 2000
  616.85′210651—dc21

                                                                00-027240

To our families and our patients—
whose gifts to us remain beyond value

and

To Dan Gottlieb, PhD, psychologist, esteemed
and beloved colleague, host of the radio
program "Voices in the Family"—who teaches
us to work together to address our personal
and collective trauma

About the Editors

Robert H. Klein, PhD, CGP, FAGPA, is Clinical Associate Professor of Psychiatry at the Yale University School of Medicine, New Haven, Connecticut, and maintains a private practice in Milford and Westport, Connecticut. An internationally recognized author, researcher, lecturer, and clinical supervisor in the area of group psychotherapy, he is coeditor of *The Handbook of Contemporary Group Psychotherapy* and has developed group psychotherapy training programs at several leading medical schools. In addition to maintaining a private practice of more than 30 years, he has directed inpatient, outpatient, and day hospital treatment programs. A Fellow of the American Group Psychotherapy Association (AGPA) and a founding member of the National Registry of Certified Group Psychotherapists, he has served as an elected member of the AGPA board of directors and the Nominating Committee. Currently, he is the secretary of the AGPA and cochair of its annual meeting, and serves on the board of directors of the Group Psychotherapy Foundation and the editorial review boards for the *International Journal of Group Psychotherapy* and *Group Dynamics*. Dr. Klein has had extensive clinical experience working with problems of trauma, grief, and loss, and has supervised therapists leading groups for incest survivors.

Victor L. Schermer, MA, CAC, is a psychologist in private practice and clinic settings in Philadelphia, Pennsylvania. He is executive director of the Study Group for Contemporary Psychoanalytic Process and director of the Institute for the Study of Human Conflict, and has sponsored three major conferences on psychological trauma. He has served as director of outpatient services at Mirmont Treatment Center, and as a faculty member of the Institute for Psychoanalytic Psychotherapies. He is coauthor of *Object Relations, the Self, and the Group*, coeditor of *Ring of Fire*, and coeditor of *Group Psychotherapy of the Psychoses*. He coauthored a chapter in *The Handbook of Contemporary Group Psychotherapy* and has contributed to journals in psychoanalysis and psychotherapy. He is a clinical member of the American Group Psychotherapy Association and has given numerous workshops and training institutes at the International and American Group Psychotherapy Associations.

Contributors

Harold S. Bernard, PhD, CGP, FAGPA, is Clinical Associate Professor of Psychiatry at New York University (NYU) School of Medicine. He ran the Group Psychotherapy Program at NYU/Bellevue Medical Center for 14 years. He coedited *The Handbook of Contemporary Group Psychotherapy* and *Basics of Group Psychotherapy,* and is the author of many papers and book chapters about group psychotherapy. He was editor of *The Group Circle* from 1995 to 1999, and book review editor of the *International Journal of Group Psychotherapy* from 1989 to 1996. Dr. Bernard is a diplomate in group psychology of the American Board of Professional Psychology, and is president-elect of the American Group Psychotherapy Association. He maintains private practices in New York City and in Westport, Connecticut.

Bonnie J. Buchele, PhD, ABPP, CGP, FAGPA, is in private practice in Kansas City, Missouri. She is president of the American Group Psychotherapy Association and a practicing psychoanalyst. She has worked extensively in treating traumatized individuals and is coauthor (with Ramon Ganzarain) of *Fugitives of Incest.*

Mark L. Dembert, MD, MPH, CGP, is currently a captain in the U.S. Navy Medical Corps and a staff member of the Psychiatry Department at Naval Medical Center, Portsmouth, Virginia (NMCP), where he heads group psychotherapy training and practice. He is assistant head of the Special Psychiatric Rapid Intervention (SPRINT) Team 2, based at NMCP. He is Assistant Professor in the Departments of Psychiatry at Uniformed Services University of the Health Sciences, Bethesda, Maryland, and Eastern Virginia Medical School, Norfolk, Virginia. He is a member of the American Psychiatric Association, the American Group Psychotherapy Association, and the National Registry of Certified Group Psychotherapists.

Catherine G. Fine, PhD, is a clinical psychologist in private practice in Blue Bell and Bala Cynwyd, Pennsylvania. She is Clinical Assistant Professor of Psychiatry at Temple University Medical School. She is the cofounder (with Nancy E. Madden) and current president of Jaria, Inc., a center for the study of dissociative disorders. She is a member of the American Psychological Association, the American Anthropological Association, the Society for the Anthropology of Consciousness, the Greater Philadelphia Society of Clinical Hypnosis (of which she is past president), and the International Society for the Study of Traumatic Stress (on whose Board of Directors she served for 3 years). Dr. Fine is a Fellow of the Pennsylvania Psychological Association, the International Society for the Study of Dissociation, and the American Society of Clinical Hypnosis (she is past president of the latter two groups). She has taught and published nationally and internationally on the topics of posttraumatic stress disorder (PTSD) and dissociative disorders, and is the author of numerous articles, book chapters, and protocols for the structured and paced treatment of these disorders.

Richard E. Gallagher, MD, is in private practice in Hawthorne, New York. He is Associate Professor of Clinical Psychiatry at New York Medical College and the director of the Comprehensive Psychiatry Emergency Program at the Westchester Medical Center's Behavioral Health Center. He is a member of the American Psychiatric Association and the American Psychoanalytic Association and is on the faculty of the Columbia Psychoanalytic Institute. He has been a faculty member at Cornell University Medical College, has lectured and published widely in the area of abuse and other trauma, and has been published in the *Journal of Personality Disorders*, the *Bulletin of the Menninger Clinic*, and the *International Journal of Group Psychotherapy*, among others.

Ramon Ganzarain, MD, CGP, FAGPA, is a training analyst at the Emory University Psychoanalytic Institute and Associate Professor of Psychiatry at Emory University School of Medicine, Atlanta, Georgia. He is a member of the International Psychoanalytic Association and the International Association of Group Psychotherapy, and has twice been elected a member of the American Group Psychotherapy Association's board of directors. He is former director of Group Psychotherapy Services of the Menninger Clinic, Topeka, Kansas. He is author of *Object Relations Group Psychotherapy* and coauthor (with Bonnie J. Buchele) of *Fugitives of Incest*. He is a frequent contributor of articles for books and scholarly journals.

Marianne Goodman, MD, has published articles in the *International Journal of Group Psychotherapy* on trauma group psychotherapy for incest survivors, and double traumata of war and childhood abuse in Vietnam veterans. She has been a faculty member at Cornell University Medical College. Currently she is Assistant Professor of Psychiatry at Mount Sinai School of Medicine, New York, New York.

Elizabeth Hegeman, PhD, is Professor of Anthropology at John Jay College of Criminal Justice, City University of New York, and a clinical psychologist in private practice in New York City. She is a member of the Council of Fellows of the William Alanson White Institute of Psychiatry, Psychology and Psychoanalysis, and president of the William Alanson White Society for 2000–2001. She is coauthor (with Michael Stocker) of *Valuing Emotions*.

David Read Johnson, PhD, CGP, is codirector of the Post Traumatic Stress Center, New Haven, Connecticut; Associate Clinical Professor in the Department of Psychiatry at Yale University School of Medicine; and former chief of the Specialized Inpatient PTSD Unit, National Center for PTSD, Veterans Affairs Medical Center, West Haven, Connecticut.

Gloria Batkin Kahn, PhD, CGP, FAGPA, has been in private practice in Hartsdale, New York, for 22 years. She is a diplomate in group psychology of the American Board of Professional Psychology, a Fellow of the American Group Psychotherapy Association (where she is cochair of the Child and Adolescent Special Interest Group), the president of the Westchester Group Psychotherapy Society, and a past president of the Westchester County Psychological Association. In 1997, she won the Westchester County Psychological Association Award for Distinguished Psychological Service.

Janis L. Keyser, PhD, has worked in the field of thanatology as a trainer, educator, grief counselor, and group facilitator for 20 years. She is director of The Center for Grieving Children, Teens and Families, and is also coordinator of the bereavement program at St. Christopher's Hospital for Children in Philadelphia, working with dying children, bereaved parents, siblings, and staff. She is director of UNITE, Inc., in Philadelphia, providing grief support after perinatal and neonatal death. She holds certificates as both a death educator and grief counselor from the Association for Death Education and Counseling (ADEC) and is chairperson of ADEC's special interest group on children's grief programs.

Howard D. Kibel, MD, CGP, DGAGPA, is in private practice in Valhalla, New York. He is Clinical Professor of Psychiatry at New York Medical College and an attending psychiatrist at Westchester Medical Center, also in Valhalla. He is a Fellow of the American Psychiatric Association, and a past president and Distinguished Fellow of the American Group Psychotherapy Association. He is a member of the board of directors of the International Association of Group Psychotherapy, and serves on the editorial boards of the *International Journal of Group Psychotherapy* and *GROUP, the Journal of the Eastern Group Psychotherapy Society.*

Robert H. Klein (*see* About the Editors).

Hadar Lubin, MD, is codirector of the Post Traumatic Stress Center, New Haven, Connecticut; Assistant Clinical Professor in the Department of Psychiatry at Yale University School of Medicine; and director of the Women's Trauma Program, New Haven, Connecticut, where she developed the interactive psychoeducational group psychotherapy model.

Nancy E. Madden, RN, MS, CS, is a psychiatric clinical nurse specialist in private practice in Blue Bell, Pennsylvania. She is the cofounder (with Catherine G. Fine) and current vice president of Jaria, Inc. She is also cofounder, with Dr. Fine, of the first outpatient psychotherapy group for adults with dissociative identity disorder (DID). She participated in designing one of the first inpatient treatment programs for patients with DID and in training the varied staff members. She is a member of the International Society for the Study of Dissociation, the Advanced Nurse Practice Group of Pennsylvania, and the American Psychological Association. She has served as a consultant to various agencies on the diagnosis and treatment of dissociative pathology, and has given presentations around the country on these issues.

Myrna Marcus, MA, MSS, is a psychotherapist in private practice in Jenkintown, Pennsylvania. A graduate of the Bryn Mawr College Graduate School of Social Work and Social Research, she is currently a PhD candidate at the Fielding Institute. She is a member of the board of directors of the Philadelphia Area Group Psychotherapy Society, and area delegate to the American Group Psychotherapy Association Affiliate Assembly. For the past 22 years, she has worked in individual and group psychotherapy with chronically and terminally ill patients.

Maureen McEvoy, MA, is in private practice in Vancouver, British Columbia, Canada, and has 20 years of experience working with childhood and adult survivors of trauma, in both individual and group settings. She has lectured and written extensively on trauma and dissociation, group work, and legal issues facing mental health practitioners. She is a long-standing instructor with the Justice Institute of British Columbia. Her group experience includes survivors of childhood abuse, war refugees, domestic assault victims, aboriginal groups, and women sexually assaulted by mental health professionals.

Victor L. Schermer (*see* About the Editors).

Kathy Seelaus, ACSW, LSW, has practiced clinical social work for 19 years in Pennsylvania and New Jersey. She has a private practice, and is Adjunct Professor of Social Work at Rutgers, the State University of New Jersey. Currently, she works with people with disabilities at Inglis House in Philadelphia. Previously, she has worked in protective services for children; with the Elder Abuse Project of Delaware County; in early intervention with children to prevent abuse and neglect; and in family counseling. Her work with bereavement includes counseling services to families that have lost children to sudden infant death syndrome; to survivors of homicide victims, and to children in the Philadelphia hospital and school systems who have experienced traumatic losses.

Edward D. Simmer, MD, is currently a lieutenant commander in the Navy Medical Corps and is a staff member of the Psychiatry Department at Naval Medical Center, Portsmouth, Virginia (NMCP), where he heads the outpatient psychiatric clinic and the division of forensic psychiatry, as well as the Navy's Special Psychiatric Rapid Intervention (SPRINT) Team 2, based at NMCP. He is Adjunct Professor of Biology at Tidewater Community College, Portsmouth, Virginia, and is a member of the American Psychiatric Association, the American Group Psychotherapy Association, and the National Registry of Certified Group Psychotherapists.

Andreas von Wallenberg Pachaly, Dipl.-Psych., Klin.-Psych., is director of the Free Counseling Center for Psychotherapy in Dusseldorf, Germany, and maintains a private group-analytic and psychoanalytic practice in Dusseldorf. He is head of the therapeutic community "Haus Steprath," and founder of the "Therapeutic Community within the Community." He is a member of Amnesty International's German standing conference of medical doctors and psychologists for the treatment of victims of torture. His special interests include therapeutic communities; sheltered living as a community-centered, group-therapeutic approach; the psychotherapy of psychosis; and the application of group dynamics to the understanding of social processes.

Daniel Weiss, PhD, is Professor of Medical Psychology in the Department of Psychiatry at the University of California–San Francisco, and director of research of the PTSD Program at the San Francisco Veterans Affairs Medical Center. He has funding from the National Institute of Mental Health to study the development of group treatments for PTSD, and has served the Department of Veterans Affairs central office as a consultant for research on the treatment of PTSD.

Agnes Wohl, CSW, is in private practice in Great Neck, New York, and specializes in issues surrounding child sexual abuse. She is former clinical director of the Queens Child Guidance Center, and (with Bobbie Kaufman) coauthor of *Silent Screams and Hidden Cries* and *Casualties of Childhood*.

Maggie Ziegler, MA, is currently in private practice in Vancouver, British Columbia, Canada. She has provided individual and group treatment to trauma survivors for 20 years in a variety of settings. Since 1990, she has been teaching in the Justice Institute of British Columbia's sexual abuse and trauma programs. Her group experience includes survivors of childhood abuse, war and political refugees, and domestic assault victims.

Foreword

This book is unique in its capacity to combine two major theoretical and clinical areas. The first of these is recognition of the multifaceted aspects of trauma and the need for a careful adaptation of treatment to ensure effective management of severely traumatized patients. The second is a deep understanding of the group environment and an appreciation of its power as well as its possible liabilities. Recent surveys clearly indicate the role of trauma in a wide variety of psychiatric conditions. This book provides a comprehensive coverage of the emerging diversity within the field.

The five chapters of Part I provide an in-depth review of the clinical concept of trauma and its manifestations, as well as the principles of treatment. The material can be applied with varying intensity to a broad range of circumstances. This parallels the "common factors" psychotherapy literature that identifies basic management strategies that form the foundation of effective treatment. The effects of trauma are found throughout the practice of psychotherapy, and the material in Part I can be usefully applied to a range of patients who may not be specifically diagnosed with a trauma syndrome.

Klein and Schermer provide a fine overview in their opening chapter, which highlights the impact of traumatic experiences on the quality of interpersonal functioning and on views of the self. This relational focus on cognitive-affective deficits is carefully distinguished from a preoccupation with intrapsychic phenomena, a theme that is pursued throughout the book. The use of the group modality is introduced with an overview of the types of groups appropriate for various phases of treatment and for a variety of patient populations. This perspective is an important one, as groups can be developed for a wide range of specific purposes. Basic themes found in trauma groups are carefully described as well as the impact of the whole group environment. This material, expanded in later chapters, forewarns the clinician with a clear set of crucial issues to be monitored in the treatment of this challenging patient population.

Chapter 2 by Goodman and Weiss focuses on various aspects of the group frame. Since trauma by its very nature implies the violation of a boundary, maintenance of a secure frame is an essential task for the trauma therapist. One aspect of the frame is a clear decision regarding the nature of the group and selection of members according to that decision. It is useful to consider a range of intensities beginning with brief structured cognitive-behavioral models, through a detailed focus on the trauma itself, and then a more general group to deal with the relational difficulty that frequently accompanies trauma. A closely related issue is the responsibility of the therapists to control the pace of disclosure and its impact both on the individual and the other group members. It is to be expected that challenges to the frame will occur and must become an important focus for therapeutic activity. These issues are common to all therapy groups but require particular attention in groups with higher levels of psychopathology. It is therefore important for therapists in trauma groups to have an advanced grounding in the general principles and techniques of group psychotherapy.

Hegeman and Wohl take a different perspective in Chapter 3, where they discuss a number of theories and techniques that are unique to the management of trauma-related conditions. These center primarily on the phenomena of dissociation and reenactment, both of which may be misinterpreted as resistance. They make the important point that responding to these predictable patterns with interpretations or seeing them as evidence of internal drives or conflicts may create an atmosphere in which the patient feels blamed and misunderstood. Rather these phenomena need to be understood as trauma-precipitated states that represent an effort to maintain control.

This material provides an important perspective on adapting group psychotherapy to the target population. The focus on mastery and the use of cognitive-behavioral strategies along with an interpersonal focus runs parallel with the current literature concerning the treatment of major personality disorder, especially borderline phenomena. The dysfunctional cognitive and behavioral patterns seen with borderline patients have a significant heritable component, which provides a rationale for a self-mastery focus rather than a purely interpretive approach. Trauma also may produce aberrant physiological and memory function. So it is interesting to see the emergence of parallel treatment strategies emphasizing the integration of cognitive-behavioral and relational therapeutic principles. A borderline disposition is likely to magnify the response to trauma when both exist, a not uncommon occurrence.

In Chapter 4, Ganzarain describes how the group as a whole can be the source or target of powerful transferential and countertransferential forces. The use of projective identification and splitting mechanisms is highlighted in particular.

In Chapter 5, Ziegler and McEvoy deal with the critical issue of therapist countertransference reactions. Trauma groups place a heavy burden on the therapist to contain and master very understandable personal reactions to abhorrent material—the therapist must be able to contain this information and manage it in a technically correct manner. The use of cotherapists is recommended for these groups since this will enable the therapists to support, criticize, empathize, and resolve tensions or errors together. This chapter also makes it abundantly clear why trauma groups require mature and experienced cotherapists who know about the trauma treatment literature. And it contains the implicit message that being a trauma recipient is not in itself an adequate preparation to lead intensive groups; indeed it places an even greater onus on mastering countertransference reactions.

Part II describes in detail the techniques developed for specialized groups adapted for the treatment of a wide range of special subpopulations within the trauma field. This format is in keeping with a broader movement in current psychotherapy toward the development of specific treatment models for specific purposes. Despite the fact that all of the models in the book deal with the treatment of trauma, the range of applications and the variation in specific techniques gives each chapter a new perspective. It is particularly gratifying to see the range of theoretical perspectives presented back to back. The treatment of more difficult patient populations is clearly moving toward an integrated approach often starting with more structure to develop a base of mastery and then moving into interpersonal or psychodynamic models to focus on relationships and stability of the self. The treatment of violent offenders, many of whom have severely traumatic backgrounds themselves, has also moved in this direction, though this population is not addressed in the book apart from brief mention by Gallagher and Kibel in Chapter 13. The increasing application of an integrated approach has had the beneficial effect of decreasing the sense of competition or alienation between cognitive-behavioral and interpersonal–psychodynamic clinicians that has unfortunately characterized the field for several decades.

This book provides a number of well-described models, many of them approaching the level of a clinical manual. The development of these is to be welcomed despite the negative reaction that the word "manual" sometimes elicits. The diversity within the material presented here indicates the importance of specific models even for the subcategories within the trauma field. Nevertheless, with a small number of exceptions, there is a disappointing absence of empirical validation for most of these models. This provides an important challenge for the field, as such validation of effectiveness is increasingly expected.

The treatment of severe trauma is a specialized area that places heavy demands on therapists. Fortunately, this book provides clinicians with clear guidelines they need to try to meet these demands.

K. ROY MACKENZIE, MD
University of British Columbia, Vancouver

Acknowledgments

For over 20 years, the editors of this book have been psychologists with a general practice in psychotherapy and clinic settings with a broad-based heterogeneous population and a special interest in group psychotherapy, object relations theory, and self psychology. Both of us have been deeply involved in the American Group Psychotherapy Association, and one of us (Klein) has held office and is a Fellow in this organization.

We did not begin our careers as trauma therapists. Rather, we are psychoanalytically trained therapists who only gradually came to see the deep and lasting impact of trauma on many of our patients, especially those with diagnoses such as major depression, substance dependence, borderline personality disorder, and narcissistic personality disorder, among others. As we strove to be true to our clinical experience, we increasingly saw the need, in particular, to bring an understanding of psychological trauma and its impact to group therapies of diverse orientations and practices. For example, our study of the work on trauma of Drs. Judith Herman, Earl Hopper, Bessel van der Kolk, David and Jill Scharff, and Leonard Shengold had a special impact on our theoretical understanding and on our clinical work. We felt it imperative that group psychotherapists incorporate this body of knowledge into their efforts so that they would not miss opportunities for healing with traumatized patients in all groups that they conduct.

We are therefore grateful to our colleagues in the fields of group psychotherapy, psychoanalysis, and psychological trauma whose work informs and inspires these pages. Colleagues such as Maurice Apprey, Christopher Bollas, Daniel Gottlieb, James S. Grotstein, Jeffrey Kauffman, Otto Kernberg, Laurie Anne Pearlman, Malcolm Pines, Therese Rando, Cecil Rice, Karen Saakvitne, John Sonne, Walter Stone, Vamik Volkan, and Stan Zuckerman come to mind especially as we think about our collegial associations over the past years.

Special thanks are due Drs. Earl Hopper and Richard Kluft for their helpful comments and suggestions. Dr. Hopper kindly critiqued a preliminary draft of the introductory chapter, with special attention to his "fourth basic assumption," and Dr. Kluft, a foremost authority on dissociative disorders, provided his thoughts from a manuscript in preparation.

We are indebted as well to the chapter authors of this volume, whose clinical and theoretical knowledge and skills are indeed awesome, for their deep devotion and commitment and for their efforts in producing this book despite their heavily committed schedules.

In creating a book, there are inevitably a cadre of unsung heroes including those who guide the authors through the creative process; edit raw copy into a polished, publishable form; and provide a variety of supports in numerous ways. In this venture, we are especially grateful to Editor-in-Chief Seymour Weingarten, our Editor, Rochelle Serwator, and production editors Anna Nelson and Laura Patchkofsky, at The Guilford Press, for their consistent support and unstinting efforts throughout the creation and production of this volume.

Above all, we would like to thank our patients, who have allowed us to witness their trauma, their wounds, and their deepest selves, and who have helped us to determine the sources of both hurt and healing that are part of all our lives.

Contents

PART II. Special Populations
and Trauma Groups

PART I

CONCEPTS, THEORIES, AND STRATEGIES

1

---<o>---

Introduction and Overview: Creating a Healing Matrix

ROBERT H. KLEIN
VICTOR L. SCHERMER

> Creating a protected space where survivors can speak the truth is an act of liberation.
> —JUDITH HERMAN (1997, p. 247)

Over the past two decades, profound interest in psychological trauma has been rekindled. This resurgence follows the better part of a century when, after Freud (1898/1962) had rejected the infantile seduction theory, trauma virtually faded into the background as a subject of inquiry and treatment—with some notable exceptions, such as work on the so-called "war neuroses" (Freud, 1920/1955; Kardiner, 1941; Grinker & Spiegel, 1945), and the writings of Ferenczi (1932/1980; see also Aron & Harris, 1993) and Lindemann (1944). Now, in the new millennium, we can expect trauma to command still greater interest as personal trauma and community catastrophes come into increased awareness within the closely linked global village, and as biological, psychological, and social research converge on new findings and treatment options.

Recent studies (Herman, 1997, p. 122) indicating that 50–60% of all psychiatric patients and 40–60% of outpatients report childhood histories of physical or sexual abuse or both (Jacobson & Richardson, 1987; Bryer, Nelson, Miller, & Krol, 1987; Jacobson, 1989; Briere & Runtz, 1987) ought to have alerted mental health practitioners to the importance of diagnosing and treating trauma. Therapists often overlook this key factor, however, partly because many traumatized patients come to treatment with a "disguised presentation" (Gelinas, 1983). They come for help because of their many symptoms or because of difficulty with relationships: problems in intimacy, excessive responsiveness to the needs of others, and repeated victimization. According to Herman (1997, p. 123), "all too often, neither patient nor therapist recognizes the link between the presenting problem and the history of chronic trauma."

As the subject of trauma had resumed importance in general psychiatry, a comparably significant and rapidly expanding interest in trauma treatment has emerged in *group* psychotherapy. This interest is evinced by the increasingly frequent appearance of articles on trauma groups,[1] as well as in the burgeoning development around the world of groups focused on victims of specific traumata: survivors of rape, sexual abuse, incest, spousal and child abuse, war, and political persecution; Holocaust victims and their children; and perpetrators of abuse (most of whom themselves were victims). The phenomena, the widening scope and more detailed knowledge of trauma sequelae, and the growing awareness of the high incidence and long-lasting impact of trauma all suggest the need for a thorough, in-depth look at group psychotherapy for psychological trauma. That is the aim of this volume. The contributors provide well-conceived group-centered and patient-oriented clinical strategies and techniques derived from a sound theoretical base, clinical experience, and a knowledge of trauma integrated with an in-depth understanding of group processes.

To orient the reader to the text, we first consider the nature of trauma and its impact upon the mind, emotions, and interpersonal relations. Knowledge of the sequelae of trauma points the way to effective treatment strategies. Then we address the group psychotherapy issues as such.

THE DEFINITION AND NATURE
OF PSYCHOLOGICAL TRAUMA

Defining Trauma

The powerful significance as well as the inherent complexity of trauma may be seen in attempts to define the concept itself. According to van der Kolk (1997), "Trauma, by definition, is the result of exposure to an inescapably stressful event that overwhelms a person's coping mechanisms" (n.p.). Such a seemingly clear-cut definition actually includes several areas of ambiguity and raises many important questions. Could "exposure" include hearing about the trauma from a patient or witnessing it on television or in a family member, in which case we could speak of "vicarious traumatization"? Was the trauma "inescapable" to a Holocaust victim who chose not to leave Germany (in cases, of course, when he or she might realistically have done so), or to a child who had an opportunity to ward off an incestuous or punitive parent but was afraid to do so?

How does one infer that a person's coping mechanisms have been overwhelmed? Does "overwhelmed" mean total immediate debilitation, or could it include an insidious social withdrawal and/or turning to self-mutilation or substance abuse some years later? Must the trauma consist of an unusual turn of life events, or can we speak of universal traumata, such as birth and the inevitability of separation, loss, and death? Variations of such definitions, which may be more or less inclusive, can be found throughout the literature on trauma. In general, for the purposes of this book, "trauma" refers operationally to a *situation-specific, severe,* and *stressful* violation or disruption that has *serious psychiatric consequences for the individual,* either soon or long after the event itself.

Trauma on a Continuum with Other Psychic Injuries

Our chapter authors see trauma as existing on a conceptual continuum with less overwhelming but nonetheless significant boundary violations, intrusions, deprivations, abandonments, absences, empathic failures, and major losses, which constitute the daily fare of so many human beings. In addition, in many families and societies, chronic dysfunction of a less catastrophic nature co-occurs with or constitutes the psychological "equivalent" of trauma. For example, one of us worked with a young adult male whose mother was often inappropriate with him in her language and touching, with sexual overtones and overstimulating physical contact. There were other disruptions in his life, such as parental quarrels and separation, and a sibling who was molested. This patient had many features of complex posttraumatic stress disorder (PTSD) (see Herman, 1997, pp. 115–129), yet there was no indication in his history of a specifically traumatic "event" as such.

On a theoretical level, a similar predicament occurs. Winnicott's understanding of "maternal impingement" (Rodman, 1990, pp. 25–26) and Kohut's (1977, pp. 116, 118) notion of "narcissistic injury," for example, are meant to address a broad spectrum of interpersonal "failures" and are not trauma-specific; yet trauma clearly involves impingements, deprivations, and narcissistic wounds (Scharff & Scharff, 1994). Therefore, clinically and theoretically a certain flexibility of definition is called for, whereas for research purposes it is important to distinguish clearly among different types of traumata and their specific effects.

Trauma-Related Diagnoses Other than PTSD

It is deceptively simple—and a common error in treatment planning—to limit the emotional sequelae of trauma exclusively to the diagnosis of PTSD. Certainly, a patient who fulfills the DSM-IV criteria for PTSD

(American Psychiatric Association, 1994, pp. 427–429) is a candidate for many of the groups described in this book. However, there exists a large population of individuals who come for treatment of other conditions (e.g., dissociative disorders, major depression, borderline personality disorder, and substance use disorders), but for whom a past or recent trauma has played a role (see especially Gallagher & Kibel, Chapter 13, this volume). Such patients frequently have long passed or circumvented the stage of full-blown PTSD; yet if the trauma is not addressed, they will remain impaired. Therefore, we have taken special care in this work to include groups not only for PTSD itself but also for syndromes where the trauma and its impact are "masked," multilayered, covered over, or transformed.

Trauma has a pervasive impact on the psychosocial life of the victim. In this volume, three broadly conceived frameworks are utilized to describe the nature of this impact and to formulate group strategies and interventions: (1) cognitive-behavioral (including social constructivist) perspectives; (2) contemporary object relations theory and self psychology; and (3) the understanding of dissociative states secondary to trauma.

THE PSYCHOSOCIAL IMPACT OF TRAUMA AND ITS IMPLICATIONS FOR GROUP PSYCHOTHERAPY

In order to provide a sense of what group psychotherapy must address, it is helpful now to summarize the impact of trauma on the psychosocial life of the individual, for the area where the psychological and the interpersonal converge is precisely where group psychotherapy can be most effective. The impact of trauma can be conceptualized under four headings: (1) PTSD symptom clusters; (2) changes in the "assumptive world" and cognitive schemata of the victim; (3) pathology of internalized object relations and the self; and (4) clinical syndromes other than PTSD. To provide a framework for the subsequent chapters of the book, we discuss each set of possible outcomes and its relevance to group psychotherapy.

PTSD Symptom Clusters

Since PTSD symptoms often occur during and between group therapy sessions, their management and treatment are discussed throughout this volume (see especially Goodman & Weiss, Chapter 2; Hegeman & Wohl, Chapter 3; and Johnson & Lubin, Chapter 6). The DSM-IV diagnostic scheme for PTSD breaks down pathognomonic symptoms into three clusters: reexperiencing, avoidance, and hyperarousal.

The reexperiencing cluster includes intrusive recollections of traumatic event, frightening dreams, sensations that the event is recurring, distress when exposed to cues of the event, and physiological reactivity to such cues.

Thus, for example, a female patient who was assaulted and robbed in the vicinity of her workplace came to treatment a week later, stating that she could not stop thinking about the event, and reporting vivid and painful memories and dreams about it. At the initial interview, she appeared anxious and tearful; she stated that she could not go near the scene of the incident, or even leave her home at times, due to anxiety. Whenever she spoke about the incident, a vivid sense memory or "flashback" occurred, and she felt overwhelmed with fear, anger, and grief.

The avoidance cluster includes attempts to avoid thoughts or feelings related to the trauma and/or situations or activities that bring on recollections of the trauma; amnesia for important aspects of the trauma; diminished interest in significant activities; feelings of detachment from others; limited range of affect; and feelings of a foreshortened future.

The patient described above had only some of these symptoms. She could not go near her workplace, where the incident had occurred. Her affect was also constricted. However, she was highly motivated to return to work, and utilized her attachments to her friends and to the therapist for support and guidance. Such adaptive responses to trauma are as important as the symptoms and need to be utilized by the therapist to facilitate the recovery process.

The hyperarousal cluster includes sleep difficulties, irritability, trouble concentrating, hypervigilance, and heightened startle response.

The above-described patient suffered from insomnia and became agitated when she perceived insignificant gestures in the behavior of strangers, which were suggestive to her of aggression.

See Johnson and Lubin (Chapter 6, this volume) and American Psychiatric Association (1994, pp. 424–429) for more detailed discussions of PTSD.

PTSD symptoms can be successfully treated in groups, often with the help of individual and family therapy and psychotropic medication. The advantages of group therapy for PTSD are its time and cost-effectiveness; the holding and support of the "mother group" (Scheidlinger, 1974); the mutual identifications among the members (Scheidlinger, 1955), which can be motivating and can relieve feelings of isolation and uniqueness; sharing of information; and, in some cases, mutual member support outside of the group. PTSD groups have long been offered at Veterans Affairs Medical Centers and other programs treating soldiers and veterans, and have become available more recently at clinics treating trauma victims in general and victims of sexual abuse in particular. It is generally recommended (see Goodman & Weiss, Chapter 2, this volume) that if PTSD is diagnosed, the patient ought to be referred to a short-term "stage 1" trauma group as part of the treatment. (See "Types and Phases of Trauma Groups," below. See also Herman, 1997, pp. 214–236; Goodman & Weiss, Chapter 2; and Johnson & Lubin, Chapter 6, for discussions of trauma group phases.) Johnson and Lubin (Chapter 6) explore the group treatment of PTSD in depth and detail, and we refer the reader to their chapter for systematic approaches to group psychotherapy of PTSD.

The response to trauma, however, goes beyond a set of distressing symptoms to the core beliefs and cognitions that govern the person's relationship to self and world.

Changes in the Assumptive World
and Social Roles of the Victim

When a person is traumatized, whether by another person or by a catastrophic life event, changes in the individual's "assumptive world" (Janoff-Bulman, 1992; see also Tedeschi, Park, & Calhoun, 1998; Brisson & Leavitt, 1995) often occur, especially in regard to interpersonal relations and a damaged sense of empowerment and mastery. Such changes often lead to further symptomatology and a restriction of the person's life.

Often there is an erosion of trust in significant others and even in life itself. The person sees the world as a dangerous place, in which survival rather than fulfillment becomes the crucial goal. The person feels helpless— a feeling that may generalize to other situations. He or she interprets the trauma as "my fault," and the self-schema becomes tainted with shame and guilt; these emotions become elaborated into a "victim role," which sometimes reverses into a "perpetrator role" in which the person identifies with the aggressor. Relationships become rigid and inflexible. Colorations of emotions and nuances of thought are diminished.

"Role formation" (Redl, 1963) is a group process in which the members share tasks and attitudes stemming from their own personality structures, interpersonal transactions, and group needs (person, member, and group roles; see Agazarian & Peters, 1981, pp. 39–45) and the group's stage of development. Roles may be structured at conscious and unconscious levels to fulfill both task and maintenance functions.

In trauma groups, roles become organized (and, all too often, distorted) around the social structure of trauma. Thus therapist and members at various times can be cast in the roles of victim, perpetrator, rescuer, and bystander. In particular, members of trauma groups utilize projective identification to cope with their emotional pain, and thus are prone to blaming and scapegoating each other, the therapist, and social institutions. A victim–victimizer mentality often prevails.

In group therapy, such a victim–victimizer configuration can gradually be defused by working through the projective identifications of the internalized pain and "badness" into the therapist and the members, who can strive to contain the projections, avoid complementary or concordant roles, observe and clarify unconscious reenactments, and restore a sense of validity and negotiability to a damaged self. Herman (1997, pp. 214–236) and others further recommend that traumatized patients "graduate" from homogeneous trauma groups, where the identification with the trauma is central, to heterogeneous groups, where a patient is regarded by his or her peers as "just another human being" and must give up the victim mentality in order to become part of the group.

Changes in Internalized Object Relations and the Self

Changes in the "assumptive world" of trauma victims may deepen into profound alterations of their core sense of self, as well as their mental representations of significant others.

"Soul Murder": The Sense of Ultimate Damage and Helplessness

Shengold (1989) calls the harm trauma inflicts on the self "soul murder," adopting that phrase from Freud's (1911/1958) case of the psychotic "Dr. Schreber," a delusional patient who was severely abused by his father in childhood. Sometimes patients themselves will describe feeling as if they or some part of themselves has been murdered, as in this example:

> A young adult patient who was sexually molested in puberty by a male relative came to treatment for relationship difficulties, stating emphatically that "I feel as if I am *forever damaged*, and that I will never be able to have a healthy relationship again." He expressed feelings of helplessness and hopelessness, which were painful for the therapist to see in a young man in his late teens. There was a sense that he had not only been violated, symbolically castrated, and rendered impotent in the sexual assault; he had also lost his ability to trust, to be intimate, and even to feel, much less to fend properly for himself in the interpersonal world.

Thus, in addition to schema changes in the person's systems of belief and expectations, trauma may induce deeper levels of harm to the core sense of self. Internalized object relations and the sense of self may undergo radical deformation, as well as a "freezing of development" at the point of the trauma. There is now evidence that the biological substrate of the self may be adversely affected by trauma (see van der Kolk, 1987b; van der Kolk & Greenberg, 1987). Specifically, the limbic system, which plays a major role in regulating affects and memories, appears to undergo significant modification (Saxe, Vasile, Hill, Bloomingdale, & van der Kolk, 1992; Bremner, Seibyl, & Scott, 1992). Thus the patient's feeling of damage and "soul murder" may reflect a biological reality of the central nervous system. This should encourage group therapists to consider that trauma patients may suffer from genuine "deficits" of cognition and affect that require special supports and empathic attunedness, in addition to intrapsychic and interpersonal conflicts that require uncovering, elucidation, and resolution.

Helplessness, Dependency, and "Annihilation Anxiety"

When a person undergoes trauma or abuse, overwhelming physical and/or emotional pain is endured. In addition, there is a terrifying experience of helplessness and entrapped dependency. Trauma-induced terror evokes the earliest, most primitive levels of "annihilation anxiety" (Winnicott, 1960/1986, pp. 243–244; Hopper, 1991, 1997)—the birth trauma, the dread of total destruction of the self, the primordial fear of disintegration of the personality. Hopper (1991) further postulates that to save the personality from annihilation, the victim compartmentalizes the trauma into an "encapsulated psychosis."[2]

Dissociation

In an effort to cope with overwhelming affect, trauma victims often utilize "dissociation," a process of segregating experiences or aspects of the self that keeps these elements at a psychological distance from other elements (Hegeman & Wohl, Chapter 3, this volume). Patients often report that while undergoing a trauma, they felt as if they had left their bodies and were observing themselves from a distance, or they engaged in physical or mental activity that distracted them. Subsequently, dissociation may combine with other defenses (e.g., denial, splitting, projective identification, regression, and/or repression) to keep painful memories and affects from consciousness. All too often, dissociation may become a pervasive mechanism leading to major intrusions and disruptions of experience, and sometimes eventuating in a dissociative disorder, where the personality becomes organized into distinct subsets (e.g., of behaviors, affects, sensations, and knowledge—the BASK model; Chu, 1998). The most extreme form of dissociative disorder is multiple personality disorder (now called dissociative identity disorder; American Psychiatric Association, 1994, pp. 484–487;

see also Fine & Madden, Chapter 12, this volume) in which the person has distinct "alternate selves" ("alters"), each of which may have a separate consciousness and memory system of its own.

In group therapy sessions, trauma patients may dissociate in trance-like fashion, drifting off and "tuning out" the group; when this happens, they need to be refocused by the therapist and group members. Hegeman and Wohl (Chapter 3) discuss dissociative defenses and their management in groups, and additional examples can be found throughout this volume (see Buchele, Chapter 7; von Wallenberg Pachaly, Chapter 11; Fine & Madden, Chapter 12). It is imperative that group therapists learn to work with dissociative defenses—a process which is related to but different from the more common situation of resolving intrapsychic and interpersonal conflicts in the group. A trauma patient may worsen if dissociated aspects of self are treated as if they represent conflicts within an intact, integrated self. It is not simply a matter of recovering and making conscious what has been repressed. Dissociated material and mental organization, if prematurely exposed, can precipitate a level of disorganization that is disruptive and potentially regressive to the self and the group.

Kluft (2000) holds that dissociation should be carefully distinguished from the "splitting" mechanisms referred to in object relations theory, in which patients divide their experiences of other persons into "all good" and "all bad" and keep these representations apart. Kluft states that in the condition known as dissociative identity disorder,

> Cohesive identity either has not been achieved or has been disrupted or has proven unable to manage stressors and has been reduplicated. However, the mind is not so much divided in any reified way as it is reconfigured to address particular stressors and adaptational tasks.... The fluctuating and inconsistent nature of the presentation made by the dissociative patient may give rise to interpersonal chaos. The alters are not unconscious in the usual sense of this term. They constitute parallel distributed processes.... [Such states are] thought to originate with the experience of being overwhelmed, usually by adverse personal experiences.

The reader familiar with Kernberg's (1975) important work on borderline personality organization will recognize similarities between his formulations about inner chaos and identity diffusion in patients with this organization and Kluft's description of the dissociative patient. However, Kernberg's early work emphasized neither trauma nor dissociative states, instead utilizing the object relations view of splitting and projective identification.

Thus the group therapist working with trauma patients will need to work not only with the regressive splitting and projective identification of object relations mentioned above and discussed in detail in what follows, but also with the dissociative states characteristic of the reorganization of the personality system resulting from trauma itself.

The understanding of dissociation pioneered by Kluft and others thus presents the possibility of an alternative view of the human personality—namely, that we all have multiple states of consciousness. Long ago, Sidis and Goodhart (1909, p. 364) asserted that "multiple consciousness is not the exception, but the law. For mind is synthesis of many systems, of many moments of consciousness." So what could be less surprising than the discovery that "I who address you am only one among several selves or Egos which my organism, my person, comprises. I am only the dominant member of a society, an association of similar members" (McDougall, 1926, pp. 546—547; see also Clark, 1996). Such a view of multiple centers of self-experience is consistent with so-called "postmodern" perspectives on the personality (see Gergen, 1991; Rosenau, 1992).

Conventional models of psychotherapy rest on the long-held assumption of a unitary consciousness. Pioneering psychiatrists such as Janet questioned this cherished paradigm (Ey, 1968; van der Kolk & van der Hart, 1991), and psychoanalysts such as Federn (1952), Fairbairn (see Sutherland, 1989, pp. 18–19),[3] and Sullivan (see Bacal & Newman, 1990, p. 33) made similar suggestions, but "mainstream" psychology is based on the notion of a single consciousness. More recently, Watkins and Watkins (1997) have offered an ego-psychological formulation of multiple states of consciousness. Such theorizing suggests that the personality may be a type of internal or mental "group" of parallel selves, so that there is a powerful isomorphism between self and group, which Agazarian (1997) emphasizes in her systems-centered approach to group psychotherapy. Agazarian's formulations about internal and external boundaries are utilized by Fine and Madden (Chapter 12, this volume) in their approach to group treatment of dissociative disorders.

Primitive Object Relations and Defenses

Over time, psychological trauma often (but not always) induces a regression[4] to or fixation at the level of primitivized object relations and defenses characteristic of what Melanie Klein (1946/1977) called the "paranoid–schizoid" and "depressive" positions of infancy. Briefly, in the paranoid–schizoid position, the primary preoccupations are with the survival of the self and with managing persecutory anxiety (feelings of an attack upon the self); in the depressive position, concerns about the well-being of significant others and consequent feelings of guilt and a need to make reparation predominate. Each position has typical defense mechanisms associated with it. Splitting and projective identification are defenses of the paranoid–schizoid position. These defenses differ from both repression and dissociation, and, importantly, can be viewed primarily as *interpersonal* (as contrasted with intrapsychic) defenses—ones that have an impact on the relational matrix of the group.

Splitting and Projective Identification

Ganzarain (Chapter 4), Buchele (Chapter 7), and von Wallenberg Pachaly (Chapter 11), all of whom have extensive backgrounds in object relations theory, cite clinical examples of splitting and projective identification in trauma groups (incest survivors, in Ganzarain's and Buchele's groups; victims of political torture, in von Wallenberg Pachaly's groups). These defenses are aspects of the matrix of all groups (Bion, 1961/1974, pp. 127–129; Ashbach & Schermer, 1987, pp. 40–42), but are intensified in trauma groups because the psychic pain and aggression of trauma are split off and projected into others for containment.

To begin with, to ward off the negative half of the split, trauma patients often go through an initial stage when their group and therapist are experienced as "all good." Such idealizations may serve a supportive function for a time. Soon, however, the group members will revert to the other half of the split and perceive each other or the therapist as "all bad" or "enemies." At such times, the members and therapist may need to contain the upsurges of blame and rage that result. Repeated successful containments of these projective identifications are healing for these patients, eventually leading to increased trust and the renewed possibility that persons and feelings can have nuanced "shades of gray." (The experienced group therapist will recognize splitting as a common collusive defense of group members with borderline personality disorder or substance abusers. The similarity may now be seen in part to be due to the fact that these populations appear to have a high incidence of childhood, adolescent, and adult trauma.[5])

Violation of the Transitional Space

The overwhelming affects associated with trauma, combined with a profound mistrust of the life process and the fixation on concretized cognitive schemata (see Fish-Murray, Koby, & van der Kolk, 1987; Fine, 1990). often lead to a diminution of the capacity for play and metaphor within the "transitional space" (Winnicott, 1951/1971)—a region of the life space halfway between reality and fantasy, a space for spontaneity and creativity. In turn, the "true self" (Winnicott, 1965), imposes a "false self" as a facade to shield it from a hostile environment. Having lost the sense of freedom inherent in the transitional realm, the true self retreats into itself; sometimes suicide paradoxically seems to be the only way to "survive."

Such a process was graphically seen in a young adult male who was depressed with suicidal ideation, complaining of feelings of emptiness and failure, and an inability to make his life and relationships succeed. Both his parents suffered from chronic depression. A traumatic outcome of his father's depression and explosive rage occurred when the patient was a child of 5. His father—flagrantly not appreciating that the play space is sacred to a child (his "not-me possession," according to Winnicott, 1951/1971), not to be challenged by the parents—impulsively destroyed his son's toys. In that act, he killed the child's transitional space, so that the boy was subsequently unable to "make" anything of his life, having no "internalized place" and "objects" with which to do so.

Interestingly, instead of growing further apart, father and son then formed a pathological bond characteristic of trauma, which was expressed in a dream in which the patient and his father were walking together on the grounds of a mental hospital that had beautiful gardens. The dream ended with a sense of catastrophic doom.

All forms of trauma challenge the transitional space, and the therapeutic process consists in large part of preserving what is left of the space and creating conditions through which spontaneous thought and aliveness may be restored (Scharff & Scharff, 1994, pp. 67–68, 332–334; see also von Wallenberg Pachaly, Chapter 11, this volume).

Loss of Self-Cohesion

The same phenomena that are understood on one level as internalized object relations may be viewed from another as self-states in relation to significant others. Bacal and Newman (1990) have explored the interconnections between object relations theory and self psychology in depth. Historically, self psychology as a distinct discipline evolved when Kohut (1971, 1977) and his students shifted their focus from object relations to the self and the developmental line of narcissism. According to Kohut, the self seeks out significant others ("selfobjects") both to mirror its narcissism and also to idealize, admire, and use as role models. When significant others fail to offer such mirroring and idealization, the self undergoes a "narcissistic injury" (a "wound" to esteem, often accompanied by shame; see Lewis, 1987) and begins to experience loss of cohesiveness (fragmentation). Such fragmentation may express itself in depression, excessive preoccupation with the body (e.g., hypochondriasis), and feelings of "falling apart." When the loss of self-cohesion is severe, the person develops compensatory structures and behaviors to restore cohesion. The use of mood-altering substances, compulsive behaviors such as gambling and sexual addiction, and experiences of an "adrenalin rush" via business risks and adulation are experiences in our culture that temporarily restore cohesion. A component of trauma is narcissistic injury, and trauma often creates a persistent vulnerability to further hurts. Therefore, traumatized persons often turn to compensatory structures and behaviors similar to those of narcissistic character types.

The cohesive spirit and mutual identifications of the therapy group play a significant role in minimizing narcissistic injury and promoting a positive sense of self. Empathy, soothing, and the therapist's consistent efforts to place him- or herself "in the group members' shoes" are of great value to traumatized patients. However, self psychology also considers that a degree of narcissistic injury due to the therapist's (and group's) failure to empathize is an inevitable occurrence in treatment (Wolf, 1988, pp. 136–165). What is important is not so much to prevent all such in-session hurts as to acknowledge and resolve them. Wolf recommends that the therapist become sensitized to the subtle wounds to esteem that occur and address them, in order to prevent patients from becoming overwhelmed and to restore their self-cohesion.

A male patient who had been repeatedly physically abused as a child seemed to become a threatening figure to the group and the therapist. He swaggered into group sessions, sometimes monopolized the group interaction, and spoke in a coarse manner. The group became increasingly intolerant of him, and the therapist experienced feelings of fear in this group of men with impulse disorders. The therapist became confrontive with the man (which only made him retaliative), and, as the tension escalated, threatened to discharge him from the group. The therapist then noticed that the patient "backed off" in fear, and—in this window of safety and compassion—engaged in introspection about his countertransference. He reflected with the patient and the group that he and the group may have been too harsh with the patient, who may have been expressing his anger at the abusive father who had punished him as a child. The group members identified strongly, verbalizing their own histories of abuse. The man expressed relief and became a highly functional group member.

Narcissistic Injury

Psychological trauma undermines self-esteem, and many of the sequelae of trauma can be viewed as fragmentation secondary to such a "wound" to the self. The familial and social mirroring and validation the person rightfully expects from others become instead seduction, boundary violation, and betrayal. The idealization is demolished, and then only recovered in a drastically compensatory way. (The victim then "admires" the person's dictatorial power over him or her, coldness, and ability to hurt.) In this connection, Fairbairn (1943; see also Sutherland, 1989, pp. 120–121), a prominent object relations theorist, observed that abused children often become *more*, not less, dependent on parents who abuse them. Paradoxically, the more such a child is hurt and deprived by a "bad" parent, the more the child *needs* a "good" parent, even if he or she must deny that parent's malevolence or lack of impulse control. Furthermore, it is safer to be "bad" in a basically "good" world than to live in a constantly threatening world, so the child blames him- or herself rather than the offending parent. As feelings of helplessness and shame gain ascendance, the victim is subject to ongoing narcissistic injury from within—blaming and shaming the self, and interpreting benign experiences as repetitions of earlier hurts.

The Development of Clinical Syndromes

Frequently, a trauma victim will present with a major mental disturbance that has "functional autonomy" from the trauma (i.e., a DSM-IV disorder that has become a primary clinical entity of its own). It may not be clear whether such a disorder has resulted from trauma or is just coincidentally present in the same person. (Our clinical experience suggests that both connections—etiology and comorbidity—do occur.) Gallagher and Kibel (Chapter 13) provide a thorough exploration of these disorders as they co-occur with trauma histories, and a discussion of their treatment in groups.

How trauma becomes transformed into a protracted mental disorder is a question that is complex and as yet not fully answered, despite a century of psychoanalytic theorizing (see Fenichel, 1945, pp. 117—128) and more recent research (see van der Kolk, 1987a). That trauma leads to biochemical changes in the central nervous system seems well established now. It can be hypothesized that such changes can then lead to endogenous biochemical alterations—changes characteristic, for example, of major depressive disorder, bipolar disorders, or panic disorder. At another level, shifts in the victim's assumptive world can be elaborated over time into the cognitive distortions (Beck, 1993; Burns, 1999) and maladaptive schemata (Young & Young, 1994) that characterize depression, or into the avoidant and anxiety-based behavior patterns typical of agoraphobia. To cope with affective perturbations, mood-altering behaviors such as compulsive overeating, gambling, or sexual acting out may occur. For example. the use of drugs and alcohol to dull the pain of trauma can escalate into substance use disorders. Furthermore, the biogenetic, familial, and or social context in which the trauma occurred may be a common ingredient fostering both the traumatic boundary violations and the mental illness. So while we do not yet know whether there are special mechanisms whereby trauma is transmuted over time into major mental illness, it is a good working hypothesis that for many patients, trauma is implicated in a variety of serious mental disorders.

This overview of the impact of psychological trauma upon the developing personality and its coping mechanisms, object relations, sense of self, and vulnerability to emotional distress suggests what a therapist might encounter in such patients and tells us something about their treatment needs. Overall, a traumatized patient presents with a broad range of intense conflicts, relational dilemmas, and cognitive–affective deficits, all of which present significant therapeutic challenges. We now explore how group treatment can best be configured to result in "therapeutic factors" (Yalom, 1995) that are most beneficial to this varied population.

ESSENTIAL CHARACTERISTICS OF PSYCHOTHERAPY GROUPS FOR TRAUMA

Group psychotherapy is utilized in clinical settings for a variety of reasons: (1) It is cost-efficient; (2) it can diffuse transference and attenuate ego regression, which may prolong or complicate treatment; (3) it provides social supports and facilitates the development of interpersonal skills; (4) it offers opportunities for acquiring new information, coping skills, and self-expectations; (5) peer feedback in some instances is easier for patients to assimilate than feedback from an authority figure such as a therapist; (6) the mutual identifications and mirroring provided by the group are potent therapeutic factors (Yalom, 1995); and (6) the exploration of the group process and dynamics by the members allows for personal growth and insight into interpersonal processes in a way that is not possible in individual treatment (Durkin, 1964).

Such a rationale for the use of group psychotherapy applies even more specifically to trauma treatment, since a substantial portion of the pain and suffering resulting from trauma stems from being existentially isolated from human contact. It has been said of the therapy group's power to bring the isolated patient back into the fold that "Together we constitute the norm from which individually we deviate." For a trauma victim, this translates into "Together we constitute the healing matrix of compassion and empowerment from which, individually, we have become isolated."

Types and Phases of Trauma Groups

The types of therapy groups utilized in trauma treatment vary across the spectrum of group theory and practice. One of the main variations is the extent to which the interpersonal relations and dynamics of the here-and-now group itself are utilized in the treatment process. Some groups are structured, educative, and cognitive, focusing on each member more than on the group as a whole (see Johnson & Lubin, Chapter 6, and Fine & Madden, Chapter 12, for stronger-boundaried educational and cognitive models); others encourage the development of transference, a tolerable degree of regression, interactions among the members, and examination of group systems and defenses/resistances (see Ganzarain, Chapter 4; Buchele, Chapter 7; and von Wallenberg Pachaly, Chapter 11). On the whole, the higher the level of patients' functioning, ego strength, and anxiety tolerance, and the more feasible it is to offer a long-term insight-oriented format, the more the latter strategies become possible.

As a working principle, trauma treatment occurs in phases. The early stages utilize approaches that are time-limited, structured, and supportive, and often provide an educational component. Such groups contain and manage the overwhelming posttraumatic affects, help the patients feel less isolated and alienated, and provide cognitive skills and perspectives that foster a sense of renewed meaning and hope for the future. Members may then "graduate" to groups in which the primary focus is on the sharing and working through of the traumatic experiences—the telling and witnessing of each patient's narrative, and the restoration of trust. Finally, some patients may move on to long-term open-ended groups in which they work out a variety of difficulties in a less structured, free-flowing setting where they can see themselves as whole persons reintegrated into society, instead of as "victims" struggling to survive a catastrophe.These stage-specific group settings are recommended by trauma specialists such as Herman (1997, pp. 214–236), Goodman and Weiss (Chapter 2), and Johnson and Lubin (Chapter 6), and are further discussed by Dembert and Simmer (Chapter 10), and Gallagher and Kibel (Chapter 13). Careful screening is crucial (see Goodman & Weiss, Chapter 2), because a patient can be retraumatized by entering a group for which he or she is not adequately prepared to function.

> For example, a female victim of repeated spousal abuse was unable to manage the "normal" verbal aggression of a relatively unstructured heterogeneous group (Herman's stage 3), after some weeks in a stage 2 support group for abuse victims. She panicked and fled treatment, most likely to engage once more in acting out with abusive men.

Because the potential for "relapse" in trauma patients is high, it should be carefully monitored and, where possible, prevented.

Healing Factors of Trauma Groups

Although the value of groups in the treatment of trauma is basically similar to that for any other clinical entity, certain group functions are particularly useful in trauma treatment. Trauma-specific problems and issues are also likely to be encountered by the group therapist. The important healing functions of group psychotherapy for psychological trauma can be inferred from our earlier discussion of the harmful sequelae of trauma. They include

(1) managing and reducing PTSD symptoms; (2) telling and witnessing the trauma; (3) grieving for the trauma and its consequences; (4) restructuring the "assumptive world" and reestablishing trust; (5) restoring the reality sense; and (6) reintegrating the personality.

Managing and Reducing PTSD Symptoms

Johnson and Lubin (Chapter 6) give a detailed description of PTSD treatment in groups, and they provide two models: their own, and Resick's cognitive processing therapy (Resick, Jordan, Girelli, Hutter, & Marhoefer-Dvorak, 1988; Resick & Schnicke, 1993), which can be used in time-limited treatment. There is strong evidence that verbalizing the trauma and managing the PTSD symptoms not only are helpful in the short run, but may prevent or aid in the treatment of complex disorders such as major depression and substance abuse. The importance of PTSD-focused interventions is highlighted by the fact that "critical-incident stress management" and other methods have evolved for working soon after an incident with individuals, families, and communities exposed to overwhelming trauma (see Dembert & Simmer, Chapter 10).

Originally, "abreaction" (recall of the trauma with full ventilation of affect) was the treatment of choice for PTSD. The dramatic Hollywood version of abreaction, in which the victim is given an injection of a "truth serum" (e.g., sodium pentothal), vividly recalls the trauma, reacts with a flood of emotions, and then processes the experience with a kindly, reflective psychiatrist, is not so far from what was actually done in many cases. In the motion picture *The Seventh Veil*, for example, a psychiatrist uses drug-induced recall and abreaction to help a concert pianist recover her ability to perform after her hands are damaged in a car accident. Today, clinicians are much more aware of the risks of emotional flooding—especially in the group setting (see Fine & Madden, Chapter 12)—and so are likely to emphasize containment, cognitive processing, and interpersonal support. Clinical judgment is crucial, and the members must of course express (rather than suppress) the hurt, fear, grief, rage, and sense of injustice they feel. Throughout this volume, the reader will find useful discussions and clinical examples of how to manage intense affects within the group therapy context (see especially Hegeman & Wohl, Chapter 3; Buchele, Chapter 7; and von Wallenberg Pachaly, Chapter 11).

Telling and Witnessing the Trauma

All psychotherapy revolves around the patient's "narrative," the telling of his or her story. Just as memory is largely a reconstruction based on bits and pieces of information colored by the person's own history and personality, so the narrative is both a telling of actual events and an interpersonal process of weaving a story that is part of the fabric of what is going on in the group. Telling this story, and having it witnessed, constitute a social process and a reparative ritual. It validates (and where necessary, corrects) the internal perceptions of the patient, helps him or her to feel less alone with the horrific experience, makes sense and meaning out of what happened, creates a feeling of at least minimal social justice via others' acknowledgment of the trauma, and restores cohesion and autonomy of the self. Furthermore, it initiates a mourning process that can help the victim to begin to let go of the trauma and focus on building a new life.

Grieving for the Trauma and Its Consequences

A considerable portion of the work of resolving trauma is to grieve for the multiple losses that trauma initiates, whether those losses are of a loved one, a part of one's body, one's possessions, one's innocence and trust, and/ or one's hope for the future. Trauma and loss overlap considerably (Rando, 1993), since all trauma leads to grief, and all major loss is traumatic. Bereavement work and trauma work are increasingly merging in the unified study of "traumatic loss," and in this respect, the treatment of trauma involves the "healing of memories" by recalling them and gradually letting go of their intense emotional charge. Traumatized individuals grieve repeatedly, and many suffer from "complicated mourning" (Rando, 1993; Volkan, 1982)—a fixation of the grieving process that keeps them locked into the past and unable to move forward.

Group therapy provides an excellent opportunity to mourn within a supportive context. Importantly, however, it is important for the members to work through the "shock" aspect of the trauma before addressing their grief. At that juncture, the interpretation of the denial of loss may facilitate the beginning of a mourning process that emerges once the "wreckage" of the trauma has been sifted through.

Restructuring the "Assumptive World" and Restoring Trust

A trauma profoundly challenges the beliefs that keep most of us "sane" and give us a sense of "going on being" (Winnicott, 1958, p. 303). When a trauma occurs, the person's basic beliefs—the conviction of a stable, orderly environment; the esteem-building assurances that one is basically good and adequate; the notion that one is loved; the trust in significant others; one's spirituality and faith; the belief that one is safe and relatively immune from harm—are all brought into question. For example, children nurture beliefs within their own cognitive schemata that are challenged by trauma. Incest, a parent's death, or a severe illness call into question the child's tenuous security (see Keyser, Sellaus, & Kahn, Chapter 9, this volume). More deeply, both children and adults need what von Wallenberg

Pachaly (Chapter 11) calls a "good internal holding group," a mental representation of significant others and the social environment, which can be contaminated or even destroyed by trauma. The group experience can help reconstruct each member's damaged "internal holding group" or, in some cases, build a new one over the ashes of the old.

The group also provides ongoing opportunities for reality testing of the members' assumptive worlds through "corrective emotional experiences" (Alexander & French, 1946), feedback from others, and (where possible) the resolution of the transference. Paradoxically, it is often through the patients' unconscious reenactments within the group that the deleterious assumptive worlds triggered by the trauma are dramatized; thus, they can be explored "while the iron is hot."

Erikson (1959) held that trust is one of the first templates of experience to be internalized by the infant. "Trust" is the conviction that one's basic needs will be provided for and that the world will proceed in an expectable, benign way, or, if not, that inner and external forces can help restore a secure state. In the trauma therapy group, the process of developing trust is often slow and has many setbacks. Later, we discuss how the slowed resolution of the trust issue can frustrate the therapist and create ongoing impasses.

As trust issues surface, group members repeatedly test each other and the therapist. Trauma victims have heightened sensitivity to nonverbal communications and feel betrayed by fluctuations in interest and attention, misunderstandings, and lapses in protective boundaries. Some therapists feel that establishing a supportive group atmosphere will provide a "corrective emotional experience" that will in time resolve the trust issue. Ganzarain (Chapter 4), however, cautions against such a tolerant approach; he holds that transference plays a major part in the mistrust and must be clarified and confronted, even if it means temporarily intensifying disillusionment and/or aggression in the group.

It is likely that at least some members will subject the therapist and group to a crucial test of trust at some point during treatment. Often it is a test to see whether the support is strong enough to counter the devastation of the trauma. Von Wallenberg Pachaly (Chapter 11), in particular, emphasizes that the therapist must be able to suspend neutrality and take a stand against the power of the perpetrator and the forces that led to the trauma, especially in the early phases of treatment.

Restoring the Reality Sense

Group psychotherapy for psychological trauma requires careful attention to (1) the reality of the traumatic event (assuming that the patient's recollection is valid), and (2) the ongoing dissociation of a portion of the patient's self. Acknowledgment and evaluation of traumatic realities and integration of such awareness with the whole personality are primary treatment needs of traumatized individuals.

Kernberg's (1975) formulations about splitting and projective identification in borderline personalities assumed that the "all bad" component of the split is a phantasy distortion of the original experience, based on the immature ego of the infant and child. With our current knowledge that many individuals with borderline personality disorder experienced actual sexual and physical abuse in childhood (Herman & van der Kolk, 1987), we can see that a patient's "all bad," witchlike, or monstrous images of significant others may be representations of the actual horrors inflicted on the patient. The "split" may be a life-saving way of preserving the goodness of self and of significant others in the face of devastating harm to the psyche. Thus, within the context of trauma, splitting is sometimes a healthy coping mechanism that must be utilized until the self has healed sufficiently to be able to tolerate "shades of gray"—that is, mixtures of goodness and badness in the same person (see von Wallenberg Pachaly, Chapter 11, this volume).

Overall, we may say that whereas other patients generally alter reality to approximate their fantasies, the trauma patient often doubts the overwhelming reality of his or her experience, engaging in "coercive doubting" (Kramer & Akhtar, 1991). Thus, while analysis of the transference as a distortion of contemporary reality has a place in trauma treatment, the recognition and acknowledgment of the reality of the actual trauma, not to mention the sometimes subtle retraumatizations occurring in the group, are crucial to restoring the reality sense. Fine (personal communication, September 12, 1999), however, cautions that the patient or group may experience the therapist's validating or questioning memories of trauma as "taking sides": "If [the therapist believes] (not necessarily overtly) that the trauma happened . . . [the group members] will internally and sometimes through acting out try to demonstrate . . . that it did not . . . all the while re-enacting." Acknowledging the reality of the trauma should occur, however, only when there is convincing evidence (to therapist *and* patient) that the traumatic event actually took place and the impact of the therapist's taking a position (sometimes experienced as omnipotence) is worked through.

Reintegrating the Personality

A difficult aspect of the group therapist's role with trauma patients is to help each member keep track of the roles played by dissociated parts of the self within the personality and in the group interaction. This imperative is most evident with dissociative identity disorder, where distinct "alters" may emerge in the course of the therapy session, and communication of disparate aspects of self must co-occur with working through of pathological patterns of interrelating in the group (see Fine & Madden, Chapter 12). In less severe cases of dissociation, such a necessity is not as obvious; however, without communication between, say, the angry part of the person and the hurt, dependent part, or between the objective recall of the trauma and the dissociated emotions of rage and grief, interpretations about the way the members relate to the therapist and each other will not lead to a resolution of the trauma. We ourselves have often seen patients who sought therapy several years after a previous treatment experience and found that the first therapy, although temporarily successful, failed to address a significant emotional component of the trauma—which was dissociated from the treatment by both therapist and patient.

SPECIAL PROBLEMS OF TRAUMA GROUP PSYCHOTHERAPY

Several issues vital to the success of trauma groups (or groups with traumatized patients in them) have been touched upon above, but they should be clarified further so that therapists will be especially alert to them. These core issues (we avoid the word "resistances," because that term too often connotes a deliberate avoidance) are (1) severe and protracted mistrust and suspicion not only of significant others, but also of the meaningfulness of the treatment process; (2) the often sudden and surprising revival of intense affects, images, memories, and dissociative states, leading to reenactments of scenes of victimization and trauma; (3) the spreading of these eruptions via group contagion effects; and (4) countertransference and vicarious traumatization of the therapist.

The Trauma Patient's Severe and Protracted Mistrust in the Group

In virtually all groups, trust is an important issue—especially at the outset, when new members are introduced and when intimate personal disclosures are made. These trust issues are partially resolved by (1) adequate group rules and boundaries; (2) discussions of the trust problem and elaboration of past violations of trust, to distinguish them from the present situation; and (3) the therapist's reliable stance. However, the traumatized patient has learned deeply to trust no one and no situation. (Conversely, he or she may overtrust and be victimized again and again, but may often trust the wrong persons and mistrust those who are genuinely supportive.)

Even if the trauma was an accident of fate and there was no actual perpetrator, the victim may subsequently be repeatedly misunderstood and inappropriately or ineffectively treated even by loving caregivers, because the phenomenological world he or she now inhabits is very different from that of his or her significant others.

For example, one patient with a residual handicap of a crippling illness, and a history of childhood hospitalizations and long-term feelings of rejection and abandonment, explained to the therapist that his
friends became annoyed with him because he often asked for favors
(e.g., help moving furniture, purchasing an appliance, or meeting people in social settings). They seemed to feel that he was overdependent
when in fact he was expressing real needs. Similarly, incest victims are
often misunderstood and rejected because of their anxieties about sexual intimacy: The husband of a rape victim felt as if his wife's fear of
sex meant that she was "cold and rejecting" and was angry with her,
despite his knowledge of what had happened.

Therapists may treat such difficulties as resistances when in fact they are
part of the everyday experience and phenomenological worlds of the patients, leaving them misunderstood, attacked, abandoned, and alone once
more.

When a group of traumatized individuals comes together as a group,
the trust issue may persist as a deeply ingrained set of difficulties with
"grouping" (forming a cohesive working group), self-disclosure, and
change. Those who have worked in groups for patients with borderline
personality disorder or substance abuse will be familiar with this protracted
trust issue, which may be at least in part explained by the traumata such
patients are now known to have extensively suffered within dysfunctional
families and in society. von Wallenberg Pachaly (Chapter 11), provides poignant examples of such mistrust in groups with political torture victims,
and it is important to see, as he does, that both past traumata and present
life circumstances contribute to the mistrust.

Addressing the trust issue satisfactorily requires active exploration of
the issue and special attention to the rules and boundary conditions of the
group. What may appear to be trivial violations may precipitate significant,
even overwhelming emotional reactions from group members, but may also
offer therapeutic opportunities.

In addition, the therapist must make a special and repeated effort to
empathize with the plight of the group members, so that he or she does not
appear to relate and interpret through the rose-colored glasses of a
noninvolved, nontraumatized observer (although at certain junctures that
perspective is paradoxically necessary!). Our chapter authors repeatedly
echo the sentiments of trauma therapists such as Judith Herman (1997)
that the detached, "neutral" role is inadequate for work with trauma. The
therapist must be strongly attuned to the struggles of these patients and
must align with them against their devastating realities and against the perpetrators of their trauma (in cases involving specific perpetrators).

As part of building trust, trauma victims will engage in a thorough examination of a therapist's personhood—a development that can be understood either as hypervigilance in the face of a potentially dangerous en-

counter (repetition of the trauma), as an attempt to address the partly projectively identified and partly real "illness" or "countertransference" of the therapist (Searles, 1975), or (which is very likely) as both. Ferenczi, one of the few early analysts to discuss the subject after Freud abandoned the trauma theory, described such a process in a seminal (1932/1980) paper entitled "The Confusion of Tongues between Adults and Children: The Language of Tenderness and Passion." Maccoby (1995) summarizes the relevant aspects of that paper as follows:

> Ferenczi argued that abuse, both seduction and punishment, can be psychological as well as physical. It can lead to identification with the aggressor and "traumatic progression" or precocious maturity in which the child becomes *finely attuned to the abusive adult and feels compelled to try and alleviate the adult's suffering. Ferenczi maintained that this attitude is transferred to the analyst.* The patient represses unconscious criticism and anger and *expresses an "exceedingly refined sensitivity for the wishes, tendencies, whims and antipathies of their analyst, even if the analyst is completely unaware of this sensitivity."* (p. 322; emphasis added)

Scharff and Scharff (1994) point out that therapists may become bored and frustrated, and feel as if they were not doing their job, when they cannot pursue the "meaning" of patients' associations but must simply be available "presences," often for long periods of time. On a group level, early phases of a group may appear slow, arduous, and bland. What may be taking place during these "slow periods" are the reestablishment of trust and the restoration of ego functions that were severely damaged by the trauma.

Within–Group Revival and Reenactment of Affects, Images, Memories, and Scenes of Trauma

Since the behaviors, affects, sensations, and knowledge (the BASK model; Chu, 1998) resulting from trauma are often split off and dissociated from one another, they have a way of surfacing in the group in "chunks" that are isolated from other components of the personality and the group interaction. A therapist is likely to observe affect storms, rage, and grief, sometimes in an apparently inappropriate context. Or a perpetrator–victim dynamic may emerge that can threaten the viability of the group. Or else the *sensations* associated with the trauma may recur in a "flashback" of one member, as another expresses trauma-related *emotions* to the group, while still another member becomes numb!

The tasks of the therapist during these difficult times are to help integrate the disparate experiences, to manage the intense affects, and to contain the potentially destructive and self-destructive energies and behaviors in the group. Examples of such events and how they may be handled by the therapist are provided in every chapter of this volume (see especially Hegeman & Wohl, Chapter 3; Ganzarain, Chapter 4; Buchele, Chapter 7; von Wallenberg Pachaly, Chapter 11). In addition, the therapist can help the group form connections between the disparate "pieces." Some of the "pieces" can be understood as having been externalized by projective identification into various members, therapists, subgroups, and the group as a whole, so that the therapy group provides a special opportunity for each member to "locate" such fragments, reown them, and place them in the proper context of the whole self. What is crucial here is to create a space in which it is safe to put all the pieces "out on the table" to permit the work of reintegration to begin.

Group Contagion Effects

Contagion is a manifestation of fusion, the group basic assumption of "oneness" (see "Group Basic Assumptions," below), overempathy, over-identification, and the loss of "reflective space" in the group. The overwhelming affects associated with trauma can make contagion particularly virulent, sometimes endangering the viability of the group itself. In addition, the weakened ego states of trauma patients, resulting from dissociative processes and feelings of helplessness and hopelessness, can make the members more susceptible to group contagion. However, trauma often gives individuals a certain courage and fortitude, which can be used to strengthen the therapeutic alliance and restore order and perspective to the group.

Group contagion may range from unboundaried empathy that leads to a shared histrionic emotionality, to episodes of acting out, to aggressive scapegoating that seeks a victim, to a subdued emotional atmosphere in which the members "numb out" and avoid the group task, to a rash of violations of group rules. Sometimes the contagion is set off by a member who seduces the group away from its task, and sometimes it is evoked by the traumatic nature of the material being explored in the group.

The Reflective Space as an Antidote to Contagion

Hinshelwood (1994) calls the mental region in which rational consideration of group issues can take place the "reflective space." The therapist must be able to maintain a reflective space even when the group members do not. Only in this way can he or she gradually restore the reflective space of the group as a whole. Hinshelwood gives an example of a scapegoating contagion attack that was initially evoked by a group member whose manipulative behavior evoked his own victimization by projective identification (the compulsion to repeat past traumatization), but quickly became a massive irrational attack by the group that would have extruded the member. In this case the therapist's maintenance of a reflective space within himself, against the intense pressures to join with the group or identify with the victim, allowed him gradually to clarify and interpret the group's behavior and to restore the "work group" mentality of attending to the therapeutic tasks.

Addressing Attacks on Linking

Gordon (1994) gives examples of "attacks on linking" (Bion, 1959/1967), in which the group members attack the bonds between them as well as the associations and connections among their diverse thoughts. The self-destructive tendencies of trauma victims are often both causes and effects of attacks on linking. When this occurs in a therapy group, the members will attempt to split the cotherapists, polarize the group, devalue the process of making connections between ideas and feelings, and/or avoid contact and intimacy. Nitsun (1996) has termed this phenomenon the "anti-group" and provided a scheme for understanding the ways in which group aims and goals are undermined. The subversion of the group is both an aim and an outcome of human-inflicted trauma. At the same time, self-destructive behavior such as substance abuse or becoming reembroiled in "sick," maladaptive relationships may occur. Attacks on linking may be addressed by systematically clarifying the painful emotions that triggered the attack, and by helping the group rediscover the linkages and restore the damaged connectedness. The role of aggression and envy must often be pointed out as well.

Emotional contagion is only one of several factors that may evoke strong countertransference reactions in therapists treating trauma in groups. In order to maintain a reflective space and a capacity to work effectively with the group, the therapist must persistently monitor and address his or her countertransference.

Countertransference and Vicarious Traumatization

"Countertransference," defined here as a therapist's total response to the group and its members, can be both a useful tool and a pitfall of treatment of trauma and traumatic loss. The therapist's empathy and internal feelings, images, memories, and responses to the group may provide useful information and guidelines about how best to respond and to stay in role despite pressures to deviate. At the same time, the often overwhelming emotions associated with witnessing the recall and reliving of the trauma can cause adverse reactions in the therapist and lead to harmful interventions.

"Vicarious traumatization" of the therapist (Pearlman & Saakvitne, 1995) occurs in response to trauma narratives and reenactments within the group. The therapist's internal conflicts in response to trauma "replays" are often masked by a "curative fantasy" of the basic assumption of dependency (Bion, 1961/1974), which expresses itself as fantasies of omnipotence, a self-idealization, and/or an intense drive to "cure." Despite such a defense, therapists who do not address vicarious traumatization either may act out with patients, may become depressed, or (in the extreme) may literally develop symptoms of PTSD or other psychiatric disorders.

In an attempt to ward off vicarious traumatization, a therapist may give up the listening stance and become more active, power-oriented, controlling, and intrusive. The most insidious of these infringements by the therapist are, of course, intimate, aggressive, and/or sexual relations with patients. Or the therapist may become easily angry and frustrated, or, worse, may form an "identification with the aggressor" and become overtly attacking. More subtly, therapist and group may collude to avoid the painful material.

We believe that all these forms of vicarious traumatization are everyday occurrences in work with these patients. To what extent they betray a therapist's own trauma (i.e., a retraumatization as opposed to a new trauma) can only be sorted out by each therapist. There is evidence that many therapists are trauma victims or at least suffered significant family dysfunction (Miller, 1981; Ganzarain, Chapter 4, this volume). The successful trauma therapist may need an ongoing or periodic course of self-analysis, self-healing, and self-care, and should not be ashamed of this fact.

Therapist Self-Care

The most important part of the therapist's self-care is the ongoing awareness of what is taking place within the psyche (subjective countertransference) and how it is related to what is occurring in the group (objective or realistic countertransference). Supervision and periodic therapy for the therapist can greatly facilitate this process. In addition, we think that a trauma group therapist should periodically review and address the following aspects of his or her daily existence: life stressors; rewarding and diverting leisure activities; life-affirming interpersonal relationships; ongoing collegial relationships to maintain a strong professional identity and commitment to the work; and stress management techniques, ranging from relaxation exercises to proper exercise and nutrition.

Attention to such details is not incidental to work with trauma groups. Indeed, it may be vital to preventing countertransference acting out and to preserving the well-being of the therapist and the group.

Countertransference and Role Relationships

Countertransference often expresses itself in the ways in which a therapist adopts a role complementary to that of a patient or group (see Racker, 1968). Problems of overidentifying with the four poles of victim, aggressor, rescuer, or apathetic bystander can occur and must be addressed (Brenner, 1999).

> In a heterogeneous, open-ended therapy group used for training psychiatric residents, the senior supervising (male) therapist made the observation to the group that one of the members seemed to be monopolizing the session. The member, a 30-year-old male with a history of sexual trauma, was at first defensive and apologized to the group, but in the next session he verbalized a series of anxiety-laden events that had occurred recently and seemed to replay his original trauma in various ways. The senior therapist had no sympathy for his "tales of woe" and once again raised the issue of monopolization. Partly because the patient had in fact raised meaningful issues for the other group members, they supported him, ignored the therapist, and verbalized their identifications with the patient. Meanwhile, the psychiatric resident therapist—a woman who usually played an active role in the group—was silent. The senior therapist tried to regain control by confronting the patient about what he (partly correctly) felt was a manipulative display, was persistently ignored, and by the end of the session was haggard and exhausted. In this example, the patient was both victim and victimizer; the senior therapist alternated countertransferentially in a complementary way between these roles; the group members were rescuers; and the psychiatric resident became a bystander. By recognizing these roles, the senior therapist could restore his empathy for the patient and adopt a more neutral yet empathic role. The psychiatric resident could identify with her own and the group's issues of aggression and authority, and restore her involved, committed stance.

Ziegler and McEvoy (Chapter 5) take up countertransference issues in considerable detail and describe instances of specific kinds of countertransference dilemmas of trauma groups. Importantly, they also provide examples of how cotherapists can work together to identify their own and each other's countertransference reactions and utilize them effectively, rather than act them out with the group.

A potent source of countertransference reactions are in response to the group as a whole, as distinct from individual members. Since group dynamics are "invisible" (Agazarian & Peters, 1991), they are frequently overlooked by therapists; yet they inevitably play a crucial "behind-the-scenes" role in group treatment outcomes.

GROUP-AS-A-WHOLE DYNAMICS
AND TRAUMA

Many group therapists, unfortunately, are merely doing individual therapy in groups, thus passing up important opportunities to utilize the group-as-a-whole dynamics themselves as therapeutic forces. Furthermore, trauma itself sheds a somewhat different light on group dynamics—a subject to which we now turn our attention.

Ganzarain (Chapter 4) examines the typical group dynamics that emerge with traumatized patients. If such dynamics are not addressed, according to Ganzarain, the group may either disintegrate or else become fixated at a stage of group development where it is difficult or impossible to work through the aggressive persecutory paranoid–schizoid and reparative depressive position elements associated with trauma; as a result, the work of therapy remains partially undone. Such truncated treatment probably occurs much more often than therapists would like to admit. For example, patients in groups that do not work through aggression and aspects of the group revolt (Bennis & Shepard, 1956; Slater, 1966) may experience symptomatic relief and a sense of being supported, but form an adaptation in which the quality of life and the sense of wholeness are significantly compromised. An understanding of what Bion (1961/1974) called "basic assumptions" can help the therapist to move through rather than around the powerful group configurations that can prevent or facilitate the resolution of deeper layers of trauma and traumatic transference.

Group Basic Assumptions

Bion's Three Basic Assumptions

A model of group dynamics that has been used extensively in group psychotherapy is that of Bion's "basic assumptions." Bion (1961/1974, pp. 93–113) posited three predominant group cultures, which he held to occur in all groups and to stem from the projection of inner objects onto the group matrix as a response to the anxiety attendant on being part of a group. In the basic assumption of "dependency," the members maintain an illusory idealization of and dependency on the leader, with a belief that the latter will do all the work and provide a magical cure. In the basic assumption of "fight–flight," the members project their "badness" into the out group or a scapegoated member, and then attack or else flee from the projected "badness." In the basic assumption of "pairing," a couple is selected to represent and contain the hopes and ideals of the group, exemplified by utopian ideas and the cultural/religious expectation that a messiah figure will be forthcoming. These basic assumptions reflect group-as-a-whole collusive resistances to insight and change, but they may also become integrated as affective themes and sources of emotional energy within a "work group" that is oriented to the group task. Thus the dependency assumption, which can be a false expectation that the therapist will do all the work, can also be manifested as support, caregiving, and nurturing by the group; fight–flight can be sublimated into an attack on the group's problem; and pairing, which can be a manic flight from depressive affect, may also represent an opportunity for the group to work together to change its norms and goals in a positive direction. Cohen, Ettin, and Fidler (1998, pp. 120–122) discuss the importance of the basic assumptions to the leadership functions of the group. They link the dependency assumption to the "nurturant" function of the leader; the fight–flight assumption to the "protective" function; and the pairing assumption to the "representational" function (the leader as representative of the group's image and goals). The importance of such leadership functions to trauma survivors goes without saying: Nurturing, protection, and the sense of meaning are profoundly damaged by trauma.

In trauma groups, basic assumptions may become intensified as aspects of trauma that are reenacted in the group, or that serve as group resistances to the task of resolving the trauma. Within such groups, the dependency assumption may incorporate trauma-based feelings of helplessness or emotional paralysis. The fight–flight assumption can reevoke the terror of the original victimization. Pairing may stir up feelings related to incest, rape, and other sexual abuse, and to lack of boundaries. These conditions can represent serious dangers to group cohesion and development, but they can also be opportunities to process and work through the pathological object relations related to the trauma. It is fair to say that with traumatized patients in a group, the basic assumptions are likely to become intensified and rigidified, and the anxieties associated with them magnified.

Bion (1961/1974), who was strongly influenced by Melanie Klein, implied, in keeping with her emphasis on innate instinctual drives, that the basic assumptions are universal manifestations of group relations (see Schermer, 1985); indeed, there is considerable evidence that such states occur often in small and large training and therapy groups, organizations, and institutions. Nevertheless, it is noteworthy that Bion's initial observations were with groups of emotionally disordered soldiers at Northfield Military Hospital in England during World War II, and we can assume that a significant number of these men may well have suffered from war stress and trauma. Since we now know that so many persons have been severely traumatized, and that almost everyone has experienced milder forms of trauma and/or vicarious trauma experiences, it is interesting to consider that the more "normal" group cultures and group regressions may be in part functions of the covert expression of trauma within the group context (given this "widened definition" of trauma).

A Fourth, Specifically Trauma-induced Basic Assumption?

Hopper (1997) is one of a small number of group theorists who have taken this possibility seriously. Hopper, a sociologist as well as a group analyst and a psychoanalyst trained in the British independent school, believes that there has been an overemphasis in psychoanalysis on phantasy; he is very interested in the impact of actual reality, including traumatic events, on individuals and groups. Trauma is a particularly intrusive and insidious reality, but to a certain extent all of reality is at first overwhelming and traumatic to an infant, who depends upon his or her caregivers for survival. This connection has allowed Hopper to integrate social theory with insights from the British independent tradition of psychoanalysis in formulating his views of a fourth basic assumption.

Hopper worked with an ongoing therapy group of Shoah (Holocaust) survivors, and also served as a consultant for businesses undergoing radical, potentially traumatic adjustments. In both contexts, he observed group climates that he takes to constitute a fourth basic assumption. He calls this assumption "incohesion," with two distinct manifestations: "aggregation" and "massification" (hence the acronym I/AM). In "aggregation," the group members behave as if each is an isolate with no contact with the others, comparable to a crustacean (a sea creature with a hard shell). In "massification," the members behave as if they are fused with each other, with an emphasis on their sameness—as if they were amoebae, which mindlessly extend their tentacles into contact with each other, or else vacuoles, which suck in everything that surrounds them. Hopper believes that these states are group defenses against annihilation anxiety, the fear of the total destruction of the self.

Hopper's work to some extent parallels that of Turquet (1974, 1975/ 1994), who posited the existence of a fourth basic assumption of "oneness" in large-group settings; Turquet attributed this to a tendency to surrender oneself to an all-powerful, encompassing entity in order to cope with the regressive forces inherent therein. Hopper, however, emphasizes the role of traumatic loss reminiscent of early abandonment and "total dependency" experiences. In this state, the group and leader are overidealized and a feeling of sameness predominates. This is a common occurrence in trauma groups, especially in the early phases of development.

Ganzarain (Chapter 4) holds that the basic assumption of oneness results from "persecutory anxiety" (the fear of retaliation by "bad" objects) and splitting. Hopper's view is different and more radical. He contends that the group state of I/AM is a regression to a presplitting, narcissistic stage of total dependency, where annihilation fears are warded off by an encapsulated psychosis. Thus, for Hopper, the fourth assumption is a distinctly trauma-based development at a deeper level of regression than the ones described by Bion.

Ganzarain (Chapter 4) relates the oneness or I/AM assumption to an early stage of trauma groups, which Lonergan (1989) has called the "pre-group." She in turn emphasizes the need of trauma patients to maintain self-cohesion and self-esteem in these early phases, and she utilizes Kohut's self psychology to understand the members' strivings to sustain self-cohesion by idealizing each other, the group, and the leader. Only in later phases, according to Lonergan (1989), can the group address narcissistic injury, loss of self-esteem, and mutual aggression, while Ganzarain (Chapter 4) suggests that they must be interpreted early in group development, albeit with sensitivity to the needs of the patients. Lonergan (personal communication, September 22, 1999) feels that the pre-group phase should be devoted to the establishment of group cohesion and a therapeutic alliance. Lonergan states:

> I wouldn't recommend that the therapist go for the underlying fear or the mistrust and hostility before there is a therapeutic alliance, and what I'm really saying is that with the pre-group you establish a therapeutic alliance and build some connection and commitment to the group, and later on, in the power phase of the group, you address the aggression.

Which of these three views of group sameness and idealization—namely, (1) preparanoid fusion as a defense against annihilation anxiety (Hopper), (2) splitting mechanisms (Ganzarain), or (3) narcissistic self-object idealization (Lonergan)—is correct is still controversial. What can be said to the therapist working with such group climates is that he or she consider the possibility that they may be related specifically to traumatic experiences and may be interpretable in that manner. Furthermore, the group, in order to grow emotionally, must eventually move beyond the fourth assumption in order to be able to deal with differences and with aggression. For underneath the blissful feeling that "we are all one and all the same" (or else "we are each safe within our individual hard shells") is severe trauma-based anxiety. The therapist's attention to the link between group-as-a-whole states and trauma is a key to unlocking the potential of the group matrix to heal trauma.

SPECIAL POPULATIONS

An important premise of this book is that attention to subtleties in and individual differences among particular patients and groups (diversity) is as important as identifying the commonalities of trauma (our common humanity). Although there are common features in the treatment of all psychological trauma, the type of trauma and the membership criteria of the group affect group initiation and maintenance, group dynamics, and transference–countertransference in particular ways. Thus we have devoted considerable space in this volume to the treatment of specific kinds of trauma and their consequences: PTSD; sexual and physical abuse; prolonged and terminal illness; traumatization and bereavement in children; catastrophic events in the community; and political persecution and torture. In addition, discussions of DSM diagnoses that are often trauma-based are provided—in particular, the dissociative disorders and complex disorders. Each chapter addresses how to apply the knowledge of trauma to the particular subpopulation, some of the logistics of the treatment process, and the specifics of treating that particular subgroup of patients in the group setting.

Due to space limitations, we have not included in this volume an exhaustive representation of the types and variations of trauma and trauma-related groups. Notably, for example, we have not considered groups specifically for victims of spousal abuse and domestic violence (although aspects of these topics are included in Buchele's discussion of physical and sexual abuse in Chapter 7); AIDS support groups (although Marcus and Bernard do address chronic illness in Chapter 8); substance abuse groups that address trauma; groups for adult children of alcoholics; adolescent groups; hospital-based crisis intervention groups; music, art, and psychodrama therapy groups; bereavement groups where trauma may play a role; and so on. We hope, however, that we have provided a sufficient range for the reader to be able to extrapolate in many instances to his or her particular groups. Of course, we strongly suggest that this book be utilized along with proper supervision in running such groups. We agree with feedback from our authors that the proper supervisor for such purposes is someone who is experienced and trained both as a group therapist and in the treatment of trauma itself.

Although most of this chapter has been devoted to a discussion of issues relevant to the remainder of the book, for purposes of orientation we now give a brief overview of each chapter devoted to a special population or set of diagnostic entities.

Posttraumatic Stress Disorder

As mentioned earlier, PTSD is the primary diagnosis of the impact of trauma. It may be full-blown, or else masked and muted for considerable periods of time. It may occur right after a trauma or years later, as the repressed memories surface. It may persist for many years, as has been the case with Vietnam veterans. PTSD is often treated in groups convened for this purpose—often, however, with mixed results. Johnson and Lubin (Chapter 6), along with their colleagues, have devoted themselves to improving the quality and results of group treatment for PTSD. As mentioned earlier, they compare and contrast a model they have developed (the interactive psychoeducational group therapy [IPGT] model) with that of a colleague, Patricia Resick (cognitive processing therapy [CPT]; Resick & Schnicke, 1993). Both techniques are structured and time-limited, and both models have empirical evidence to support their usefulness. As Johnson and Lubin (Chapter 6, p. 165) say,

> Group therapy can serve as a primary treatment for PTSD symptoms when the group format is specifically designed toward that end. Two models of group therapy have been described that hold promise as means of decreasing PTSD symptomatology. . . . The essential feature of these treatments is their attention to the symptom pictures of individuals in the context of their psychosocial functioning, as well as a relentless pursuit of distorted traumatic schemata and confrontation of faulty cognitions (CPT) or lack of differentiation (IPGT).

The IPGT approach utilizes an object relations model for helping the patients reown their projective identifications and overcome role formations such as victim–victimizer, which have a negative impact upon their functioning.

Physical and Sexual Abuse

Both physical abuse and sexual abuse occur in epidemic proportions in the United States and worldwide. In certain respects, they can be considered "concealed norms" of a society that "paints a pretty picture" of the family unit and of interpersonal relations, while the "dark side" of human nature manifests itself "offstage" (Goffman, 1959). Incest, physical beatings of children, "date rape," assault, domestic violence, and spousal abuse occur at alarming rates, as shown by police reports, courtroom data, and other sources. In Chapter 7, Buchele provides a concise overview and in-depth discussion of group psychotherapy for victims of such severe boundary violations. She stresses that the primary goal for such patients is to recover from the betrayal of trust and the abuse of power implicit in such acts. Since many of these traumata take place in childhood and adolescence (and also, we now know, in old age, with the phenomenon of elder abuse), Buchele also emphasizes the importance of the stage of psychological development at which such a trauma occurs, and the impact of developmental stage upon the ego regression triggered by the trauma. She focuses on the revival of the emotional pain of trauma in the group, which evokes primitive defenses in the members as they interact with each other. And she provides vivid examples of reenactments of trauma and shows how they are managed.

Chronic and Terminal Physical Illness

A much-neglected population for group therapists to treat consists of patients with severe chronic and/or terminal illnesses. Many of the groups that do exist are set up by medical personnel, and the facilitators often lack group psychotherapy training. Thus these patients' emotional conflicts and deeper layers of feelings may never be addressed. Marcus and Bernard take a step in Chapter 8 toward helping group therapists to engage in this much-needed service (which can also enhance their practice!) by presenting a group therapy perspective on the types of groups to be made available, the problems and issues that arise, and the dynamics of these patients in the group context. They utilize Yalom's (1995) "therapeutic factors" as a scheme for conceptualizing the potential benefits of group treatment for physically ill patients, and they give lucid examples of the struggles of the group members and the benefits they gain.

An issue that often needs to be addressed in these groups is the impact on a patient and the group of disruptions caused by relapses of the physical illness, which may overwhelm the patient and family and/or prevent the patient from coming to the group for a period of time. In addition, the patient may know that his or her condition is terminal or else progressive and ultimately disabling. In these cases the aim of the group is the acceptance of the inevitability of future pain and loss (grieving for the future), whereas in groups for other types of trauma (e.g., childhood incest), the prospects for recovering can look considerably brighter. It is interesting that so little attention has been given to the patient's projected future and its effects on the therapy process. Work with the chronically and terminally ill can give us a better perspective on what "adjustment" means when the trauma is bound to recur and even intensify during and after treatment.

Traumatization and Bereavement in Children

In Chapter 9, Keyser, Seelaus, and Kahn take up a subject that is infrequently dealt with in the literature: group psychotherapy for children. The group setting would seem to be a natural place for children to work through their conflicts and emotions; yet the difficulties can be daunting, given their relatively short attention span and tendency to act out rather than "put into words." On the other hand, most children naturally gravitate toward their peer group, and they are relatively open and receptive to growth and change when given a modicum of attention, support, and boundaries.

Keyser et al. present an effective and deeply compassionate protocol for group psychotherapy with traumatized and bereaved children. Importantly, they take up details of how to arrange such groups in a context where "little things mean a lot." They discuss the group processes and roles that develop, and ways of managing them to therapeutic advantage. Their case examples both of individual children and of a sequence of group sessions are very vivid and illustrate the principles they espouse in a very palpable way. We would characterize their overall approach as a combination of ego-supportive and interpersonal modalities. A great deal of emphasis is placed on helping the children to give a narrative of what happened and to verbalize their innermost feelings and thoughts in a safe atmosphere. Simple rituals familiar to children are used to create a sense of community and to reinforce the main therapeutic factors. This approach seems to us to incorporate basic "mental hygiene" principles and to be consistent with the ego-psychological formulations of Anna Freud and the Hampstead Clinic in London (see Freud, 1999; Freud & Dann, 1951). We believe that Keyser and colleagues have made a unique contribution to the group psychotherapy literature, and hope that their model will provide an impetus and guide to the creation of these much-needed groups in children's hospitals, child guidance centers, schools, and other settings throughout the world.

Catastrophic Events in the Community

To call up an example of the large-scale disasters that affect our local and global communities on a daily basis, all one has to do is consult the daily news releases about such events as the ongoing conflicts in the former Yugoslavia and USSR; earthquakes in Turkey and elsewhere; devastating airplane crashes; and the shooting of high school students (most notoriously at Columbine High School in Littleton, Colorado) by their peers. Mental health workers are increasingly being called upon to provide "on-the-spot" psychiatric interventions to individuals, families, groups, and whole communities affected by such disasters. Group treatment is a significant part of the armamentarium of therapeutic measures—notably, acute interventional debriefing groups and medium- and long-term support groups.

In Chapter 10, Dembert and Simmer describe critical-incident stress management (CISM), which includes a range of approaches designed to support individuals and communities soon after an incident—often at the site of the event or at a nearby location. Victims, their families, community members, and crisis/emergency workers may be offered "debriefings," which help to address their emotional lability, PTSD symptoms, and practical concerns. Dembert was in fact called upon while writing this chapter to support the U.S. Navy SEALs in their recovery work following the crash of SwissAir Flight 111, near Peggy's Cove, Nova Scotia, on September 2, 1998. CISM training is now available through various organizations and practitioners, and Dembert and Simmer provide some resources for the reader. These authors also describe several types of support groups that have been offered to the victims of various disasters for considerable periods after these events.

Political Persecution and Torture

The appearance of a new biography of Helen Bamber (Belton, 1998)—a courageous member of Amnesty International in England, who has worked extensively and devotedly with victims of torture—highlights the contemporary attention being given to this horrific means of exercising political control. As

Bamber discovered, the suffering of torture victims for years after the event is unspeakable yet must be repeatedly spoken! Although in the United States, at least, there are not yet many groups for victims of political persecution and torture, we offer von Wallenberg Pachaly's sensitive and compassionate presentation of his work (with victims who come to Germany, his home country) in Chapter 11. We do this because we believe that (1) more such groups will be forming in the coming decades as a function of immigration patterns; (2) political persecution highlights the sociopolitical matrix of all trauma (von Wallenberg Pachaly calls it the "large-group system"), which is often neglected by the practitioner; (3) torture is an extreme form of trauma that involves an attempt by the perpetrator to obliterate the victim's personality and its social matrix, and therefore provides a magnifying glass, if you will, for understanding the dynamics and impact of all trauma; and (4) its treatment in the group setting illustrates the rebuilding of the personality from the ground up, which is essential to the treatment of some traumatized patients.

Like Buchele, von Wallenberg Pachaly emphasizes the reestablishment of trust via the group process, and the sorting out and reduction of the "victim–victimizer" mentality manifested in the members' projective identifications into each other, the therapist, and significant others. In addition, he stresses the nature of the group as a "good," nurturing, "maternal" object (Scheidlinger, 1974), and as a transitional space and object within which the members can have a safe space, a sanctuary in which literally to recreate their inner worlds by introjecting the healthy aspects of the group matrix.

In addition, as noted above, von Wallenberg Pachaly stresses the importance of the "large-group system" (the network of social workers, lawyers, family members, courts, etc., involved in rehabilitating the victim). The therapist, in von Wallenberg Pachaly's view, must work with the patient's network to reestablish the patient's trust and to prevent the sabotage of the curative work accomplished in the therapy group. In this respect, the therapist does not remain "neutral," but is a source of genuine concern and empowerment. In addition, the therapist does not remain entirely a detached analytical observer, but must take the side of the patient against the forces of victimization—a point also emphasized by Herman (1997, pp. 133–154).

Dissociative Disorders

As mentioned earlier, dissociative disorders (American Psychiatric Association, 1994, pp. 477–491) include a spectrum of long-term psychopathological outcomes of trauma that involve the persistence of severe dissociative states. These may range from trance states to compartmentalization and sudden resurfacing of ego states (e.g., the person may undergo a personality change or a change of mood) to dissociative amnesia, dissociative fugue, dissociative identity disorder (formerly multiple personality disorder), and depersonalization disorder (American Psychiatric Association, 1994).

As we have pointed out earlier, the study and treatment of dissociative disorders have led to a new paradigm of mental states and psychopathology (see Fine & Kluft, 1993; Putnam, 1989). Fine and Madden, the authors of Chapter 12, are thoroughly steeped in the new paradigm, but they retain a strong interest in "mainstream" cognitive-behavioral and psychodynamic psychotherapies.

Fine and Madden established the first outpatient group for dissociative identity disorder. They do not "pull punches" about the difficulties inherent in treating dissociative disorders in groups. For an approximation to the management issues involved, consider that it is equivalent to treating "groups" of internal alternate selves within the group, which exponentially increases the number of possible interactions! Furthermore, dissociative patients are prone to acting out, reenacting, and (of course) dissociating. Therefore, Fine and Madden recommend extensive training in treating dissociative disorders before conducting such groups. They also advise very thorough screening and consider that individual treatment may be the primary treatment approach, with group therapy providing a useful adjunct.

Fine and Madden utilize insights from group systems theory (see Agazarian, 1997) to formulate an approach that emphasizes cognitive restructuring as opposed to affective expression, the latter of which tends to become chaotic for these patients. Like the real estate agent who says that the three most important things about a property are "location, location, location," Fine and Madden stress "boundaries, boundaries, boundaries" with dissociative patients, pointing out the absence of semipermeable boundaries that selectively permit an exchange among different parts of the personality and with the outer environment.

Axis I and Axis II Disorders

Burton and Marshall (1999) have provided a case report illustrating the difficulties that can accompany the evaluation and treatment of an individual with a history of psychological trauma. They review the history of an adult female patient who initially presented with symptoms of major depression, PTSD, and borderline features (such as impulsivity, affective lability, and substance misuse), and who subsequently underwent a series of psychotherapeutic and pharmacological treatments at several inpatient and outpatient facilities. Diagnoses included the three mentioned above, as well as adjustment disorder (!) and bipolar I disorder. Treatment efforts were largely unsuccessful, even regressive, and the patient became a treatment recidivist until she encountered a therapist who made the trauma-based diagnosis (what Herman, 1997, pp. 199–222, calls "complex PTSD") the focus of treatment, without denying the comorbid diagnoses. The patient subsequently made significant progress toward becoming a significantly more functional and symptom-free individual.

This patient is one of innumerable patients who constitute a large percentage of the "bread-and-butter" caseload at both inpatient and outpatient facilities. Their various diagnoses may include mood disorders, substance use problems, eating disorders, personality disorders, and various combinations thereof. They sometimes bring up their trauma histories in treatment, but all too often treatment of the trauma itself is not systematically addressed, despite its being placed on the agenda by the patient.

Gallagher and Kibel (Chapter 13) forthrightly and systematically confront the problems and prospects inherent in treating these complex disorders in group psychotherapy. They take a conservative but cautiously optimistic stance on whether the traumata themselves can be properly addressed in groups. Pointing to the fact that both overwhelming affects and untoward behaviors may be released at times when neither the individual nor the group is able to deal with them, they place great emphasis on ego strength and external support systems, as well as adjunctive therapies, medication, and proper preparation—all of which increase the probability that the patient can benefit from the group experience. The capacity of the other members in these often heterogeneous groups to identify with the traumatized patient and to support him or her through the process is also an important factor.

Now that we have gone over specific subpopulations of traumatized patients in group psychotherapy, we hope that we have given the reader a thought-provoking "bird's-eye view" of a most important endeavor. However, what we have written is only an overview and is colored, of course, by our own biases. We invite the reader to partake of the rich lode of clinical insight and specialized knowledge that our highly experienced authors have brought to the ever-expanding field of group psychotherapy for psychological trauma. We believe our readers' efforts will be richly rewarded.

ACKNOWLEDGMENTS

We would like to thank Drs. Catherine Fine, Earl Hopper, Richard Kluft, Elaine Lonergan, and Andreas von Wallenberg Pachaly for their helpful comments and suggestions.

NOTES

1. A computer search of *Psychological Abstracts* (PsychINFO) revealed that in the 1970s there were only 3 articles abstracted on trauma groups with "trauma" and "group" in the title, while in the 1980s there were 8, and in the 1990s (excluding 1999) there were 19! In the same period, there were over 970 citations on trauma and groups with "trauma" and "group" anywhere in the citations or abstracts. The literature on trauma and groups has increased exponentially over three decades.
2. An "encapsulated psychosis" is a state of delusion, hallucinosis, and/or lack of reality testing that, instead of taking over the whole personality (as in schizo-

phrenia or bipolar disorders), is dissociated or split off from the main body of the personality—in a sense, preserving the self from total madness and annihilation.

3. "Fairbairn prefers [in contrast with Freud—Eds.] to regard the organizations that are repressed as more extensive and so more akin to a 'secondary personality' as investigated by Morton Prince and others" (Sutherland, 1989, p. 19).

4. If a brief, limited trauma occurs, prompt attention to the trauma and PTSD symptoms may minimize or reverse such regression. It has also been found that children who have an opportunity to verbalize a traumatic experience soon after it occurs suffer fewer long-term consequences than those who remain silent. These observations provide a rationale for addressing trauma, whenever possible, soon after it occurs.

5. The correlation between trauma and splitting is consistent with the finding of Herman and van der Kolk (1987) that many patients with borderline personality disorder—whose transference involves considerable splitting and projective identification (Kernberg, 1975)—have trauma and abuse histories. These reports echo our own group experiences. One of us (Klein), for example, found that in a group consisting of women diagnosed with borderline personality disorder, five of the six women reported histories of trauma and abuse.

REFERENCES

Agazarian, Y. M. (1997). *Systems-centered therapy for groups.* New York: Guilford Press.

Agazarian, Y., & Peters, R. (1981). *The visible and invisible group.* London: Routledge.

Alexander, F., & French, T. M. (1946). *Psychoanalytic therapy.* New York: Ronald Press.

American Psychiatric Association. (1994). *Diagnostic and statistical manual of mental disorders* (4th ed.). Washington, DC: Author.

Aron, L., & Harris, A. (Eds.). (1993). *The legacy of Sandor Ferenczi.* Hillsdale, NJ: Analytic Press.

Ashbach, C., & Schermer, V. (1987). *Object relations, the self, and the group: A conceptual paradigm.* London: Routledge.

Bacal, H.A., & Newman, K. M. (1990). *Theories of object relations: Bridges to self psychology.* New York: Columbia University Press.

Beck, A. (1993). *Cognitive therapy and the emotional disorders.* New York: New American Library. (Original work published 1976)

Belton, N. (1998). *The good listener: Helen Bamber, a life against cruelty.* New York: Pantheon.

Bennis, W. G., & Shepard, H. A. (1956). A theory of group development. *Human Relations, 9,* 415–437.

Bion, W. R. (1967). *Second thoughts: Selected papers on psycho-analysis.* London: Heinemann. (Original work published 1959)

Bion, W. R. (1974). *Experiences in groups, and other papers.* New York: Ballantine. (Original work published 1961)

Bremner, J. D., Seibyl, J. P., & Scott, T. M. (1992, May). Depressed hippocampal volume in posttraumatic stress disorder (New Research Abstract 155). *Proceedings of the 145th Annual Meeting of the American Psychiatric Association.

Brenner, I. (1999, April 30). *The therapist's countertransference response to traumatized patients.* Workshop presented at the conference Phoenix Rising: Healing Trauma through Resilience and Transcendence, Thomas Jefferson University, Philadelphia.

Briere, J., & Runtz, M. (1987). Post sexual abuse trauma: Data and implications for clinical practice. *Journal of Interpersonal Violence, 2,* 367–379.

Brisson, K. J., & Leavitt, S. C. (1995, December). Coping with bereavement: Long-term perspectives on grief and mourning. *Ethos, 23*(4), 395–400.

Bryer, J. B., Nelson, B. A., Miller, J. B., & Krol, P. A. (1987). Childhood sexual and physical abuse as factors in adult psychiatric illness. *American Journal of Psychiatry, 144,* 1426–1430.

Burns, D. D. (1999). *Feeling good: The new mood therapy* (Rev. ed.). New York: Avon.

Burton, J. K., & Marshall, R. D. (1999). Categorizing fear: The role of trauma in a formulation. *American Journal of Psychiatry, 156*(5), 761–766.

Chu, J. (1998). *Rebuilding shattered lives: The responsible treatment of complex post-traumatic and dissociative disorders.* New York: Wiley.

Clark, S. R. L. (1996). Minds, memes, and multiples. *Philosophy, Psychiatry, and Psychology, 3,* 121–128.

Cohen, B. D., Ettin, M. F., & Fidler, J. W. (1998). Conceptions of leadership: The "analytic stance" of the group psychotherapist. *Group Dynamics: Theory, Research, and Practice, 2*(2), 118–131.

Durkin, H. (1964). *The group in depth.* New York: International Universities Press.

Erikson, E. (1959). *Identity and the life cycle (Psychological Issues,* Monograph No. 1). New York: International Universities Press.

Ey, H. (1968). Pierre Janet: The man and his work. In B. B. Wolman (Ed.), *Historical roots of contemporary psychology.* New York: Harper & Row.

Fairbairn, R. W. D. (1943). The repression and the return of bad objects. *British Journal of Medical Psychology, 19,* 327–341.

Federn, P. (1952). *Ego psychology and the psychoses* (E. Weiss, Ed. & Trans.). New York: Basic Books.

Fenichel, O. (1945). *The psychoanalytic theory of neurosis.* New York: Norton.

Ferenczi, S. (1980). The confusion of tongues between adults and children: The language of tenderness and passion. In M. Balint (Ed.) & E. Mosbacher (Trans.), *Final contributions to the problems and methods of psychoanalysis* (pp. 156–167). London: Karnac Books. (Original work published 1932)

Fine, C. G. (1990). The cognitive sequelae of incest. In R. P. Kluft (Ed.), *Incest-related syndromes of adult psychopathology* (pp. 161–182). Washington, DC: American Psychiatric Press.

Fine, C. G., & Kluft, R. (Eds.). (1993). *Clinical perspectives on multiple personality disorder.* Washington, DC: American Psychiatric Press.

Fish-Murray, C. C., Koby, E. V., & van der Kolk, B. (1987). Evolving ideas: The effect of abuse on children's thought. In B. van der Kolk (Ed.), *Psychological trauma* (pp. 89–110). Washington, DC: American Psychiatric Press.

Freud, A. (1999). *Selected writings of Anna Freud.* Harmondsworth, England: Penguin Books.

Freud, A., & Dann, S. (1951). An experiment in group upbringing. *Psychoanalytic Study of the Child, 6,* 127–168.

Freud, S. (1955). Beyond the pleasure principle. In J. Strachey (Ed. & Trans.), *The standard edition of the complete psychological works of Sigmund Freud* (Vol. 18, pp. 3–64). London: Hogarth Press. (Original work published 1920)

Freud, S. (1958). Psycho-analytic notes on an autobiographical account of a case of paranoia (dementia paranoides). In J. Strachey (Ed. & Trans.), *The standard edition of the complete psychological works of Sigmund Freud* (Vol. 12, pp. 3–84). London: Hogarth Press. (Original work published 1911)

Freud, S. (1962). Sexuality in the aetiology of the neuroses. In J. Strachey (Ed. & Trans.), *The standard edition of the complete psychological works of Sigmund Freud* (Vol. 3, pp. 261–285). London: Hogarth Press. (Original work published 1898)

Gelinas, D. (1983). The persistent negative effects of incest. *Psychiatry, 46,* 312–332.

Gergen, K. J. (1991). *The saturated self: Dilemmas of identity in contemporary life.* New York: Basic Books.

Goffman, E. (1959). *The presentation of self in everyday life.* Garden City, NY: Doubleday.

Gordon, J. (1994). Bion's post-*Experiences in groups* thinking on groups: A clinical example of—K. In V. L. Schermer & M. Pines (Eds.), *Ring of fire* (pp. 107–127). London: Routledge.

Grinker, R. R., & Spiegel, J. J. (1945). *Men under stress.* New York: McGraw-Hill.

Herman, J. (1997). *Trauma and recovery* (Rev. ed.). New York: Basic Books.

Herman, J., & van der Kolk, B. (1987). Traumatic antecedents of borderline personality disorder. In B. van der Kolk (Ed.), *Psychological trauma* (pp. 111–126). Washington, DC: American Psychiatric Press.

Hinshelwood, R. (1994). Attacks on the reflective space: Containing primitive emotional states. In V. L. Schermer & M. Pines (Eds.), *Ring of fire* (pp. 86–106). London: Routledge.

Hopper, E. (1991). Encapsulation as a defence against the fear of annihilation. *International Journal of Psycho-Analysis, 72*(4), 607–624.

Hopper, E. (1997). Traumatic experience in the unconscious life of groups: A fourth basic assumption. *Group Analysis, 30,* 439–470.

Jacobson, A. (1989). Physical and sexual assault histories among psychiatric outpatients. *American Journal of Psychiatry, 146,* 755–758.

Jacobson, A., & Richardson, B. (1987). Assault experiences of 100 psychiatric inpatients: Evidence of the need for routine inquiry. *American Journal of Psychiatry, 144,* 908–913.

Janoff-Bulman, R. (1992). *Shattered assumptions: Towards a new psychology of trauma.* New York: Free Press.

Kardiner, A. (1941). *The traumatic neuroses of war.* New York: Hoeber.

Kernberg, O. (1975). *Borderline conditions and pathological narcissism.* New York: Aronson.

Klein, M. (1977). Notes on some schizoid mechanisms. In M. Klein, *Envy and gratitude and other works: 1946–1963* (pp. 1–24). New York: Delacourt Press. (Original work published 1946)

Kluft, R. (2000). *A vademecum for the treatment of dissociative identity disorder.* Manuscript in preparation.

Kohut, H. (1971). *The analysis of the self.* New York: International Universities Press.

Kohut, H. (1977). *The restoration of the self.* New York: International Universities Press.

Kramer, S., & Akhtar, S. (Eds.). (1991). *The trauma of transgression: Psychotherapy of incest victims.* Northvale, NJ: Aronson.

Lewis, H. B. (1987). Shame and the narcissistic personality. In D. L. Nathanson (Ed.), *The many faces of shame* (pp. 93–132). New York: Guilford Press.

Lindemann, E. (1944). Symptomatology and management of acute grief. *American Journal of Psychiatry, 101,* 141–148.

Lonergan, E. C. (1989). *Group intervention: How to begin and maintain groups in medical and psychiatric settings,* Northvale, NJ: Aronson.

Maccoby, M. (1995). [Review of *The Legacy of Sándor Ferenczi* (1993), edited by L. Aron and A. Harris]. *Psychoanalytic Psychology, 12*(2), 321–323.

McDougall, W. (1926). *Outline of abnormal psychology.* London: Methuen.

Miller, A. (1981). *Prisoners of childhood.* New York: Basic Books.

Nitsun, M. (1996). *The anti-group.* London: Routledge.

Pearlman, L. A., & Saakvitne, K. W. (1995). *Trauma and the therapist: Countertransference and vicarious traumatization in psychotherapy with incest survivors.* New York: Norton.

Putnam, F. W. (1989). *Diagnosis and treatment of multiple personality disorder.* New York: Guilford Press.

Racker, H. (1968). *Transference and countertransference.* New York: International Universities Press.

Rando, T. (1993). *Treatment of complicated mourning.* Chicago: Research Press.

Redl, F. (1963). Psychoanalysis and group psychotherapy: A developmental point of view. *American Journal of Orthopsychiatry, 33,* 135–147.

Resick, P., Jordan, C., Girelli, S., Hutter, C., & Marhoefer-Dvorak, S. (1988). A comparative outcome study of behavioral group therapy for sexual assault victims. *Behavior Therapy, 19,* 385–401.

Resick, P., & Schnicke, M. (1993). *Cognitive processing therapy for rape victims.* Newbury Park, CA: Sage.

Rodman, F. R. (1990). Insistence on being himself. In P. L. Giovacchini (Ed.), *Tactics and techniques in psychoanalytic therapy: Vol. 3. The implications of Winnicott's contributions* (pp. 21–40). Northvale, NJ: Aronson.

Rosenau, P. M. (1992). *Post-modernism and the social sciences.* Princeton, NJ: Princeton University Press.

Saxe, G. N., Vasile, R. G., Hill, T. C., Bloomingdale, K., & van der Kolk, B. A. (1992). SPECT imaging and multiple personality disorder. *Journal of Nervous and Mental Disease, 180,* 662–663.

Scharff, J. S., & Scharff, D. (1994). *Object relations therapy of physical and sexual trauma.* Northvale, NJ: Aronson.

Scheidlinger, S. (1955). The concept of identification in group psychotherapy. *American Journal of Group Psychotherapy, 9,* 661–672.

Scheidlinger, S. (1974). On the concept of the "mother group." *International Journal of Group Psychotherapy, 24,* 417–428.

Schermer, V. L. (1985). Beyond Bion: The basic assumption states revisited. In M.

Pines (Ed.), *Bion and group psychotherapy* (pp. 139–150). London: Routledge and Kegan Paul.

Searles, H. (1975). The patient as therapist to his analyst. In P. L. Giovacchini (Ed.), *Tactics and techniques in psychoanalytic therapy: Vol. 2* (pp. 95–151). Northvale, NJ: Aronson.

Shengold, L. (1989). *Soul murder: The effects of childhood abuse and deprivation.* New Haven, CT: Yale University Press.

Sidis, B., & Goodhart, S. P. (1909). *Multiple personality.* New York: Appleton.

Slater, P. (1966). *Microcosm: Structural, psychological, and religious evolution in groups.* New York: Wiley.

Sutherland, J. (1989). *Fairbairn's journey to the interior.* London: Free Association Books.

Tedeschi, R. G., Park, C. L., & Calhoun, L. G. (Eds.). (1998). *Posttraumatic growth: Positive changes in the aftermath of crisis.* Mahwah, NJ: Erlbaum.

Turquet, P. (1974). *Leadership: The individual and the group.* In G. S. Gibbard, J. J. Hartmann, & R. D. Mann (Eds.), *Analysis of groups* (pp. 349–371). San Francisco: Jossey-Bass.

Turquet, P. (1994). Threats to the identity in the large groups. In L. Kreeger (Ed.), *The large group: Dynamics and therapy* (pp. 87–144). London: Karnac Books. (Original work published 1975)

van der Kolk, B. A. (Ed.). (1987a). *Psychological trauma.* Washington, DC: American Psychiatric Press.

van der Kolk, B. (1987b). The separation cry and the trauma response: Developmental issues in the psychobiology of attachment and separation. In B. van der Kolk (Ed.), *Psychological trauma* (pp. 31–62). Washington, DC: American Psychiatric Press.

van der Kolk, B. (1997). Post-traumatic stress disorder and memory. *Psychiatric Times* [Online serial], *14*(3). Available: http://www.mhsource.com/pt/p970354.html

van der Kolk, B., & Greenberg, M. S. (1987). The psychobiology of the trauma response: Hyperarousal, constriction, and addiction to traumatic reexposure. In B. van der Kolk (Ed.), *Psychological trauma* (pp. 63–88). Washington, DC: American Psychiatric Press.

van der Kolk, B., & van der Hart, O. (1991). Pierre Janet and the breakdown of adaptation in psychological trauma. *American Journal of Psychiatry, 146,* 1530–1540.

Volkan, V. (1982). *Linking objects and linking phenomena.* New York: International Universities Press.

Watkins, J. G., & Watkins, H. H. (1997). *Ego states: Theory and therapy.* New York: Norton.

Winnicott, D. W. (1958). Primary maternal preoccupation. In D. Winnicott, *Collected papers: Through paediatrics to psycho-analysis* (pp. 300–305). New York: Basic Books.

Winnicott, D. W. (1960). The theory of the parent–child relationship. *International Journal of Psycho-Analysis, 41,* 585–595.

Winnicott, D. W. (1965). Ego distortion in terms of true and false self. In D. Winnicott, *The maturational processes and the facilitating environment: Studies in the theory of emotional development* (pp. 140–152). New York: International Universities Press.

Winnicott, D. W. (1971). Transitional objects and transitional phenomena. In D. Winnicott, *Playing and reality* (pp. 1–25). New York: Basic Books. (Original work published 1951)

Winnicott, D. W. (1986). The theory of the parent–infant relationship. In P. Buckley (Ed.), *Essential papers on object relations* (pp. 233–253). New York: New York University Press. (Original work published 1960)

Wolf, E. S. (1988). *Treating the self: Elements of clinical self psychology.* New York: Guilford Press.

Yalom, I. (1995). *The theory and practice of group psychotherapy* (4th ed.). New York: Basic Books.

Young, J. E., & Young, J. S. (1994). *Reinventing your life: How to break free from negative life patterns and feel good again.* New York: Plume Press.

2

◄O►

Initiating, Screening, and Maintaining Psychotherapy Groups for Traumatized Patients

Marianne Goodman
Daniel Weiss

Group treatment is a powerful therapeutic modality for traumatized patients, but the formation and maintenance of a therapeutic group require careful consideration. This chapter describes various aspects of how to start a trauma group, with an emphasis on determining the most appropriate type and stage of group treatment for the population to be aided. In addition, the importance of adequate screening and preparation of group members for the therapy task is discussed, along with strategies to keep a trauma group viable and functioning.

GROUP VERSUS INDIVIDUAL TREATMENT

Numerous treatment strategies are available to clinicians treating traumatized people. Dye and Roth (1991) reviewed individual approaches for incest survivors and Vietnam veterans with posttraumatic stress disorder (PTSD), including systematic desensitization, implosive therapy, stress management, hypnosis, gestalt therapy, pharmacotherapy, and stress-oriented psychotherapy. Although their study focused on individual modalities, it is relevant to group psychotherapy, in that it points out the diversity of approaches that may be used in treating trauma. Dye and Roth also concluded that, regardless of the form of therapy chosen, questions pertinent to "uncovering" or to "shoring up of defenses" remain paramount, and that most treatments use aspects of both.

Individual therapy is indicated when a detailed examination of the trauma is necessary, and when retrieval of lost memories needs to be conducted in the safest arena possible and in the context of a trusted relationship. During individual treatment, a referral to trauma group treatment is indicated in the following circumstances: (1) Trauma work threatens to overwhelm the original focus of individual treatment, which may not be the trauma itself, so that there is a need for an additional venue to address the trauma issue; (2) the patient desires more in-depth trauma-focused experience; (3) the patient wishes for a more complete memory of the traumatic event; (4) the patient needs to combat the social isolation, feelings of shame, and self-deprecation associated with the trauma; and/or (5) the patient needs to mend disrupted interpersonal relations stemming from a traumatic incident.

A number of clinicians consider group psychotherapy the treatment of choice for traumatized individuals (Herman, 1992; Koller, Marmar, & Kanas, 1992; van der Kolk, 1993). Trauma group psychotherapy shares many qualities with group treatment in general, including the provision of support and empathy, the goal of developing an observing ego, the ability to help others, and the importance of peer feedback (Courtois, 1988; Yalom, 1985). However, a distinctive feature is its focus on each patient's constructing a narrative of the traumatic incident and having this narrative validated by others. The understanding and identification with others who have shared a similar misfortune mitigate the shame associated with secrecy.

In addition, group treatment allows for an *in vivo* experience of seeing how the traumatic experience affects interpersonal relating—a domain that is often negatively impacted. The other members in the group help to lessen guilt and correct distortions (Kanas, Schoenfeld, Marmar, & Weiss, 1994).

Many therapists advocate concurrent individual and group treatment for maximum benefit. Trauma group treatment ranges from being an ancillary component of individual treatment to being the primary modality, depending upon the severity of the patient's symptoms, as well as the degree of psychic pain and dysfunction originating from the trauma. Ideally, a patient enters individual treatment with a trustworthy therapist first and is then referred to concomitant trauma group psychotherapy for specialized services. Other treatment modalities, including medications, family treatment, couple therapy, and/or Twelve-Step groups, are often necessary and complement the healing process.

INITIATION OF PSYCHOTHERAPY GROUPS
FOR TRAUMATIZED PATIENTS

When therapists are forming a trauma group, the choice of a model for intervention is a function of target population, theoretical orientation, and stage of group treatment. Various structural parameters must also be considered.

Target Population

In defining a target population, therapists must consider the degree of similarity and difference among members. Traumatized patients feel more connected to others who have shared a similar misfortune. Overly disparate types of traumata or large gradients in the severity of trauma may hamper the formation of group cohesion, a critical component of group treatment (see below). However, the traumata need not be identical. Consider this example:

> A group for women with a history of childhood sexual abuse contained individuals who also suffered from adult tragedies of rape, muggings, and wife battering. These later traumata were discussed and were understood to stem from an inability to detect danger adequately, which in turn arose as a consequence of childhood abuse. These connections facilitated group cohesion.
>
> However, when one member of this group developed lung cancer, her descriptions of the medical procedures, the pain, and the details of chemotherapy, although traumatic, deflected from the group process. This woman ultimately left the group in search of a more medically focused supportive venue.

In initial group treatment, it is expected that members will measure their experiences of trauma against those of others. Variations in the severity of the incident, protective forces, quality of supports, and level of premorbid functioning all contribute to the degree of maladaptive response. These expected differences become the material for the group to discuss. It is therefore important that the target population forming the group have a common defining element from which to explore differences.

> In a trauma group for survivors of childhood sexual abuse, one discussion centered on the perpetrators of the abuse. Members talked of their traumatic betrayal by either a parent, uncle, teacher, brother, or minister. Examination of these different relationships with the abusers led to increased disclosure about these connections. Ms. M's abuse by her brother, although initially innocent, progressed to his visiting her at night to play "doctor." This was contrasted with Ms. P's memories

of an inebriated father forcing himself upon her. Ms. L and Ms. T shared common ground as "students" to their abusers. However, the added elements of religion and of confusion over "right" and "wrong" were imperative for a full understanding of Ms. T's traumatic story.

Members of the group, although unified by the shared trauma of unwanted sexual acts, came to appreciate the unique experience of each member and the variability in childhood sexual abuse.

Types of Group Therapy for Traumatized Individuals

As with individual treatment, there are numerous theoretical approaches to trauma group treatment, including psychoeducational, cognitive-behavioral, psychodynamic, rap, and trauma-focused. Psychoeducational trauma groups are highly structured and helpful in early stages of treatment; they inform the patients about PTSD symptoms, illness course, and available treatment. A cognitive-behavioral paradigm focuses on changing negative behaviors and on the teaching and practicing of new skills (Linehan, 1993). A psychodynamic approach stresses insight and promotes more adaptive coping through the understanding and resolution of trauma-related conflict (Lindy, 1993). Rap groups originated in the 1970s with the purpose of providing Vietnam veterans a forum to discuss their war experience in a peer group without an authoritarian leader (Scurfield, Corker, Gongla, & Hough, 1984). More recently, the concept of trauma-focused groups has emerged; these groups have the explicit goal of examining the trauma and giving each member the opportunity to reconstruct the history of what happened (Rozynko & Dondershine, 1991). When a trauma group is being formed, the selection of a theoretical backing anchors a clinician and guides the types of interventions made. It is, of course, important that the conceptual base be relevant to the patient population and setting.

Stages of Trauma Group Treatment

Herman (1992) has proposed a three-stage model of group treatment for traumatized individuals. Patients move in sequence from one group to the next. Her three stages include (1) a crisis-oriented group; (2) a short-term, trauma-focused group; and (3) a relationship-focused group that is not specifically targeted for trauma victims. Stage 1 treatment focuses on establishing safety and self-care, encouraging discussion, and providing a cognitive framework for each patient's traumatic event. Psychoeducational and cognitive-behavioral approaches are often applied (Srein & Eisen, 1996). Stage 2 is conceptualized as a time-limited, trauma-focused intervention with a homogeneous population, with the explicit goals of creating a narrative of each patient's traumatic event, retrieving lost memories, and beginning to experience appropriate affect. Lastly, stage 3 has an interpersonal focus, achieved through a long-term general psychotherapy group treatment.

Applying Herman's model to examples from the literature allows one to appreciate how different interventions are necessary during the course of recovery. An example of a stage 1 group is provided by Najavitas, Weiss, and Liese (1996), who describe an outpatient cognitive-behavioral therapy group targeted to women with PTSD and a substance use disorder. Their group approach aims to minimize symptoms, encourage abstinence, teach coping skills, and educate patients about PTSD. They do not explore the trauma or promote insight; these are elements of stage 2 and stage 3 groups. Their treatment lasts for 24 sessions and utilizes the following techniques: visual aids, a syllabus, memory enhancement exercises, and homework assignments. Sessions are structured; include role play; and are divided into behavioral, cognitive, and relationship units.

Rozynko and Dondershine (1991) report on a stage 2 trauma-focused inpatient group therapy for male veterans with PTSD. They propose that such a group should have 12–18 members and last approximately 3 months, with the implicit goal of having each veteran share his war trauma experience with the group. (Inpatient groups with a 3-month duration are rarely feasible in the managed care environment, but this model may still be practical in Veterans Affairs Medical Centers and in long-term residential programs in the community. In addition, these authors' findings are partially relevant for outpatient groups.) Through creating a narrative, each participant is helped not only to remember and examine his traumatic experience, but to challenge the problems and distortions resulting from the trauma that affect his current life. The authors note the importance of creating a safe, supportive environment for this process to occur successfully.

A group combining stages 2 and 3 is described by Tyson and Goodman (1996), who discuss a weekly, long-term psychodynamic psychotherapy group targeted to women with a childhood history of sexual abuse. The goals of the group extend beyond just telling the traumatic "story," and include understanding how current and past interpersonal connections have been affected by the trauma. An exploration of behavioral reenactments and of transference between group members is stressed. All members have had previous or concurrent individual psychotherapy.

Factors that influence the choice of theoretical underpinning and trauma group stage include the patient mix that is available, as well as the degree of dysfunction, current symptomatology, and treatment goals of prospective members. For many patients with PTSD, symptom control of nightmares, flashbacks, or affective illness may be the goal, which is best achieved by a stage 1 or stage 2 group. A more psychodynamic exploratory approach is more advanced and potentially difficult, requiring patients to possess adequate coping skills and the desire for more complete healing.

These issues are expanded upon below in the "Screening Patients for Trauma Groups" section.

Group Structural Parameters

Structural parameters to consider in initiation of trauma group treatment include time frame, open versus closed enrollment, degree of heterogeneity in the members' traumatic experience, group composition and size, degree of structure in the format, number of therapists, and cohesion. Each of these topics is addressed separately.

Time Frame

In the structuring of a trauma group, the time frame deserves attention. Will the group be time-limited or open-ended? Time-limited groups serve to focus the patients and are usually more structured and supportive, whereas open-ended groups are geared for later stages of treatment and higher-functioning patients. Koller et al. (1992), in their outpatient program for Vietnam veterans with PTSD, utilize a flexible short-term approach to provide additional treatment for those who require it. The trauma group psychotherapy is divided into 16-week blocks. Patients can either "graduate" or opt to continue for the next 4-month segment.

The length of treatment for short-term approaches varies, depending upon the goals and objectives of each group. An informal survey of the literature reveals that most time-limited stage 1 or stage 2 groups range from 10 weeks to 6 months in duration.

Open versus Closed Enrollment

Another consideration is whether to permit enrollment in the group to remain open or to keep it closed. In closed enrollment, all members start together and new members are not added. In open enrollment, members join the group as needed or as they become available. Groups with closed enrollment have less disruption in the group process, but require sufficient numbers at first to keep the groups from becoming too small if members drop out prematurely. Longer-term psychodynamic groups benefit from adding members as additional transference relationships become possible. Shorter-term stage 1 and stage 2 groups, where safety and trust are paramount issues, will have greater difficulty with an open-enrollment policy.

Homogeneous versus Heterogeneous Composition

A frequent concern when therapists are setting up a treatment group is the degree to which the members' traumata should be homogeneous. A guiding principle is that earlier-stage groups are more successful when they are composed of similarly traumatized individuals, in order to facilitate bonding and a sense of belonging (i.e., group cohesion; see below). In later-stage groups, a more heterogeneous population is indicated, to challenge overidentification with victim status and to fully integrate the traumatic experience into everyday living. However, one must be aware that there are considerable individual differences within a given category of trauma (e.g., war, sexual abuse, rape, political persecution), and that group treatment of psychological trauma is more successful when the composition of group members is similar in terms of age, gender (especially for sexual abuse and rape), previous treatment history, level of PTSD pathology, and concurrent Axis I diagnoses.

Group Size

Trauma groups vary in size. In the general group psychotherapy literature, eight is the optimum number of members (Yalom, 1985). However, in the trauma group literature, outpatient stage 2 and stage 3 groups usually run smaller, because of the intensity of the work and increased likelihood of dropouts.

Degree of Structure in Format

The degree of structure within the group format will depend upon the theoretical orientation and the particular goals and objectives of the group. Shorter-term groups tend to be more structured and may even follow an agenda or schedule of topics predetermined by the therapist (see Najavitas et al., 1996, for examples). Later-stage psychotherapy groups may be unstructured, and material for discussion may be generated by the patients.

Use of Cotherapy

The use of cotherapy in conducting the group is another factor to evaluate. Cotherapists are more costly in terms of time and personnel, but offer various benefits: potential parental transference figures; assistance in difficult countertransference reactions; and minimization of disruption centering around therapist absence, vacation, or burnout. Consider this example:

> In a group for Vietnam veterans suffering from the effects of war and childhood abuse, one member developed a strong paternal transference to the male coleader. As a child, the patient had been brutally beaten by a stepfather and abandoned by his biological father. In the group, a pattern developed that any perceived criticism or lack of attention by the "father" of the group was experienced by this patient as

"being destroyed." Slights felt like "slaps in the face" and triggered flashbacks of beatings. Support from the female cotherapist enabled the patient to recognize his distortions and continue his work in the group.

Cohesion

Individuals are attracted to others whose values, backgrounds, and attitudes are similar to their own. This perception of homogeneity is a defining aspect of group cohesion, which is vital for attachment of individuals to the group and for development of acceptance and support (Marziali, Monroe-Blum, & McCleary, 1997; Yalom, 1985). It is therefore imperative for group leaders to factor this concept into their definition of the target population and selection of individual members.

SCREENING PATIENTS FOR TRAUMA GROUPS

Once the target population for the trauma group is established, along with the basic structure, theoretical orientation, and treatment strategy, then screening for the group may proceed. Appropriate and thorough screening of potential group members is essential to ensure viability of the group. The general group psychotherapy literature provides data supporting this notion (Friedman, 1989; Piper & Perrault, 1989).

A screening interview serves multiple purposes, in addition to gathering information and history. The data collected highlight any potential problems, help determine a diagnosis, and indicate whether the patient is appropriate for the group. The screening also ensures a stronger commitment; prepares the individual for the group and lets him or her know what to expect; helps delineate treatment goals; and provides a forum for reviewing group policies regarding fees and absences, as well as other rules. It is imperative to determine whether there is a match between group stage and the patient's needs.

The content of a screening interview consists primarily of questioning regarding the nature of the trauma, premorbid functioning, subsequent coping style, and problems. A history of previous traumata, current and past physical and mental illness, presence of substance use, legal history, educational and vocational level, quality of relationships, past treatment, and current goals is also elicited.

In addition to factual information, consideration of the following questions will help assess the patient's ability for change: Is this individual ready for a group? Are the treatment goals feasible and realistic? How verbal is the patient? How does he or she view healing? Does he or she show a capacity for empathy and an ability to reflect? How will this person fit into the group? In addition, a critique of the patient's acting-out tendencies, impulse control, psychological-mindedness, motivation for change, overall ego strength, capacity to manage affect, and anxiety tolerance will highlight potential problems and help identity patients for whom group treatment is not an appropriate choice, or who require a different stage of group treatment.

The screening interview can vary in length between one and four sessions, depending upon the type of group and the needs of the therapist or patient. If the group is led by two therapists, then both must meet the prospective group member. For more psychodynamically focused group treatments, a longer screening process is helpful. Those who are less committed will not complete the several-session screening, thereby protecting the group from premature dropouts.

Depending on the stage of treatment and type of trauma group, inclusion and exclusion criteria will vary; however, the focus should be on the extent and success of previous treatment, concurrent therapies of any kind, comorbid Axis I diagnoses, presence of any current or recent suicidal or homicidal ideation, degree of outside supports, and concurrent alcohol or other substance abuse. Elsewhere, we (Goodman & Weiss, 1998) have noted that concurrent polysubstance use was a major source of dropouts in an outpatient stage 2 trauma-focused group for veterans. We now advocate that patients have at least 3–6 months of abstinence prior to attending such a group. Additional factors of concern include the presence of dissociation as a coping mechanism, sociopathy, or severely limited intellectual functioning.

Patients who have poor impulse control and limited ego strength coupled with high anxiety are better suited for a stage 1 or early stage 2 group. More advanced stage 2 and stage 3 groups require more psychological-mindedness, a capacity to handle pain, the ability to manage affect, and the ability to utilize outside supports (including an individual therapist). Inappropriate placement in a more advanced group treatment is potentially damaging to the group process and harmful to the patient, who may become overwhelmed, anxious, and potentially retraumatized.

A detailed examination of trauma and trauma symptomatology is crucial not only in the formation of trauma groups, but in clinical practice generally. For a thorough compendium and discussion of assessment and screening processes and protocols for trauma, see Wilson and Keane (1997).

Once the screening process is complete, a decision is made as to whether the patient is appropriate for the group. If the patient is satisfactory, than a start date is arranged. If not, than a list of referrals and reasons for the decision are warranted.

MAINTAINING PSYCHOTHERAPY GROUPS
FOR TRAUMATIZED PATIENTS

Once a group is established, the most important factor in maintaining its viability is to provide a safe framework and working environment in which difficult trauma treatment may proceed. Group rules and appropriate pacing of disclosure are paramount. Also of great importance are keeping several types of behaviors—tuning out, acting out, and overidentifying with victimization—to a minimum.

Group Rules

Group rules form the basis of the group's structure. These often include policies on absences, fees, and need for confidentiality of group material. Ideally, these rules are discussed in screening interviews and initial group meetings. In addition, some group leaders distribute a written list of group rules.

Excessive absences can be detrimental to both the group process and the individual's treatment, and need to be avoided. A feeling of safety cannot be maintained if there is not stable group membership. A firm policy toward absences, with consideration of the number of allowable missed appointments, whether the person will be charged, and what notification is needed, must be set. This conveys the message that each member's presence and commitment to the group are important.

Payment and money issues constitute another potential area for boundary violation and acting-out behavior, and thus another arena for clear policy formation. Group leaders need to decide how individual financial concerns will be handled and whether these issues will be group material or not. A billing and payment strategy needs to be arranged and adhered to reliably. One method is to distribute bills once a month with the expectation of payment that session. Deviations become clinical issues as well. The exact payment schedule is not as important as the need for consistency.

Confidentiality is a vital component of group safety, and of particular importance to individuals whose trauma experience has damaged their trust. Members need to be assured that the content of group sessions will never leave the room. Exceptions will include disclosure of material to members' individual therapists and on insurance company clinical reports. Serious ramifications are indicated for anyone who breaks this rule, and these can include removal from the group.

Other group rules include no violence, being on time, respect for others, no foul language, and no eating during sessions.

The issue of whether or not to allow members to have contacts with one another outside group sessions differs among groups. For trauma-focused groups and groups containing individuals with poor socialization skills, outside contacts among group members may be therapeutically helpful and may diminish social isolation. However, such encounters should be discussed in the group. For psychodynamically oriented groups, outside contacts should be discouraged, as they dilute the power of the group process and promote opportunities for secrecy, special relationships, and acting out. There is, however, the capacity for a therapeutic outcome if boundary violations are handled successfully within the group. This is especially important with personality-disordered individuals or with group members for whom boundary violation was an essential aspect of the trauma, and who may use behavioral reenactment to tell their story (Tyson & Goodman, 1996).

The establishment of rules and of a structure within which to run the group lays the groundwork for a successful treatment. However, maintenance of this safety structure throughout the life of the group is vital for the therapeutic process to continue. Any disruptions to this structure and to group rules need to be pointed out, understood, and corrected, or the potential for damage to the group process can occur. In more advanced group treatments with a psychodynamic approach, rule breaking itself is often regarded as clinically relevant and as a statement about the individual's traumatic experience, to be examined by the group.

> In an advanced stage 2 group for incest survivors, the group rule of no outside contact between group sessions was established, discussed, and agreed upon by all members. If contact happened, it was to be mentioned in the next group meeting. After one session, a member was waiting for the bus in the rain. Another member asked whether she would like a ride home, to which she agreed. Not realizing they were breaking the rules, they shared aspects of their personal lives, feelings about the group, and dreams about the future. The following week, neither member disclosed their contact, and they left together after the group session. This continued for 4 weeks. Eventually another member introduced the topic of secretive relationships and spoke eloquently about the turmoil of keeping hidden from her mother a sexualized relationship with her father. This propelled a guilty confession by the two members whose liaison after group meetings had progressed to coffee and dinner. Group members expressed jealousy, anger, and envy, while the rule breakers explored the connection with their incest experience—noting feelings of entitlement, "specialness," and power, but also guilt and shame.
>
> In this example, the rule breaking permitted the exploration of a behavioral reenactment of a boundary violation. These actions, once interpreted, allowed aspects of the two patients' traumatic stories to be understood. If the surreptitious outside meetings had continued, both the individuals involved and the group as a whole would have suffered.

Appropriate Pacing of Disclosure

With growing security in the group process, individuals will begin to relate details of their traumatic experiences. One of the most challenging aspects of running trauma psychotherapy groups is the successful regulation of how the traumatic material is disclosed. A group with no disclosure is not therapeutic. A group with overly rapid and lurid accounts of traumatic details without affect is potentially traumatizing to others. It is a therapist's role to pace the disclosure and to ensure that it is done in a therapeutic manner. This includes the goal of connecting affect to the traumatic story line rather than simply retelling "war stories," but it also includes preventing emotional overload through the use of check-ins, deep breathing exercises, or other relaxation exercises. A "check-in" is an interruption of the group process, in which the therapist stops the discussion and asks each member how he or she is coping with the material being discussed. This allows patients to reconnect with their emotions and helps those who are in distress to regain composure.

Minimizing Tuning-Out Behaviors

Although it is important for traumatized individuals to tell their stories of what happened to them, and to be heard, this needs to be balanced with the reactions and discomfort felt by other members who are listening. In order to maintain the integrity of a trauma group treatment, tuning-out behaviors must be minimized. "Tuning-out behaviors" are any maladaptive actions that numb or obfuscate feeling.

The most serious numbing mechanism is illicit drug use. Assessing the degree of use and the potential for and precipitants of intoxication, and requiring or recommending adjunctive treatment (e.g., a Twelve-Step group or rehabilitation), will minimize the chance of a relapse and a disruption to the group process.

Another form of tuning out is dissociation, a very common form of coping in patients with a history of childhood abuse. Although dissociation is not actively disruptive to a group, because many people cannot recognize it when it is happening to another individual, it is counterproductive. If a member is dissociating, he or she is unable to handle the emotional tenor of the group or to cope with his or her feelings, and thereby is communicating that the group feels unsafe. As safety is paramount to the group process, a break in the safety structure of the group has occurred. The group process needs to be interrupted, and all members must be made to feel safe. This may disrupt another member's disclosure of his or her traumatic story, but the speaker may continue once the elements of discomfort are addressed and ameliorated. For the individual with strong dissociative tendencies, additional treatment—including the identification of "triggers" for dissociative episodes; dialectical behavior therapy skills (Linehan, 1993); and attempts to substitute more adaptive, active coping strategies, including the use of words and a hand gesture to signify "stop"—may be necessary. If these are unsuccessful, then a referral to a less advanced or more ego-supportive stage of group treatment may be indicated.

Other maladaptive means of handling intense emotion and feeling include splitting and projective identification. Both defensive mechanisms serve to ward off intolerable affective states. With projective identification, a more severe form of splitting, other group members experience the feeling state that is unacceptable to the patient—a process that can be disturbing and uncomfortable for the group as a whole. In a stage 2 or stage 3 group, therapeutic goals include the ownership of these unwanted affects by the patient in a safe and metabolized form. A clinical example of how such projective identifications can be resolved with benefit to the patient and the group can be found in the example of Ms. M in a stage 2 group (see below), in which she projected elements of both the internalized "victim" and the internalized "abuser" into the group as a whole. (Additional examples can be found in other chapters of this volume. See Hegeman & Wohl, Chapter 3; Ganzarain, Chapter 4; Buchele, Chapter 7; von Wallenberg Pachaly, Chapter 11; and Gallagher & Kibel, Chapter 13.)

Handling Acting-Out Behaviors

Another tenet in maintaining trauma group treatment is the appropriate handling of acting-out behaviors (Silverstein, 1997). Dangerous actions that place a patient or others at risk for harm, such as cutting, self-destructive acts, suicidal preoccupation, or threats of violence, must be stopped. Less serious acting-out behaviors (e.g., rule or policy violations, tuning-out behaviors) may be understood as behavioral reenactments and used clinically to help the patient recognize maladaptive patterns. In addition, as noted earlier, the interpretation of behavioral reenactments may be an important aspect of the trauma narrative (Tyson & Goodman, 1996). The trauma story can be told not only in words, but also through actions and behaviors. Understanding these nonverbal expressions, and determining their effects on interpersonal relationships and level of functioning, are important therapeutic goals in an advanced group. In a stage 1 or early stage 2 group, these reenactments are curtailed and pointed out, and limits are set.

The following clinical example demonstrates these principles.

In a stage 2 group for women who had suffered from childhood sexual abuse, one of the participants, Ms. M, a teacher, relayed shockingly vivid accounts of her abuse history on repeated occasions. Despite feedback from other participants regarding their discomfort, and the precipitation of flashbacks in two other members, the patient continued to offer graphic details. This served to create a group-wide abused–abuser dynamic, where sadistic and masochistic thoughts and feelings dominated the group process. Herein lay the potential for dropouts and harm to the feeling of safety in the group. Attendance faltered, other members' dissociative tendencies intensified, and the viability of the group itself was threatened. Safety was reestablished by the therapists' intervening to stop the "war stories" and to explore Ms. M's behavior and the connection with her trauma history. She revealed that she felt "big and strong" when others were frightened with her stories, and that she believed no one could hurt her when she dominated the group. Her behavior was an identification with her abuser, an older brother who would intimidate her and force himself upon her—an act he had learned from his own encounters with an abusing father. The cowering, frightened group members were identifying with the abused child who had few options available to her—a similar dynamic in several of the other members' traumatic past. Over time, Ms. M shared her traumatic background with greater compassion for others and acknowledged her vulnerable, "weak" side. The group regained its safety, allowing valuable work to continue.

Another aspect of minimizing damaging acting-out behavior is the appropriate management of anger. This is especially relevant with male trauma victims and with patients with borderline personality disorder or polysubstance use who exhibit the potential for escalation to violence. It is important in the screening process to assess for a history of anger dyscontrol and violence, and to identify at-risk individuals. Within the course of the group treatment, factors that may facilitate an expression of violence need to be identified and monitored (e.g., anything that increases impulsivity, such as drugs and alcohol; also, mention of weapons, especially guns or revenge fantasies). Techniques such as anger management skills, facilitation of a mourning process, and encouragement of a fuller array of affect beyond anger may prove helpful (Reilly, Clark, Shopshire, & Lewis, 1994). However, concomitant treatment or hospitalization for substance misuse may be necessary if behaviors become dangerous.

Discouraging Overidentification with Being Victims

One pitfall of running trauma group therapies is when patients become overidentified with being victims. Although being with others who have suffered from a similar fate is necessary for stage 2 trauma-focused work, and facilitates rapid cohesion within the group, never moving beyond victim status denotes incomplete healing. The ability to explore group differences and "intragroup aggression" (van der Kolk, 1993) promotes an identity beyond victimization. For these reasons, Herman (1992) recommends that stage 3 group work be done in a general psychotherapy group with a heterogeneous population.

> For example, in a group of female survivors of incest, one member—despite 18 months of group treatment—remained unable to discuss anything beyond her incestuous past. Her outside reading focused on ritual abuse, and her television watching centered on talk shows detailing childhood abuses. Members grew tired of her and were frustrated by her inability to progress. Her identity had crystallized as a victim, and she was using the group to reinforce this self-concept. The therapists believed that this was a resistance to examining her deeper losses, involving being "given up" and placed for adoption—traumas that were too painful to address. Her identity as an incest survivor was preferable to no identity, and being inappropriately desired was preferable to being abandoned.

For some patients, maintenance of a victim role that is self-supportive and assertive against future victimizations may be a significant achievement. Others may have the resilience to reintegrate with society as a whole. Heterogeneous groups facilitate this process of moving beyond a role that may have been initially adaptive to one that allows full participation in here-and-now interpersonal experience.

Termination

The ending of a trauma therapy group requires careful consideration. Many traumatized individuals have minimal experience in saying goodbye in a healthy manner, as their earlier relationships were often severed or abandoned. Thus termination becomes an opportunity for a more positive experience of farewells in a controlled setting, where reactions and feelings can be monitored and expressed. Elements of a successful termination include chances to process feelings of loss, to review progress and change, to say goodbye to each member individually, and to plan for the future with tools and skills acquired from the group experience (Rice, 1996). Some trauma groups ritualize the ending with goodbye cards and a party.

SUMMARY

In summary, group psychotherapy is an effective modality for treating individuals with PTSD and other sequelae of trauma. Considerations of target population, theoretical orientation, group stage, and structure are necessary before initiating a group. Structural parameters, rules, and other policies serve to create a safe haven for the therapy. Maintaining this framework through appropriate pacing of disclosure, minimizing tuning-out behaviors, preventing dangerous acting out, and discouraging overidentification with victim status ensure a secure and productive milieu in which to treat these individuals. Group psychotherapy offers patients with traumatic experience a forum in which to tell their stories, receive validation, and relieve their secrecy and shame in a context that allows direct examination of the trauma's effect on interpersonal relating.

REFERENCES

Courtois, C. (1988). *Healing the incest wound: Adult survivors in therapy.* New York: Basic Books.

Dye, E., & Roth, S. (1991). Psychotherapy with Vietnam veterans and incest survivors. *Psychotherapy, 28,* 103–120.

Friedman, W. (1989). *Practical group psychotherapy: A guide for clinicians.* San Francisco: Jossey-Bass.

Goodman, M., & Weiss, D. (1998). Double trauma: A group psychotherapy approach for Vietnam veterans suffering from war and childhood trauma. *International Journal of Group Psychotherapy, 48*(1), 39–54.

Herman, J. (1992). *Trauma and recovery.* New York: Basic Books.

Kanas, N., Schoenfeld, F., Marmar, C., & Weiss, D. (1994). Process and content in a longterm PTSD therapy group for Vietnam veterans. *Group, 18*(2), 78–88.

Koller, P., Marmar, C., & Kanas, N. (1992). Psychodynamic group treatment of posttraumatic stress disorder in Vietnam veterans. *International Journal of Group Psychotherapy, 42*(2), 225–246.

Lindy, J. (1993). Focal psychoanalytic psychotherapy of post-traumatic stress disorder. In J. Wilson & B. Raphael (Eds.), *International handbook of traumatic stress syndromes* (pp. 803–809). New York: Plenum Press.

Linehan, M. M. (1993). *Skills training manual for treating borderline personality disorder.* New York: Guilford Press.

Marziali, E., Monroe-Blum, H., & McCleary, L. (1997). The contribution of group cohesion and group alliance to the outcome of group psychotherapy. *International Journal of Group Psychotherapy, 47*(4), 475–497.

Najavitas, L., Weiss, R., & Liese, B. (1996). Group cognitive-behavioral therapy for women with PTSD and substance use disorder. *Journal of Substance Abuse Treatment, 13*(1), 13–22.

Piper, W., & Perrault, F. (1989). Pretherapy preparation for group members. *International Journal of Group Psychotherapy, 39*(1), 17–34.

Reilly, P., Clark, W., Shopshire, M., & Lewis, E. (1994). Anger management and temper control: Critical components of posttraumatic stress disorder and substance abuse treatment. *Journal of Psychoactive Drugs, 26*(4), 401–407.

Rice, C. (1996). Premature termination of group psychotherapy: A clinical perspective. *International Journal of Group Psychotherapy, 46*(1), 5–24.

Rozynko, V., & Dondershine, H. (1991). Trauma focus group therapy for Vietnam veterans with PTSD. *Psychotherapy, 28*(1), 157–161.

Scurfield, R., Corker, T., Gongla, P., & Hough, R. (1984). Three post-Vietnam "rap/therapy" groups: An analysis. *Group, 8,* 3–21.

Silverstein, J. (1997). Acting out in group therapy: Avoiding authority struggles *International Journal of Group Psychotherapy, 47*(1), 31–45.

Srein, E., & Eisen, B. (1996). Helping trauma survivors cope: Effects of immediate brief cotherapy and crisis intervention. *Crisis Intervention and Time-Limited Treatment, 3*(2), 113–127.

Tyson, A., & Goodman, M. (1996). Group treatment for adult women who experienced childhood sexual trauma: Is telling the story enough? *International Journal of Group Psychotherapy, 46*(4), 535–542.

van der Kolk, B. (1993). Group psychotherapy for posttraumatic stress disorder. In H. Kaplan & B. Sadock (Eds.), *Comprehensive group psychotherapy* (3rd ed., pp. 550–560). Baltimore: Williams & Wilkins.

Wilson, J. P., & Keane, T. M. (Eds.). (1997). *Assessing psychological trauma and PTSD.* New York: Guilford Press.

Yalom, I. (1985). *The theory and practice of group psychotherapy* (3rd ed.). New York: Basic Books.

3

-◄O►-

Management of Trauma-Related Affect, Defenses, and Dissociative States

ELIZABETH HEGEMAN
AGNES WOHL

With the resurgence of interest in traumatized populations, therapists have been confronted with a new set of challenges to their training in verbal psychotherapy. In addition to the dynamic formulations based on repression and defenses against awareness of internal conflicts, we now understand that there are several types of defensive adaptations to traumatic experience—including "dissociation," which can be defined here as a discontinuity either between psychic structures within the self, or between the self and the external world (Bromberg, 1998, p. 130). Dissociation is a "glitch" or a dead spot inside the self, or between the person and the world, that arises when the self is overwhelmed by terror, dread, or the perception of malevolence or danger. Dissociation blocks verbal access to experience and disrupts coherent self-experience. It may take the form of trance, of a sudden numbing or loss of feeling, or a flashback of intense experience. Memory for traumatic events, the feelings and sensations that go with them, and crucial aspects of self can be unintentionally blocked in what appears to be an attempt to preserve functioning. Awareness of the feelings of terror, helplessness, betrayal, and pain often returns in uncontrolled bursts of reenactments, nightmares, and flashbacks, only to be blocked off again as the dissociating person returns to a frozen state of affectless numbness. "Empty," "zoned out," and "dead" are common descriptions of the latter.

The diagnosis of posttraumatic stress disorder (PTSD) relies on the presence of both numbing and intrusive symptoms. Most often, traumatized patients alternate between being flooded by panic and painful affect on the one hand, and avoiding the pain and terror in a way that keeps it from being processed and symbolized on the other. This alternation leaves little room for development of a cohesive, integrated, flexible sense of self, adapted to more ordinary life experiences.

Two keys to effective therapeutic work with dissociative experience are (1) the recognition that no matter how odd or emotionally jarring events in therapy might be, they often mean that dissociated material is being returned to awareness; and (2) the analytically informed assumption that what is being relived or enacted means something, and that the patient is the one who must decipher the meaning in the supportive setting provided by the therapist and the group. We are now finding that it is possible to decipher repetitive patterns in patients' lives (often very self-defeating patterns) by using the assumption that unrecognized traumatic experiences and relationships often lie behind these patterns.

Because traumatic experiences have often been encoded differently from normal experiences, and often at a nonverbal level, they may need to be retrieved differently—to be lived through rather than talked through. Trauma theory requires a shift in the conventional therapeutic point of view, which now makes it possible to work successfully with patients who might not benefit from therapy without it. Many events in which a patient was unable to adhere to the customary requirements of a therapy group (e.g., regular attendance at sessions, bringing up problems early in the group session) used to be regarded as "resistance." Viewing these events as the return of dissociated traumatic affect or relationships makes it possible to work therapeutically with formerly unworkable clients and issues, especially in the group setting.

Because traumatic dissociation is the last-ditch defense of a desperate person, patients come to therapy having adjusted to their dissociative patterns and knowing no other way to live, even though they almost always feel mortified and undermined by these uncontrollable aspects of self. For example, people who use dissociative defenses heavily often think that they are not intelligent, or even think they are learning-disabled, because their functioning is uneven. Dissociative patients have become accustomed to being taken over by flashbacks, numbing, or (most often) both, and the very idea that these symptoms can be transcended or outgrown is foreign. It is important for a therapist working with dissociative patients to be able to hold out the hope that dissociative patterns can gradually be brought under the patients' conscious and intentional control, and to work actively for that goal by proposing techniques and reminding the patients to try them.

As Bromberg (1998, p. 132) describes, "presymbolized experiences too intense to be cognitively processed by the forming self were forced to be re-

tained as traumatically unbearable mental states that were then dissociated
. . . to preserve other areas of functioning and sometimes sanity itself."
These states can then hover around the edges of awareness until they are
evoked by something that triggers them, or they can stay hidden for years.

This chapter is organized into three parts. The first consists of a discussion of some aspects of dissociation; the second has to do with issues
that arise in dealing with dissociation in groups; and the third describes the
handling of specific affects.

SOME ASPECTS OF DISSOCIATION

The Continuum of Dissociation

Dissociative experiences fall somewhere on the continuum between the ordinary (e.g., "spacing out" at a traffic light, or the feeling that "this isn't
really happening to me" during a traffic accident) and the extremely complex layering and compartmentalization of the multiple personality. Usually
the more chronic and bodily intrusive the trauma has been, the more extreme the dissociative defensive operations become. Since there is a tendency for dissociative operations to become more and more pronounced
over time, once the personality has come to dissociate almost automatically
in the face of anxiety, it becomes a disorder. The anxiety avoidance may
lead to extreme behavior, such as the "compulsion to engage in state-alter-
ing behavior" (Spiegel, 1994, p. 204)—self-cutting, substance misuse, sex,
violence, thrill seeking, gambling—or loss of impulse control, as in eating
disorders. Realization of how important this pattern can become has led
trauma clinicians to change their view of responsible treatment; now,
achieving stability and preserving optimal functioning are the primary
treatment goals. After years of encouraging abreactive reconstruction of
traumatic events, trauma experts have realized that the danger and likelihood of such a patient's becoming "addicted to abreaction" has led to an
emphasis on enhancing mastery and current functioning rather than abreaction as the center of the treatment.

Reenactments

Tyson and Goodman (1996) define "reenactment" as "the unconscious
reexperiencing and behavioral re-creating of past events in the current therapy setting and in the person's daily life" (p. 536). A traumatized person
can relive chunks of dissociated traumatic experience in startling ways.
These disruptions in awareness and self-regulation come on suddenly and
unpredictably in any social setting, leading to shame and eventually isolation, avoidance, and even social phobia. They are inexplicable both to the
trauma sufferer and to observers until they are decoded. The therapy group

can promote this decoding when the therapists take the position that reenactments are a valuable form of communication, and when they model exploration and acceptance of whatever feelings or expectations a patient brings.

Tyson and Goodman (1996) illustrate this therapeutic position with an example of reenactment that took place early in the development of their group. One group member, Meg, "barraged people with words in a loud, insistent voice, and started topics without regard for the interactive flow of the conversation" (p. 538); she attacked the therapists during the second group meeting. The therapists listened and encouraged her expression of feelings, and restated what they heard as her legitimate concerns. They interpreted her behavior as testing whether the group would be safe enough for her to trust. "The therapists proposed this as a group topic: How did others test and learn to trust?" (p. 538). As the group developed, Meg's understanding of her own behavior deepened. With the group's assistance, "she was able to notice that her loud and demanding manner covered her fears that she would not be heard" (p. 538). Eventually, group exploration reached an even deeper level, which revealed that Meg's behavior was a reenactment of dangerous and traumatic harangues she had endured from her manic father. She had internalized both positions in the traumatic relationship, but the formulation of reenactment placed her in the active role. Through seeing her patterns unfold in the group, Meg became aware of how she drove away and provoked others.

In an example of reenactment from our own group work, Michelle came to group sessions expecting to be ignored and excluded. As a child she had been silenced through neglect, and ignored when she cried. Although the other group members did not usually allow any member to be excluded, and the structure of the group routine of "checking in" at the beginning and "closing" at the end prevented her being left out, Michelle still dreaded that her needs for empathic attention would not be met. During one session, she talked about feeling ignored by a girlfriend; when it came time for the group "closing," in which each member shared what had been important to her during the session, the therapist "forgot" and passed over her. In tears, Michelle expressed her feeling that the dreaded ignoring had finally taken place, and that she was indeed "forgettable."

This reenactment turned therapeutic through the therapist's insistence on exploring her own mistake, in the spirit of understanding what was being communicated. Michelle's fantasies included that the therapist was being intentionally provocative, so that Michelle would become angry, because her anger was more bearable to the therapist than her despair. This disclosure led to exploration of how Michelle was ignored in other contexts, and how the way she communicated her despair made her hard to be around. This material would not otherwise have been available for therapeutic work, because it was dissociated. Michelle was even able to consider how she induced "forgetting" in others, as in the therapist, and to do a thorough review of her impact; the group supported her by giving her honest feedback and by challenging her conviction that she would never be fully accepted by others.

Tyson and Goodman (1996) suggest that "It may not be curative just to tell the traumatic story" (p. 541), and that work with reenactments is necessary for maximum benefit from a therapy group. Therapeutic use of reenactments depends on a therapist's ability to recognize what is happening while it is happening, and on the therapist's nondefensiveness in exploring his or her own motivations and behavior. As these examples show, reenactments take everyone by surprise and are not at first seen for what they are! The language of dissociation and reenactment provides a blame-free framework for discovery and recognition of previously hidden aspects of self.

Reenactments Centering around Disclosure

Disclosure can be the occasion for reenactment of some of the internalized dynamics that surrounded the original trauma, even if it was not based on betrayal. Gold-Steinberg and Buttenheim recommend that in screening interviews for groups for female incest survivors, a screening therapist ask about a survivor's previous experiences of telling the story of the trauma (To whom has it been told? What happened in connection with the telling?) and about her expectations about telling in the group. They point out that there is often an implicit expectation that each survivor will "tell her story," meaning that there will be a detailed sharing of personal historical events around the trauma, but that given the anxiety and ambivalence that surround telling, "a positive outcome is by no means assured" (p. 175). Survivors have often had disastrous experiences when they have tried to tell their stories, if they have ever tried. It is frightening to relive the trauma and get in touch with intense feelings, with no guarantee that other group members will respond therapeutically (or at all). Survivors often fear that the group will recreate the disappointing emotional environment of the original family, or the shocking betrayal of the trauma itself—and may thus unwittingly bring this about. That is, they may find the group unresponsive or critical, or may feel betrayed in some way that replicates the original neglect or emotional failure of the family, or the terror and helplessness of their abuse. At the same time, they may feel endangered by the chance to give up their emotional isolation and risk trusting again, so they may stop themselves from speaking fully, or unwittingly drive others away (as Meg and Michelle did in the reenactments discussed earlier).

The Therapeutic Task

The challenge for the group and the therapist in working with dissociated ego states is to find ways to recognize, observe, describe, give meaning to, and finally integrate these states into a person's awareness and ongoing life. The empathic stance of the therapist makes it possible for the trauma victim to internalize structures that will allow him or her to observe and communicate about experience, and to increase access to those unbearable mental states within. Again, the therapist's conviction that there is a reason for every feeling, even for experiences that seem inexplicable, lays the groundwork. Finding meaning in these baffling and overwhelming experiences, and allowing these raw affects to be processed symbolically, constitute a synthetic function of the self that allows the patient's life and self to be disrupted less and less as time goes on.

Since dissociative defenses are not voluntary, bringing dissociated states under a patient's control and helping the patient become more self-regulating are challenging tasks indeed. These defenses feel essential; they are the only way the person has had of coping with the trauma, and they have become part of his or her identity. And since the alternation between numbing and intrusive symptoms is beyond the control of a person's will, it undermines self-confidence, judgment, and the ability to make reliable plans. "I can't even count on myself any more!" exclaimed a frustrated Vietnam veteran who resented being stuck on disability because of his hypervigilance, sleep disorder, and flashbacks. Group treatment brings with it the possibility of the restoration of meaning in social participation; connection with community has often been swept away as a person swings between feeling empty and being flooded with overwhelming affects. The restoration of a sense of connection to others that comes with increased trust and communication with self and others is the greatest gift therapy can bring to someone in despair (Herman, 1992).

Not all patients who are traumatized come to rely heavily on dissociative defenses, and it may be that not all dissociators have been traumatized, though the presence of dissociation certainly suggests the possibility of trauma. Recognition of numbed and hypervigilant states, knowledge of how they disrupt the self, and awareness of their possible connection to trauma are important tools for the therapist. It is especially important to work with the sequence of clinical events in the session—that is, what took place just before the dissociative defense came into play. This kind of work trains the patient in observing ego, and demonstrates convincingly the way the defensive system actually works. That is, dissociation doesn't "just happen," but is about something, and is an attempt to preserve something of importance in the patient.

The BASK Model

James Chu (1998) has offered the descriptive scheme of the BASK model, according to which any one or any number of the following may be dissociated: behaviors, affects, sensations, and knowledge. The model can be used to conceptualize the aspects either of self or of traumatic experience that are affected by the dissociative defenses. For example, a woman may give a factual and full account of the accident she suffered, her injuries, and what she did, but may tell the story like a robot because she does not have access to the affective dimension of the terror or pain she felt. In such a case, affect is dissociated while knowledge is not. Or, in a more dramatic instance of dissociative fugue, a man may recollect getting on the train to Chicago and what it was like, but may not have a clue as to how he wound up in Syracuse in bed with a stranger. In such a case, all of the BASK elements are dissociated for the period of amnesia. Most therapists are trained and accustomed to rely heavily on their intuitive empathic knowing, derived from affective contact with their patients. This way of understanding doesn't work when a dissociative patient doesn't have self-experience to empathize with, so the therapist may feel lost or inadequate without understanding why. For this reason, the BASK model is useful: It enables the therapist to be able to ask and think about what part of the experience is missing, and to work cognitively to reconstruct the missing parts of the self as well as the experience.

Multiple Memory Systems

Recent models of memory identify at least two distinct and separable systems. "Explicit" or "declarative" memory for facts and events calls for effortful recall, in which a person can usually remember where he or she first acquired the information. "Implicit" or "procedural" memory taps skills that can be accessed in a more visceral way, without someone's knowing how he or she learned the skill (Putnam, 1997, p. 104–105). A coherent, functioning personality relies on a relatively smooth integration of the different memory systems. Trauma changes the neurophysiology of the body and seems to break links between different memory systems, making it harder to integrate sensations into a coherent narrative. Explicit memory seems to fail more easily during conditions of terror or pain; this leaves a person baffled and overwhelmed as to how he or she came to have these feelings, and confused as the person was in the original experience. Although the construction of a narrative is helpful, van der Kolk (1996b, p. 289) points out that traumatic memories still return as sensory perceptions or as affective states even after a verbal narrative has been formed. Gartner (1999) has described the hallucinatory quality of a patient's vivid inner image of being surrounded by yellow roses—an image that would arise in connection with certain triggers. The image later came to be understood as representing the wallpaper in the setting in which the patient was originally abused. The patient had taught himself (as many abused children do) to focus on the roses very intensely, to the point of "losing himself" in the image. We may speculate that since the image of roses once helped him cope, the image might return in a way that felt arbitrary and intrusive when triggered by cues that might signal he was in danger again. The failure of the explicit memory system left him baffled as to why he was seeing the image at that time.

Flashbacks

The finding of van der Kolk (1996b) and Putnam (1997) that flashbacks may diminish over time but do not go away completely contradicts a central assumption in many forms of treatment that flashbacks can be eliminated by verbal therapy. It also suggests that a realistic goal of trauma therapy should be to help the patient understand the meaning of the flashbacks, and to give the patient sensory and emotional tools to stay grounded in the present and work actively against being carried away by the dissociative memory element in a flashback, rather than to have the patient expect to get rid of flashbacks completely.

In addition, memory for shocking experiences may be encoded and recovered in unusual ways, different from those for ordinary events, perhaps because the body is in a different physiological state or because the nature of focal attention is different. Traumatic memories may return "in the form of mental imprints of sensory and affective elements" (van der Kolk, 1996b, p. 280). In trauma people experience "a significant narrowing of consciousness, and remain focused on only the central perceptual details" (Putnam, 1997, p. 285). One way of coping with overwhelming affect is to focus dissociatively on a sensory detail of a scene—the sound of an airplane, the pattern of the wallpaper, or the leaves on a tree outside the window—in order to ward off painful feelings. These visual or auditory stimuli may then become powerful triggers for flashbacks when the dissociative defense breaks down, because they have become associated with the original feelings.

Nancy Napier (1993, pp. 76–77) calls flashbacks "pockets of time" and describes the therapeutic task of turning flashbacks into memories: "When you get triggered, all the feelings and thoughts from that unprocessed pocket of time suddenly flood into your awareness, bringing with them the responses you had back then" (p. 76). Once this experience has a name, it can be talked about, talked through, and put in its proper place as a memory. The new understanding of memory systems suggests that this work of talking about trauma transforms dissociated material from implicit (or visceral and childlike) memory to explicit (or more adult and cognitively mediated) memory.

Trauma and Addiction

Another reason why traumatic memories may be encoded and retrieved differently from more ordinary experience is that the hyperaroused body generates "endorphins," or opiate-like substances that plug opiate receptors and temporarily dull the body's experience of pain. These neurochemical changes may activate different neural pathways for memory processes, which may then only be recoverable when that physiological state is reestablished. This may account for the observation that patients can get addicted to reliving trauma, as well as to behaviors such as eating disorders, and to substances that can bring relief from inner pain.

The fact that implicit memory systems hold up better than explicit ones in the face of trauma may tie in with the finding that most patients find it "grounding" and stabilizing to establish a routine, and to perform familiar activities like cooking or cleaning when they are in shock or flashback. Nancy Venable Raine (1998) painstakingly scraped the floors in the attic where she was living in the months following her rape, digging the dirt out from between the cracks one by one. She had had trouble sleeping for months, but "the day I started working on the floors, I slept soundly through the night for the first time and my nightmares stopped" (p. 104). Though far from healed, she felt calmed by asserting herself in this physical way, and by exerting control over her surroundings.

Relationships as Triggers

Contrary to expectations, when a traumatized patient enters either individual or group therapy, he or she may "get worse" for a while rather than better right away. This should not be surprising, since many traumatized people have difficulty trusting, and have managed to function by isolating themselves or limiting the degree of their relatedness to others. Since many have been hurt in relationships, they will naturally bring into the therapy the expectation or fear of being hurt or betrayed again in the same way. In the case examples given earlier, both Michelle and Meg were reacting to the expectation of trust within the group and with the therapists. Or, in psychoanalytic terms, they each experienced a transference reenactment triggered by something in the new relationship, such as a growing sense of trust.

Breaking through into genuine feeling can be shocking and feel "wrong" or "too much" for someone who has been used to "faking" relatedness or living in the numbness and partial isolation of dissociative defenses. When she began to feel again in her group, one woman said, "What's wrong with me? I'm crying!" Fortunately, the therapist and the group were able to help her to recognize and eventually rejoice in the restoration of her capacity to feel.

Repression versus Dissociation

"Repression" and "dissociation" are alternative conceptual schemes for picturing how someone can be unaware of aspects of experience. In the field of trauma work, the group of defensive structures that arise to cope with shocks outside the scope of "normal" development is called "dissociation." According to Davies and Frawley (1994), repression and dissociation can be understood as different processes, with repression as an active process "in which the ego gains mastery over conflictual material," while dissociation is "the last ditch effort of an overwhelmed ego to salvage some semblance of adequate mental functioning" (p. 65). They further differentiate repression as a response that adds to a sense of mastery because it allows for ongoing internal psychic work, making the material potentially available for rediscovery in therapy, whereas dissociation "is experienced as an inadequate response, a submission and resignation to the inevitability of overwhelming, even psychically deadening danger" (p. 65). Repression applies to material that has been in awareness and can potentially be remembered and thus linked with other experiences, contributing to a coherent sense of self; traumatic dissociation (like trauma itself) breaks connections between groups of events and their internal representations, with the apparent function of warding off awareness of trauma.

Hidden Strengths

A further difference of dissociation from repression is that repression is conceived of as hiding an undesirable aspect of the self from the self, whereas dissociation describes splits around desirable aspects in the self as well as in the object. This is especially true of initiative, assertiveness, intelligence, creativity, and spontaneity. Typically, in a chronically abusive or otherwise traumatizing family, a person has had to hide from self and others the recognition of valuable qualities (such as autonomy or initiative) that would have challenged or threatened abusive figures. Joyousness, loving feelings, and sensuality may have become dissociated from the self when they triggered sexualized or otherwise inappropriate attention from adults. Members of a group can be especially helpful in seeing these hidden strengths, and in relabeling these capacities as wanted rather than unwanted; the group provides a context for the linkages within the self to reconnect and assert ownership of desired qualities.

Trauma-induced dissociative defenses produce an unevenness in functioning that complicates the accurate screening and assessment of level of functioning. It is not uncommon for someone with even a severe dissociative disorder to hold a highly responsible, demanding job, for example; dissociative patients have often become adept at "faking it" through the development of false self as well. Thus, if trauma is known to be in the picture, it may be wise to include a measure of dissociation such as the Dissociative Experiences Scale (DES; Putnam, 1997) or the Structured Clinical Interview for DSM-III-R—Dissociation (SCID-D; Steinberg, 1995) so that both therapist and patient can be alerted to the possibility of a potentially intrusive "return of the dissociated." Such screening can also give valuable feedback to the person who is unaware of his or her talents or strengths, as well as of areas of dissociation.

Dissociation as a Protective Defense

Dissociative defenses are often essential in helping patients survive overwhelming and intrusive events by keeping the self separate from the awareness of noxious and damaging feelings. Briere (1995) points out that such defenses can be called "solutions" rather than a "disorder." Unfortunately, this survival happens at the cost of becoming adapted to toxic conditions; when this has happened at an early age, it may have substituted for ordinary development, leaving the child without strategies or ability to contain the strong feelings associated with trauma that are still encapsulated in the self. Self-soothing and self-regulating behaviors of an ordinary kind may not have been learned, and until they are, the person is at risk for "feeling worse before feeling better." If someone is flooded with anxiety and intense feelings before he or she has methods of containing them, that person may be retraumatized and turn to self-destructive or compulsive behaviors.

Gartner (1999) cites Briere in adopting the model of the "therapeutic window," which exists because people defend themselves somewhat more than they have to. He points out that it is important neither to overshoot nor to undershoot this "window," which allows the patient to talk more deeply and fully about the trauma without being flooded by it. Gartner gives examples of how the therapist can choose the level of abstraction or specificity of questions about the trauma so as to maintain the maximum of therapeutic effectiveness while preserving the patient's internal stability.

Dissociation or Resistance?

A dissociative defensive style can interfere with effective group participation in many hidden ways.

One patient, Sally, had trouble "shifting gears" to be emotionally present at the beginning of group, during the "check-in" time, and often did not become aware of her own anguished concerns until the group was well underway. By that time, the group was usually deeply absorbed with the issues of one or another member who had been able to ask more openly for attention during the check-in. Sally's belated bids for group time then felt intrusive to the other members, who viewed her as insensitive. In this way, Sally unwittingly recreated the environment of her early family life, in which her needs had been passed over. Her experience in the group replayed the dissociative pattern of alternation between numbing and flooding: She lived out of touch with her needs, until she was flooded by them. Sally came to dread the group sessions; she felt blamed, resentful, and deeply lonely, as she had for much of her life. The group leader felt annoyed at her and called her "resistant," rather than looking deeply at what Sally might be communicating in her pattern of not using the check-in.

Once the group came to observe and understand Sally's pattern as having meaning for all of them, they were able to ask questions about the pattern. How had Sally gone about getting attention in the family? (She hadn't. Getting attention was dangerous; it had precipitated her incest. She had tried to be as invisible as possible.) Was there something she needed to avoid by not speaking up? (Yes—competition with other women, and being noticed.) What was she aware of feeling about the group between sessions? (Wistful longing.) Did she have fantasies about the group in between? (Yes—of being enthusiastically appreciated and supported.) Recognition of this pattern as a reenactment showed the way for Sally to learn to accept her needs for emotional contact and to present them in a way more likely to lead to an affirmative connection.

Tyson and Goodman (1996) discuss another instance in which a group member's behavior appeared to be "resistance," but masked a deeper dynamic. Although Diane was a member of a group formed to explore incest experience, she focused instead on her feelings of guilt as a bad mother. In addition, she often missed group meetings and neglected the group in this way. As a life pattern, she tended to set up repetitive situations in which she felt guilty; this guilt then served as a cover for more deeply shameful guilt over the secret that as a child, she had waited for her perpetrator and looked forward to the contact with him. In the group, Diane was carrying on her pattern of creating a more manageable form of guilt to obscure the more painful one connected with her early abuse. Over time, Diane was able to begin to think of herself as an abuse survivor, rather than sticking with her cover story of identifying with the abusing adult. Eventually group members were able to confront her with their feelings of abandonment and powerlessness generated by her absences, and she became more able to connect with her own frightening sense of vulnerability as a child.

These examples illustrate the importance of looking deeply into frustrating or challenging behavior. Starting with the premise that symptomatic behavior is meaningfully related to trauma, dedicated therapists are able to bypass shallow interpretations of "resistance," to reconstruct trauma-related patterns, and to challenge even entrenched habits and character.

ISSUES IN DEALING
WITH DISSOCIATION IN GROUPS

Breaching the Trauma Barrier

As a person continues to develop after a trauma, much of the traumatized person's defensive structure can shift to the goal of blocking out awareness of the shocking reality. Often the traumatized patient has achieved a compromised level of adaptation, which continues as long as the "trauma barrier" is not breached. Once it has been breached, however, emotional and cognitive flooding may take place (as with other PTSD patients), threatening the patient's coherent sense of self as well as stable routines of job and family life. When memory has become encapsulated, trauma-focused treatment is especially problematic because it is diphasic: At first, it means getting a patient to confront what the patient has been doing his or her best not to be aware of! Once memories come flooding back, good treatment means finding ways of wrapping up the very feelings that therapist and patient were probing for earlier. This can be especially problematic in a group, since group members will undoubtedly trigger each other as they discuss their painful experiences of abuse or neglect.

Dissociative defenses can play havoc with a patient's identity and ego functions, such as attention and emotional flexibility. Because the dissociated traumatic experience has not been verbally encoded or internally processed in any way, it can be as terrifying and overwhelming when it reemerges into awareness as when it first occurred. Strategies to support ego functioning and promote orientation can take many different forms, but all emphasize coping and grounding in the present rather than deepening the experience of the traumatic memory.

One of the earliest theorists who dealt with trauma and its effects was Henry Krystal, who pointed out not only that anxiety regulation is essential to self-regulation, but that tolerance for intense emotions is equally likely to be disrupted by traumatic experience. He led the field in shifting an emphasis in models away from issues of internal drive regulation to a consideration of the attempts of the overwhelmed organism to reestablish some control and regulation with the environment, including other people. We now understand that the challenge intense emotions present to the developing self depends very much on the level of maturity of the emerging ego. Thus the younger a person is when flooded by trauma, the more likely that person will be to dread affective experience, leading affects to be "mostly somatized, poorly verbalized, and poorly differentiated" (Krystal, 1974, p. 183). Dissociative defenses may arise as primitive attempts to preserve some form of regulation in the swamped person, and may only become disorders over the course of years because they eventually come to interfere with functioning instead of facilitating it. The developing self must be capable of mourning the losses intrinsic in each shift in growth. Only if this mourning work is possible can a person develop "self-awareness of one's affects as signals to oneself" (Krystal, 1974, p. 200). This mourning work, done in the presence of others within the group, can be all the more powerful and healing because it is shared with these others.

Body Memories

Some people who have dissociated memory for trauma are overcome by bodily pain and sensations for which there is no medical basis. These seem inexplicable unless and until they are understood as memories of intrusive abuse. Karen Hopenwasser (1998) vividly describes her work with a patient who felt odd bodily sensations in a "not quite asleep" state: "It was becoming clearer to me that these episodes at night were dissociated flashbacks that during the daytime were often not remembered or were remembered without the intense terror reported in association with them" (p. 222). Although it is important for the therapist to be aware of the ethical obligation not to overinterpret such feelings, and not to infer abuse with certainty unless there is external corroboration, it is just as important to consider all possibilities in coming to understand the meaning of this bodily experience.

A group member reported with intense embarrassment that at times during the group sessions, her breasts would tingle in a painful and unpleasant way; she was both mortified and bewildered as to what this meant. Over time the group helped her to track these experiences, and it became clear that she had these unpleasant feelings when another member was talking about her abuse. This led her to consider the meaning for herself, with group support, of what the feelings represented. Over time, she came to believe that the tingling feeling represented her dread and repulsion at having been fondled during several episodes of abuse.

The role of the therapist in such a case should, of course, be that of encouraging exploration of meanings by the patient, rather than imposing interpretations.

Supportive Interventions for Dissociation

The most fundamental coping strategy for a dissociating patient is to achieve "grounding," or maintenance of contact with current reality. Maintaining good lighting in the room, making visual contact with cues in the environment, and perhaps making eye contact with the therapist all help to diminish dissociative escape from a flashback while promoting awareness of current safety. The therapist can ask, "Do you want me to remind you where you are right now, and that you're safe?" Chu (1998) emphasizes that the therapist's tone should be firm and reassuring, but not hypnotically soothing. Relaxation techniques, hypnosis, and guided imagery are helpful for therapists who are comfortable and skilled in these techniques, but Chu (1998) emphasizes that these should be used for stabilization and containment, not for exploration of traumatic experiences that would deepen awareness of the trauma. An example of the use of imagery in this way might be suggesting to a patient who is in the grips of a flashback, "Imagine that you are seeing the scene on a TV screen, and then that you can change the channel if you wish, or even turn off the set. Or you can imagine that you are reading a book, and can turn the pages as you choose."

Another image for containment of intense memory material is the use of an imaginary safe that needs two keys to be opened; the group has one key and the patient the other. Thus only the group and patient together can open and close access to the dissociated material. This image conveys the message that it is "safe" to feel and remember intensely during the group sessions, but that those feelings can and must be left in the sessions. Supplying the context that makes sense of intense feelings can also be grounding: One group member coined the expression, "You are having history feelings."

Every dissociative patient, intentionally or not, has discovered and developed his or her own dissociative triggers and should be encouraged to bring them under intentional personal control. This use of self is similar to what athletes do to promote peak performance in an athletic event. Visual stimuli and the use of eye muscles are often important in regulating dissociative states; people often focus on a spot on the wall or a knickknack in the office when putting themselves into trance. Curiously enough, this can go both ways: Either people can organize themselves by bringing their surroundings back into focus, or they can go (intentionally or unintentionally) into trance in order to numb painful feelings or ward off anticipated trouble. Chu (1998, pp. 109–111) feels that darkness—either inadequate lighting of the office or the darkness of evening—facilitates dysfunctional disengagement from visual grounding, and conveys acceptance of disorientation. He suggests that this be vigorously opposed in partnership with the patient for management of dissociation. Work with eye muscles can also be helpful: To restore trance-free focus and full access to the self, the patient can imagine looking at a distant flagpole though a split-image lens of a camera, while gradually bringing the top and bottom half of the flagpole together through the viewer. This exercise brings the image into focus, and brings the visualizer into grounded contact with the outside world.

A basic stabilization technique that can be helpful for anyone who dissociates is to ask the patient to imagine his or her own "safe place"—a place in the real world where the patient has experienced safety, but that also exists inside the self, where he or she is completely protected. Describing the details in the image of this safe place, even drawing it, and anchoring the feeling of safety to a texture that can be rubbed or felt are all calming. Remembering that the place is always there when the patient needs it, because he or she carries it inside the self, conveys the message that each of us has the power to calm and soothe ourselves when we need to by thinking about safety, hope, and healing. Adding physical relaxation sensations such as stomach breathing increases the sense of control over anxiety. The group and the therapist may suggest rituals to promote self-soothing, such as making a tape a member can play at home, or giving the member a candle to keep by the side of the bed to light if he or she is waking up at night.

Finding Ways to Be with Someone Who Is Dissociating

In group sessions, members may notice another member going into trance; if this is stated, it may help pull the dissociating member out. Or, if the member is not ready to give up the trance state, the group may need to provide a holding environment by tolerating the member's trance and finding ways to be with him or her. Reading a children's book aloud might be a way for the group to be together with the patient while he or she is in trance. Group discussion based on this issue can usefully raise questions for other members, while still including the member in trance: "What are your triggers? What helps ground you? What is it most useful for the group to do when a member enters trance? How would you like people to be with you when you are dissociating?"

It can be helpful to have modeling clay and other art materials freely available in the office; these nonverbal modalities often reveal themes for exploration. One member unconsciously modeled dice with the clay in her hands while speaking of her father, who was a compulsive gambler.

Trauma or Transference?

The development of theory in the history of psychology has set the stage for a split in theoretical approaches between trauma theory and internal conflict theory. Since Freud's emphasis on the seduction hypothesis and the importance of internal fantasy life, psychoanalytic theory has tended to overlook traumatic origins of symptoms. But interpreting symptoms as resulting from internal fantasies rather than as stemming from a traumatic source (when that is the case) runs the risk of blaming the victim; the most familiar instance of this is when rape has taken place. Still, some psychoanalytically trained therapists are likely to conceptualize issues in terms of inner conflict, and thus implicitly to underestimate the importance of trauma in many ways. For example, a classically oriented therapist might view a patient who shied away from the developmental tasks of adolescence as avoiding erotic experience, while a more interpersonally oriented therapist might feel that family dynamics and early abuse may have left the patient unable to integrate his or her own initiative and autonomy because these were too closely connected to trauma.

Guided imagery that is intended to help a client contain painful feelings can backfire, unless it is introduced carefully and treated as a tool placed at the disposal of the client. An image of a "locked box" to contain thoughts and feelings can become a cage, or the "soothing surf" can become a tidal wave, unless issues of power and dependency between therapist and client have been worked through thoroughly and the client is willing to relinquish any claims for dependency that the dissociative symptoms may represent. When the patient slips into trance in a session, or reacts fearfully to an image supplied by the therapist, this may represent hypervigilance stemming from the trauma rather than transference resistance, as the psychoanalytically trained therapist might assume. If the therapist explores the meaning of the behavior with the patient and extends the working alliance to bring the symptom into the relationship, rather than slipping into treating it as defiance or evasion, unnecessary power struggles can be avoided. The group may also help defuse such transferential dependency conflicts, since the transference is spread among group members and therapist.

Traumatic Transference

Although access to the traumatic experience may be important for full access to a functional self, during the last decade the field of trauma treatment has shifted away from a focus on reconstruction or reliving the trauma through "planned abreaction," as we have noted earlier. Therapists discovered that reliving the trauma can in itself be addictive and can take over the therapy, as it has often taken over patients' lives. Often a tug of war has developed between a therapist who wants to focus on daily functioning and strengthening the self, and a patient who seems only to want to relive the trauma, claiming to gain relief from that process. We now know that through the physiology of intense fear, endorphins are released and fill opiate receptors during an abreaction, so that the "relief" the patient may feel comes from a physical flooding with opiate-like substances. But the effects of adaptation to trauma go beyond physiological addiction to the whole issue of character development; Bessel van der Kolk has written insightfully that some patients "seem to organize much of their lives around repetitive patterns of reliving and warding off traumatic memories, reminders, and affects" (1996a, p. 183). These patterns have often acquired a central meaning in patients' lives.

A safe way to recover and process trauma can be through the transference derivatives that get stirred up in group sessions, even without direct recall.

> For example, a patient suddenly flashed on the word "therapist" as being identical to "the rapist," and reported that her thought triggered intense feelings of fear and rage. The fantasy embodied in this condensed word play was one in which the possibility of trauma was recreated in the word imagery, and the condensation allowed both patient and therapist access to the possibility that they might somehow recreate the trauma and all the fear, rage, and other affects in it.

Cognitive-behavioral training to promote affect tolerance, thought replacement exercises, and challenges to dysfunctional beliefs such as self-blame can certainly strengthen patients who feel overwhelmed. These techniques must, however, be well grounded in a therapeutic relationship and jointly undertaken, or they will precipitate despair that others really do not want to know about the horror and terror a patient has been living with. Other group members can powerfully convey educational messages.

> For instance, when one member was having trouble feeling entitled to set boundaries for others in her world, another member who worked as an exotic dancer told her that she believed that no one had the right to touch her while she was dancing, even though she was dressed in a revealing way. This was a vivid and meaningful message, and the fellow group member successfully modeled and conveyed the feeling of healthy entitlement to one's own boundaries.

The Group as Container

The group can provide an especially powerful sense of containment. The therapist may supply a basket for helpful objects, and members may bring in contributions as they are able. In the basket may be art supplies, a special box, a music box that plays "Tea for Two," favorite bedtime books, or music and story tapes for children. When a member anticipates stress between group meetings, or is still visibly upset at the end of a group meeting, the member can be invited to choose an object to take home from the basket. If someone begins to withdraw dissociatively during a group, and the usual grounding strategies do not work, the therapist may read from a book brought in by another member because it has been meaningful.

In ongoing groups, breaks for vacation or summer can feel very disruptive for members who have come to rely on the group. The therapist can suggest a ritual, or ask the group to help design one. A piece of paper for each member can be passed around, with members being invited to write messages to the therapist about him- or herself and about what the therapist means to them. Or the therapist can buy each member a candle, and instruct members to light it every week at the usual time of the group sessions. Or the therapist can hand out a piece of pretty stationery for each week the group will not be meeting, and instruct members to write something on each piece once a week, to be shared with the group or not, as each member chooses when the group meets again. Members can be invited to leave painful issues or feelings in the group room, corked up in bottles, until the group resumes. Group members can each be given a matching bracelet.

One group member wrote the following poem for another:

Let our love be an umbrella to shelter you from life's rain.
Let us hold you close until the storm around you subsides.
Let our voices whisper gently
to shut out all the noise and confusion.
Let us help stop the chaos while you find the peace.
Let us be beside you ... behind you ... to reassure you that we'll
never be farther away than your nearest thought.
Let us convince you that as long as we're in the world,
you'll never be alone.

DEALING WITH SPECIFIC
AFFECTS IN GROUPS

Trust and Vulnerability

Trust is undoubtedly the most difficult emotional capacity for trauma survivors, especially if they have become adapted to chronic trauma. For many, the dread of vulnerability and the need to destroy it have reached the proportions of attachment disorder. We might safely say that for many, the ability to trust marks the completion of the therapeutic work.

The feelings that are not present may be as important as the ones that are in group sessions. Harrison and Morris (1996) propose that certain common issues in life—such as "asking for help, expressing oneself, setting limits, confronting perpetrators, experiencing a feeling of being protected, trusting others, and accepting care and protection from other men" (p. 346)—are particularly difficult for male abuse survivors, because their coping styles have led them to distance themselves from the feelings involved.

They recommend prescriptive exercises for groups of male survivors. For instance, the group might stand behind a member who is imagining and putting into words a confrontation with his perpetrator, putting their hands on his shoulders. If a man is having trouble finding his "voice," another group member might speak for him and allow him to add to and correct what is said. These exercises help group members to identify patterns of avoidance of certain feelings in their lives, to overcome these patterns, and to gain needed skills.

Fear

Gartner (1999) describes a group member's experience of intense fear upon being triggered by a sensory impression.

> Andreas had learned to carry out adult roles by dissociating himself from all forms of feeling, and by avoiding situations in which he might feel vulnerable or anxious. He hated "checking in" at the beginning of the group meeting, in which members told the group how they were at the moment, and often arrived late to avoid it. When a new member joined the group, Andreas became terrified and unable to sleep; "his terror had broken through his dissociation" (Gartner, 1999, p. 164). While it was difficult for Andreas to identify the trigger for his terror, he finally realized that the new member's hands looked to him exactly like the hands of one of his abusers. "Seeing Seth's hands had plunged Andreas back into the panic state he had endured as a boy. Never having allowed this dissociated panic into awareness before, he was now terrified in exactly the same ways he had been at age eight" (p. 164). Having identified the source of his terror in intensive individual therapy sessions, Andreas was able to go back to the group, to enlist group support for his fear of vulnerability, and to examine some of his emotional distortions.

Despair and Hope

Despair is one of the affects likely to be introduced into a group with which the group can be most effective. A member of one group said, "I used to be able to tell myself that I could at least get by, one day at a time, and now I don't feel that way." The therapist responded, "Maybe being in the group makes you feel that just 'getting by' isn't enough."

Watching others make progress and participating in that progress provide hope, even for a member who feels blocked or has reached a plateau him- or herself. Herman (1992) states, "The solidarity of a group provides the strongest protection against terror and despair, and the strongest antidote to traumatic experience" (p. 215).

Anger

Although nondefensive exploration of angry affects may always be recommended for groups, it may be especially important for groups of dissociative patients, since the perceptions that trigger anger are often part of important dissociated reenactments of an original trauma, as in the examples of reenactment discussed earlier in this chapter.

> In an especially useful example of the continuation of buried feelings about trauma and victimization, a member expressed fury at all the obligations of the group—at having to come on time every week and having to pay for sessions, when her perpetrator wasn't in therapy, didn't have to pay anything, and didn't have to go through any of the painful work that she was having to do. The therapist interpreted that the group was being experienced at that moment as a continuation of her abusive situation, and of the unfairness of having been victimized. In this way, the therapist led recognition and acceptance of her ongoing but hidden anger at being exploited, and reopened an understanding of the meaning of the rage, while tolerating its verbal expression.

Grief

Almost all successful work with dissociative defenses at some point involves strengthening the patient to be able to bear the painful feelings of loss. Therapeutic work with trauma involves loss at many levels: actual concrete losses (of income, achievement, or health); loss of the kind of life that can now never be, or of the person one might ideally have become had the trauma not taken place; and loss of the idealized "good" parent or abuser. Nancy Napier (1993), Yvonne Dolan (1991), and Christine Courtois (1988) have described detailed exercises to help patients develop compassion for themselves, such as writing condolence letters to themselves for the losses caused by the trauma.

Group co-constructed rituals are an especially powerful means of expressing feelings connected with endings and loss. For example, when a member completes his or her work and leaves, the other members can each be given a helium balloon and instructed to release it in space with a good wish for the departing member, as well as a goal for themselves.

Shame and Isolation

A person in this culture who has dissociative experiences is isolated. Not only the trauma but also the symptoms developed to cope with it must be hidden, since both are shameful. The experiences of "hearing voices," "losing time," amnesias, depersonalization, and derealization have historically been grounds for social rejection and stigma. Only recently has the coping aspect of these symptoms become clear, so the need is great for group experience to help with shame. Wright, O'Leary, and Balkin (1987) point out the curative factors in group treatment that enable the shame-ridden or antisocial patient "to shift from a self-absorbed position in life a to position of greater social awareness, and also help increase self-esteem" (p. 243). Quoting Bacal (1985), Wright and colleagues discuss the potential for the narcissistic group member to fulfill the need for selfobject experience in ways that are impossible in dyadic therapy because of the simultaneous but incompatible need for idealization of the therapist. Positing that shame rather than guilt motivates altruism, Wright and colleagues also point out the advantages of a group for a shame-ridden patient in providing a milieu for altruistic experience to alleviate feelings of shame and inadequacy. In helping others, a person can—and should—come to feel greater self-worth.

Finding Ways to Be with a Group Member Who Is Experiencing Intense Affects

Sometimes it is a new experience simply to be with others who are supportive, and to learn that intense emotions can be talked about and responded to.

> One group member who sobbed for 40 minutes about a painful memory was worried that she was taking up too much of the group's time. Drawing on the idea that the group is a connected whole, the therapist pointed out that the grieving member was freeing others in the group by having that feeling for all of them. This gave the patient the room she needed to sob, and it let the group know that they were playing a role in her healing. This interpretation also paved the way for all to understand that suffering has a wider meaning for all, and does not just have to enforce isolation. At the next meeting, the group was very quiet after one member spoke of a particularly horrible memory, and one member voiced anxiety about "just leaving her alone" after such intense feelings had been brought up. The therapist responded, "Maybe she needs to rest now too." This interpretation gave all the group members needed permission just to be together without having to do something. The therapist can model the value that just "being with the feelings" is a valuable task in itself.

Trance

It is likely that discussions of emotional material will trigger trance in some group patients. This may be very obvious, as when someone "spaces out," or it may be less obvious: The therapist may experience countertransferential feelings of sleepiness, boredom, emptiness, nothingness, or restlessness. Such feelings are sources of "vital communication in relation to early life objects" (Scharff & Scharff, 1994, p. 332). The Scharffs point out that this form of countertransference, concordant with a patient's dissociative states, is harder to recognize and value than more clearly trauma-identified internal states, but they emphasize the importance of these states in understanding such a patient's experience. As with intense affects, it is necessary for the group and the therapist to find a way of being with someone who is in trance. It may be helpful for the therapist to allow the patient to determine whether he or she wants to be grounded and pulled away from the trance, or whether the patient just needs to be in that state for now. The therapist may ask members to share what it feels like to be with someone who is dissociating, or elicit members' fantasies about what the dissociating person is feeling. The Scharffs call this welcoming "going-on-being," and understand that it is a defense for survival as well as a communication about early life. It is helpful to use the patient's own metaphor for the experience, such as "having trouble focusing" or "zoning out."

Supportive exercises using other modalities such as writing and drawing, can be helpful for patients who are trying to manage affective flooding. The Sidran Foundation has a number of self-help publications such as *Managing Traumatic Stress through Art* (1995), by Barry M. Cohen, Mary-Michola Barnes, and Anita B. Rankin, which are especially helpful for work with dissociation. Nancy Napier's *Getting Through the Day* (1993) is readable and very useful.

Trance Contagion

Affectively powerful material may even trigger a number of people in the group to dissociate at the same time. The therapist can speculate on what might have made group members slip into trance. It is advisable for therapists who want to work with visualizations and hypnotic techniques to do so after training and under supervision, but it may be helpful for all therapists who work with dissociative patients to explore their own feelings about trance and their capacity for it. Phillips and Frederick (1995), Watkins and Watkins (1997), and Jarrett (1991) agree that "Achieving a positive countertransference trance state with dissociative patients can result in an enhanced 'holding' environment—attached yet individuated, separate yet connected and engaged" (Phillips & Frederick, 1995, p. 224).

From Affect to Political Awareness in Groups

Jones (1993, pp. 14–23) points out that from a feminist perspective, power-based violence within the nuclear family is normalized by the culture. Without group validation of a woman's right to be free from violence, it will be difficult for a female abuse survivor to stop blaming herself for the abuse and to achieve a level of awareness of the social and political significance of what she has been through. It is difficult for such survivors to feel entitled to be treated decently, and to behave in ways that elicit being valued rather than being victimized, unless the collective meaning of their abuse is addressed. Dolan (1991) agrees that "hearing another's story of victimization can be a powerful way—sometimes the only way—for a client to recognize that the abuse was not her fault" (p. 29). The meaning of witness has been an important part of healing from trauma, because it gives a public meaning to the traumatic experience and establishes norms about justice, placing the victimization in a context that overcomes the isolation and secrecy often surrounding trauma. This is especially true for the dissociative patient, who has suffered from self-doubt as well as from the original trauma. Thus the meaning of connectedness within the group is especially important for this population.

REFERENCES

Briere, J. (1995, October 5). *Treating male survivors of sexual abuse.* Workshop presented at the Sixth World Interdisciplinary Conference on Male Sexual Victimization, sponsored by the National Organization on Male Sexual Victimization, Columbus, OH.

Bromberg, P. (1998). *Standing in the spaces: Essays on clinical process, trauma, and dissociation.* Hillsdale, NJ: Analytic Press.

Chu, J. (1998). *Rebuilding shattered lives: The responsible treatment of complex post-traumatic and dissociative disorders.* New York: Wiley.

Cohen, B. M., Barnes, M. M., & Rankin, A. B. (1995). *Managing traumatic stress through art.* Lutherville, MD: Sidran Press.

Courtois, C. (1988). *Healing the incest wound.* New York: Norton.

Davies, J. M., & Frawley, M. G. (1994). *Treating the adult survivor of childhood sex abuse: A psychoanalytic perspective.* New York: Basic Books.

Dolan, Y. M. (1991). *Resolving sexual abuse: Solution-focused therapy and Ericksonian hypnosis for adult survivors.* New York: Norton.

Gartner, R. B. (1999). *Betrayed as boys: Psychodynamic treatment of sexually abused men.* New York: Guilford Press.

Gold-Steinberg, S., & Buttenheim, M. C. (1993). "Telling one's story" in an incest survivors' group. *International Journal of Group Psychotherapy, 43*(2), 173–190.

Harrison, J. B., & Morris, L. A. (1996). Group therapy for adult male survivors of child sexual abuse. In M. P. Andronico (Ed.), *Men in groups: Insights, interventions in psychoeducational work* (pp. 339–356). Washington, DC: American Psychiatric Press.

Hopenwasser, K. (1998). Listening to the body: Somatic representations of dissociated memory. In L. Aron & F. S. Anderson (Eds.), *Relational perspectives on the body* (pp. 215–236). Hillsdale, NJ: Analytic Press.

Jarrett, K. (1991). Ericksonian hypnotherapy and sexual addiction. *American Journal of Preventive Psychiatry and Neurology, 3*(1), 43–46.

Jones, E. (1993). *Family systems therapy: Developments in the Milan–systemic therapies*. New York: Wiley.

Krystal, H. (1974). Affect tolerance. In H. Krystal (Ed.), *Massive psychic trauma* (pp. 179–217). New York: International Universities Press.

Napier, N. J. (1993). *Getting through the day: Strategies for adults hurt as children*. New York: Norton.

Phillips, M., & Frederick, C. (1995). *Healing the divided self: Clinical and Ericksonian hypnotherapy for post-traumatic and dissociative conditions*. New York: Norton.

Putnam, F. W. (1997). *Dissociation in children and adolescents: A developmental perspective*. New York: Guilford Press.

Raine, N. V. (1998). *After silence: Rape and my journey back*. New York: Crown.

Scharff, J. S., & Scharff, D. (1994). *Object relations therapy of physical and sexual trauma*. Northvale, NJ: Aronson.

Spiegel, D. (1994). *Dissociation: Culture, mind, and body*. Washington, DC: American Psychiatric Press.

Steinberg, M. (1995). *Handbook for the assessment of dissociation: A clinical guide*. Washington, DC: American Psychiatric Press.

Tyson, A. A., & Goodman, M. (1996). Group treatment for adult women who experienced childhood sexual trauma: Is telling the story enough? *International Journal of Group Psychotherapy*, 46(4) 535–542.

van der Kolk, B. A. (1996a). The complexity of adaptation to trauma: Self-regulation, stimulus discrimination, and characterological development. In B. A. van der Kolk, A. C. McFarlane, & L. Weisaeth (Eds.), *Traumatic stress: The effects of overwhelming experience on mind, body, and society* (pp. 182–213). New York: Guilford Press.

van der Kolk, B. A. (1996b). Trauma and memory. In B. A. van der Kolk, A. C. McFarlane, & L. Weisaeth (Eds.), *Traumatic stress: The effects of overwhelming experience on mind, body, and society* (pp. 279–302). New York: Guilford Press.

Watkins, J. G., & Watkins, H. H. (1997). *Ego states: Theory and therapy*. New York: Norton.

Wright, F., O'Leary, J., & Balkin, J. (1987). Men, shame, and antisocial behavior: A psychodynamic perspective. *Group, 11*, 238–246.

4

‐◄◦►‐

Group-as-a-Whole Dynamics in Work with Traumatized Patients: Technical Strategies, Their Rationales, and Limitations

RAMON GANZARAIN

The purpose of this chapter is to describe the typical dynamics and roles that occur when traumatized patients are treated in psychotherapy groups, including the characteristics of their transferences and of our countertransference reactions. I rely primarily on my observations when doing analytic group psychotherapy with incest victims (Ganzarain, 1991; Ganzarain & Buchele, 1988, 1993), but I also discuss group therapy with persons suffering from other kinds of trauma—parental abandonment (Ganzarain, 1989), physical abuse, confinement during mental illness, and police brutality, for example. Each specific trauma has peculiar characteristics, different from those of others; however, certain common denominators are present in every kind of trauma.

In general, "trauma" is a frightening event defined by its overwhelming intensity, by the victim's helplessness to respond adequately, and by its disturbing and long-lasting effects on the person's mental organization (Laplanche & Pontalis, 1973). The feelings of helplessness are experienced as a metaphorical loss of maternal protection. The defenseless inability to respond to the threat of annihilation of the self seems to validate the fears of being annihilated by powerful persecutors—the so-called "paranoid anxieties." In other words, trauma reactivates and intensifies the basic human anxieties about losing the mother's caring help and of suffering the annihilation of the self.

In addition to the reactions to trauma usually described as posttraumatic stress disorder, traumatic experiences may leave indelible "emotional scars." Recently traumatized patients still feel acute mistrust upon entering a new emotional relationship (including one with a psychotherapy group). The delayed effects of old traumas appear instead as personality disorders or as chronically difficult interpersonal relationships. I refer metaphorically to these effects as "emotional scars."

Groups for traumatized individuals are experienced as offering helpful support to their members. Individuals often attribute maternal functions to the groups with which they are affiliated. Hence, experiencing the loss of one's group supportive feedback and attention may trigger "depressive anxieties" associated with the loss of maternal care. The terror of being annihilated by powerful persecutory elements is also rekindled and ever-present in these groups; such "paranoid anxieties" are easily stirred up when individual self-assurance is challenged. Both types of anxieties—depressive and paranoid—are reactivated in an individual's mind upon entering a group and negotiating membership. The defenses against these fears are loosely organized as the group "basic assumptions" (Bion, 1961).

Since traumata trigger extremely intense anxieties, the group defenses against them are formidable. Such defenses create typical transference paradigms, which I discuss below.

THE GROUP AS A MATERNAL METAPHOR

The group as a whole may become an unconscious metaphor representing innumerable aspects of human life. Among the negative are the flaws of society; the mental misery of dysfunctional families; the limitations of parents, such as the unavailability of a depressed mother; and various aspects of the divided self, such as a cruel, ethically overdemanding superego, or a traumatized person's "ego ideal" imposing expectations to assume the role of an omnipotent survivor and rescuer. Such infinite versatility of multiple unconscious metaphors allows the exploration of complex layers of the unconscious in analytic group therapy when it is focused primarily on the transferences to the group as a whole. Work on group-as-a-whole phenomena can be very productive without necessarily excluding the interpersonal transferences, which do expand and supplement the group-oriented ones. The feelings for the "mother group" are universally essentially ambivalent, but are intensified in persons who have experienced trauma. However, groups often deny the "bad" features of "our" group, using splitting and projection as defenses to push them far away. In addition, they resort to confusion, blurring their perceptions of "Who is 'bad'?" by displacing and diffusing the "badness" from the group to either the leader, some scapegoated member, or another group. There is consequently a limited expression of anger toward or hatred of the negative attributes of "our" group, "instead of accepting that the unpleasant qualities belong to 'our' group and to every member, as well" (Ganzarain, 1991, p. 158).

I wrote (Ganzarain, 1991, p. 158) that "the 'bad' mother-group is perceived as overdemanding, devouring, intrusive and lacking in reciprocity." It is seen as overdemanding when imposing the group values on the individual, leaving no freedom to be one's self (Bion, 1961). It is viewed as devouring because it takes away the member's personal credits and possessions, thus threatening the member with what Freud (1921/1955) called a "loss of individuality." It is perceived as intrusive when inquiring with hostile, controlling curiosity about private, even secret matters, attempting to influence members, or ruthlessly subjecting them to public ridicule. Finally, it is seen as lacking in reciprocity because the group can survive socially without any given member (just as mothers do not need their infants to survive biologically), whereas members need their status as group members to define themselves socially. Each member feels that "the group can do without me." And most groups do survive after losing any one member, in spite of the fact that a group will not be the same "without any one of its members" (Ganzarain, 1991, p. 158). Briefly, the group is experienced as "bad" when it takes away from its members. The loss of its life-giving supportive feedback becomes traumatic (Hearst, 1981).

As I have noted elsewhere, "The 'bad' mother group images have multidetermined, confusing meanings, undergoing disguising condensations and far-fetched displacements across several transferential targets. What unifies those multiple 'bad' group images is a psychotic-like schizo–paranoid and sadomasochistic style of relationships between the self and its objects" (Ganzarain, 1991, p. 172), which are dramatically intensified by trauma.

In group psychoanalytic therapy, significant hidden negative transferences can be explored by following the complex metamorphosis of the "bad" mother group images, thus overcoming the group's prevailing schizo–paranoid anxieties and the primitive defenses against them: splitting, projection, and projective identification. "We can help the patients to work through and to achieve maturing integrations of the 'good' and the 'bad' mother images, allowing the mental reality of human ambivalence to be fully experienced" (Ganzarain, 1991, p. 172).

GROUP BASIC ASSUMPTIONS AND THE
TRANSFERENCES THEY GENERATE

In psychoanalytic group therapy, the transference is targeted in the patient's mind at the internalized images of the "group as a unit," at the images of the other members, and at that of the therapist(s). Feelings are also interpersonally experienced and expressed externally for the therapist(s) and other group members. Those transference feelings focused on given persons are manifested in interactions with those individuals, whereas the feelings transferred to the group as an entity are less explicit. They are often confused with those simultaneously related to a psychotherapist who is using the group as his or her professional tool to help the members.

The transferences to the group as a whole offer a perspective of the group dynamics and role assignments at any moment in a specific group. Such transferences express mainly the activity of primitive defense mechanisms protecting the group against the prevailing unconscious psychotic anxieties. "Such [fears] derive from conflicts with aggression in the fantasied exchanges between the self and its objects, perceived as a threat, either of annihilation of the self (schizo–paranoid anxiety—as illustrated by the example below about the South American mayors)—or of destruction of the loved objects (depressive anxiety)" (Ganzarain, 1992a, pp. 205–206). In the same context, I defined Bion's "basic assumptions" (abbreviated in later text as BAs) in relation to group anxieties as follows:

> Bion's "basic assumptions" are clusters of defenses organized to protect the group from psychotic anxieties. Paranoid anxiety refers to the feared anticipated annihilation of the self by persecutors. Splitting is the defense against it, leading to the fragmentation of both the self (making it appear as weaker) and the objects, which may appear as even more threatening. By contrast, the depressive anxiety is the fear that one's own aggression could eliminate (or has already destroyed) one's good maternal object: the "good" mother [as exemplified by Laura's reaction, reported later in this chapter, when I canceled a group session]. The ego feels also threatened in identification with the attacked object. After attacking the ambivalently loved mother, the self experiences her loss, which gives rise to pain and guilt. These anxieties culminate during infancy, but they are not exclusive of a passing phase (for example the "oral" stage), but persist through life as specific configurations of Melanie Klein's "positions" of object relations and anxieties. (Ganzarain, 1992a, p. 207)

The focus on group–centered transferences leads the therapists to examine the defensive dynamics determined by such underlying psychotic group anxieties. To protect itself from annihilation, the group resorts typically to Bion's "fight–flight" BA to deal with an "enemy" (see the vignette on the South American mayors, below). A group member, a therapist, or the entire group may be cast in an enemy role. Ambivalent hate of the object may bring up dependency upon an idealized object (Bion's "dependency" BA); again, the whole group, a therapist, or a fellow member can be seen as "ideal" reliable providers to gratify the group's needs. Manic contempt leads to the devaluation of the object, while the self feels triumphantly omnipotent, denying any dependency upon or any guilt related to the worthless object (again, see the vignette on the South American mayors, below). Guilt about having damaged the once valued and loved object is denied, since if the manic group's omnipotent reparatory capacity to love (Bion's "pairing" BA) is mobilized, it is felt as "magic." Two members or any couple may become the agents of this fantasized magic love, which reassures the group about its future and generativity. "Love" in this context extends beyond its genital, sexual aspects. In my earlier discussion of the BAs, I continued:

> The group members defend themselves against psychotic anxieties, by using projective identification. Hence each member disowns the basic assumptions [as] feelings, claiming no personal participation in them, perceived as "not me." Paradoxically the same individual simultaneously believes those basic assumptions are an active and powerful part of the group to which he or she belongs; hence each member perceives them also as part of "us." In other words, the group as an object is neither self nor other, but subsumes both of them, as does a transitional object (Winnicott, 1951[/1974]). Because the basic assumptions are the disowned parts of the individual group members, they are anonymous and function ruthlessly (no one is personally responsible), which is why members fear them. (Ganzarain, 1992a, pp. 206–207)

A FOURTH BASIC ASSUMPTION?

Turquet (1974) and Hopper (1997) have each postulated a fourth BA of groups, in addition to the three described above. Turquet observed in large groups what he called the BA of "oneness," which he considered a result of an individual's feeling traumatized by a large group's behaviors toward him or her. Hopper has described Holocaust victims in a small long-term therapy group as developing a culture of "group incohesion," apparently instead of resorting to fight–flight, when they felt abandoned by their therapist's absence from a group session.

Large groups are not really used "therapeutically" in working with traumatized patients, but rather in quasi-administrative/educational ways in the so-called "community meetings" run by mental health institutions. Nevertheless, the questions about a possible fourth BA are still relevant, because observers such as Hopper see "oneness" in small groups with traumatized patients. The description of being "at one" with the group is related to the idealization that makes the group so protective and appealing. It should be kept in mind that idealization happens after the objects are split into "bad" versus "good." Hence "being one" with the powerful, "good" group seems to fit simultaneously either the fourth BA or the fight–flight BA, after splitting occurs (see the example below with a group of medical students). Likewise, Hopper's term "incohesion" seems to overlap with "fragmentation," after repeated splittings that leave either the self or the object divided into multiple small parts.

As mentioned above, Turquet's (1974) postuation of the BA of "oneness" in large groups stemmed from his systematic study of such groups, and especially of their significant differences from small groups. Anzieu (1975, p. 80) proposed conventional numbers of members (e.g., 25 to 60) as defining a "large" group. Members of a large group, according to Turquet (1974, p. 357), "seek to join in powerful union with an omnipotent force, to surrender the self for a passive participation [in power], thereby [to] feel well being and wholeness." As a result, "The group member is lost in oceanic feelings of unity" and "becomes a part of a salvationist inclusion" (Turquet, 1974, p. 360). Hopper (1997, pp. 446, 448) barely acknowledges that Turquet viewed the fourth BA in large groups as a response to the trauma of finding oneself isolated and ignored. Hopper, in my opinion, also omits any consideration of the significant differences between small and large groups, insofar as large groups present specific threats to a person's identity through surrounding the individual in an atmosphere of emotional isolation (limited face-to-face interactions) and anonymity, to the degree that participating in a large group constitutes an emotional trauma that is in itself "a transient experience of depersonalization" (Turquet, 1975/1994, p. 80). The absence of social feedback in large groups evokes feelings of loss of maternal protection; participants often feel there as if they are "suffering from a fracture of their personality" (Anzieu, 1975, p. 80). The threat to one's identity experienced in a large group may bring a "conversion" response of "magically feeling at one with the group as a whole"; thus members may come to believe in a homogenization, with absolute sameness of belief and no role differentiation among members. The leaders of oneness are "charismatic." Homogenization is the source of the BA of oneness.

Hopper (1997) discusses Turquet's ideas but seeks an alternative theory based on the fear of annihilation, which leads him to a different view of the fourth BA. He argues against Turquet's ideas, disagreeing "in principle" and stating his belief that envy and annihilation fear "are not inevitable" (Hopper, 1997, p. 448). He describes his own views on annihilation extensively, using sociological terminology, such as redesignating the fourth BA "incohesion/aggregation and massification." He argues that deep regression "follows loss, abandonment and damage" not simply from the "stimuli and response bombardment of the large group situation" (p. 450).

He has tried to complete an "exhaustive inventory of the roles and character types associated with the two styles of leadership called: aggregation or massification" (p. 45).

When reading Hopper's (1997) paper, one wishes for more clinical observations (only one is provided) as the basis for his theory, as well as clearer clinical relevance for each of his different sociological terms. Hopper describes his opposition to Melanie Klein's ideas, but attempts to bring the ideological disagreement into his sociological territory without enough consideration of intrapsychic conflict or contents.

A third approach to this issue has been provided by Lonergan (1989), who has elaborated on how to treat the traumatized self-esteem of the medically and psychiatrically ill, building up on her observations about what she labels the "pre-group dynamics" (p. 150). She uses terms from self psychology to describe a transient idealization, comparable to the defense mobilized by the fourth BA:

> Severely disturbed patients are usually self-involved and have a tenuous capacity for object relations; they spend considerable time in the narcissistic phase of development being in the same room but ignoring each other. The pre-group has a stage of "parallel" talk which ends when members recognize each other's existence, and a stage where members use each other and the group for a narcissistic purpose. . . . In order to enter the trust phase, they need to face the fact that fellow members are strangers and could be hurtful, as opposed to . . . being an extension of themselves and present to fulfill their narcissistic needs. The pre-group is a collection of individuals whose thought and actions are primarily motivated by narcissistic needs. (Lonergan, 1989, pp. 149–150)

The leader's understanding of how the group "can help the patients achieve . . . their self-esteem and psychic stability" defines his or her task as helping "the patients to use the group for their own narcissistic needs, so that the group [becomes] useful and meaningful for each member" (p. 151). Use of denial is common during the pre-group; it seems to cultivate the notion that "we're all the same; there are no differences between us" (p. 151). Lonergan's approach seems to leave little room for early exploration of envy/jealousy or competition. Exploring aggression is avoided.

Lonergan (1989, p. 150) continues: "Grandiosity and idealizing can take many forms. . . . Those who maintain their own grandiosity in a group have a harder time staying in the group. They can do so, however, by identifying with the leader." Such members often enact the role of "doctor's assistants." They find "an equal" and proclaim themselves "cotherapists." In the power phase of group development, these members will "face the hostility" of their group mates. "Their characteristic grandiosity makes them the target of other members' attacks."

Just as their peers' fury at those group members who act as "doctor's assistants" is sooner or later expressed by these peers, so also there will occur other postponed expressions of hostility. Anger is an important and often neglected element in trauma, because traumatized persons' helpless inability to respond adequately to the harm they have received elicits both a reactive impotent rage and a continued fear of being annihilated by powerful forces that seem "to be after them"—either as imaginary, godlike, revengeful persecutors, or as envious peers whose "evil eye" has already hurt them before. Hence traumatized patients' expressions of hostility should not be indefinitely postponed, because their ever-present fear of being harmed again is closely connected with their anger. In addition, the potential enemy becomes the recipient of the victims' projected hostility. Their aggression is communicated nonverbally through the web of projective identifications; they send wordless, angry messages that put pressure on their group mates and therapists and attempt to control them from inside. Such unspoken exchanges may sustain or mute the paranoid mistrust and sadomasochistic interactions typical of the schizo–paranoid mentality.

SPLITTING AND PROJECTIVE IDENTIFICATION IN TRAUMA GROUPS

The anxious mistrust of traumatized patients seriously undermines their capacity to initiate new emotional relationships, including those involved in psychotherapy. Whether we use the terms "paranoid anxiety," "incohesion," "pre-group dynamics," or other words pointing in the same direction, we are referring to these patients' basic mistrust, which informs these groups' schizo–paranoid mentality. The idealization of such a group may act initially as a stabilizing factor, helping members to feel transiently protected from "bad" objects. Splitting is the underlying defense through which objects are rigidly divided into "persecutors" and "benefactors." The traumata shared by these patients bring them together against their "common enemies" while they use the group as their emotional shelter, feeling "really understood" there, as if they were among "identical twins." The idealizing and twinship transferences (Kohut, 1968, p. 89) fuse them together as if they had no differences among them. Yet such a comforting situation has a price: the quasi-delusional, rigid splitting that prefers the predictability of the "bad" object over the unreliability of the "possibly good" one, because such a systematic view of the world offers constancy and stability, instead of the anxious, uncertain unpredictability of the relationship with "possibly good" objects who may fail again.

The pre-group dynamics, which may set in as the denial of differences among group members, promotes the development of group-level twinship transferences (Kohut, 1968, p. 89). Such a process initially facilitates group cohesion. However, the group needs to acknowledge the trauma-based mistrust sooner or later. The therapists can help the group members to observe in themselves or in one another the use of their defenses: splitting (both of parts of self and of objects) and projective identification (Ganzarain, 1992a), in order subsequently to deal with their mutual mistrust. Splitting leads them to differentiate themselves from their externalized bad objects and to oppose them with their internalized good objects. Good objects become idealized, while the bad ones are vilified and felt as persecutors.

An understanding of projective identification is useful in treating traumatized patients, because this represents another major defense for them. The effects on the recipients of such projections consist of feeling pressured, almost forced to assume some specific roles (see the section "Further Roles Elicited by Traumatized Patients in Groups," below). Bion (1962) described as effects of projective identification his feelings of being invaded "by fantasies alien" to him, while Schafer (1997) has written of being "colonized" by the projector. Sandler (1976) wrote instead about the recipient's "role responsiveness." I myself have stated elsewhere:

> Projective identification is both an intra-psychic defense mechanism (Klein, M., 1946[/1952]) and a vehicle for interpersonal communication (Bion, 1962). As a defense, projective identification can be used by the anxious self (after splitting and projection) to protect itself from annihilation fears through fantasies of entering the objects and omnipotently controlling them. Klein labeled this aspect as an "intrusive identification fantasy of defense" which also elaborates wishes to get rid of, to evacuate, unacceptable mental contents onto objects. (Ganzarain, 1992c, p. 15)

The following vignettes illustrate the operation of these defenses in groups. The first example comes from a training group; the second comes from a therapy group for incest survivors with a schizophrenic member. Although the first example is not an example of a trauma group as such, both vignettes vividly illustrate the dynamics of splitting and projective identification.

A group of eight medical students had elected to become group patients in order to learn about psychotherapy while attending the department of psychiatry. As their group therapist, I had canceled one of their planned sessions and offered them a replacement meeting, which they accepted. During that replacement session, there was a medical emergency in my family, and my secretary had to interrupt the meeting and request me to answer a phone call. I did. Before the interruption, the students were praising highly "the quality of our teaching," stating that I was their "best teacher." When I returned to the room, the group looked at me and kept silent. Various members told Bob, "You have to tell him!" (pointing to me). They said that Bob had had an important association/fantasy while I was out. He hesitantly said that when I left, he was reminded of another instructor in our school who used to mislead his students by letting them believe that he had briefly left their meeting room, but instead he stayed by the door, eavesdropping on what the students said about him. Whoever criticized him had his or her name written in that instructor's pocket notebook, and thus included on his "blacklist." During the final oral examination, that instructor took revenge against his critics. Bob wondered whether I had really gone to answer the phone or was eavesdropping. When I left the room, the group was idealizing me. When I came back, Bob was the spokesman for the group's paranoid anxieties and the negative half of the split. In his fantasy, I was vilified. Before I left, splitting was silently operating. When I returned, it became obvious that the previous idealization was a defense against acknowledging their mistrust of me. Idealization may appear as "so objective" (our narcissism is at stake!) that it may become difficult to accept its unconscious defensive function to protect from persecutory anxieties.

Bob's role as the group's spokesman for their paranoid fears was not a matter of chance, but indeed overdetermined. He had told us before of his deep ambivalence toward psychiatry after being himself a psychiatric patient at age 11. He had suffered from extreme anorexia nervosa, which required force-feeding him. He hated the whole experience of the psychiatric unit and the gastric intubation. He also felt betrayed by his mother, with whom he had a hateful relationship. He considered becoming a psychiatrist, but finally decided not to. His previous history of traumatization provided the basis for his becoming the spokesman for the group's persecutory fears. His fellow group members contained his anxiety and helped him and themselves to bring it up to be openly examined. The group dealt with their paranoid mentality by first idealizing me and later demonizing me. Idealization was used by this group as a defense against their persecutory fears.

A contrasting situation is illustrated in the second case.

In a group of incest survivors, Vivian had to face her peers' consensus in hating their male abusers. Since for Vivian her brother/sexual abuser was her only emotional support against her delusion of persecution, she experienced the other members' hatred of their offenders as an attack against her still-ongoing relationship with her brother. We discovered that although Vivian had been hospitalized with paranoid schizophrenia, she had managed to use his visits to continue their sexual contacts. The idealization of him was, for her, the only emotional shelter available in her family, since her mother had rejected her as an unplanned baby. Eventually we had to remove Vivian from the group, which was not helping her. Vivian's hospital psychiatrist, after our group "discovery," asked her brother to stop having sex with her. His hallucinated voice defended and protected her from the "mean" accusations of her female delusional persecutors, claiming incest as a loving experience. Splitting defended her from her extreme anxiety.

Buchele and I (Ganzarain & Buchele, 1988) described the extreme vilification of us as group psychotherapists while we treated incest victims. An acting out of power and sadism occurred when the group members transferred to us the hatred of their parents and implemented fantasies of finding other parents, "a better family":

> Betty was vocal in describing us therapists as "uncaring, arrogant, and stupid." She doubted our credentials and criticized our techniques. Wilma then agreed, claiming that "whatever good was coming out of the group came actually from the other group members who were giving to each other, but nothing good was coming out of the therapists' interventions." The devaluation of us as therapists culminated in Betty's calling other agencies and inquiring about group therapy programs for incest victims. The patients were ready to leave as a group for another agency, because they considered us unqualified to treat them. In our own words, "During this bitter power struggle we felt cornered and controlled, fearful that anything we said would be construed as a sadistic attack on them. Communication was distorted to such an extent that at times it seemed impossible. We began doubting our ability to use our clinical skills in helping the group through this intense paranoid crisis." (p. 44)

This group cast us as the therapists in the role of "bad" objects, whom they wished to "fire" while idealizing the help offered by the group members. The splitting consisted of "us versus them." The members envied our power and attacked us, devaluing our skills. Betty became the "rescuer," based on personal circumstances in her life. She began studying to become a mental health professional, competing with us. As a result she also had the power to treat mental patients, thus eliminating in her mind the differences and envy between her and us therapists. She could now lead the group away from us. Incest victims often dream about assuming the function of "rescuer" in their own families of origin. Betty's abuser had been an older brother, who had also taught her how to survive; hence she identified herself with him in becoming "streetwise."

I now turn to a group example involving police brutality, which can take many forms. For example, traffic violations, substance use cases, and drug dealing have at one time or another led in the United States to scandalous accusations against the police in New York City, Los Angeles, and New Orleans. In South America, police abuses have frequently been related to repressive military governments' spying on, torturing, or murdering citizens for their political activities and ideologies in opposition to dictatorships. Although the most talked-about police brutalities are significantly different in the United States and in South America, the chronic fear of being taken to a police station to be interrogated and possibly abused or tortured is not necessarily a rare occurrence. In the United States, if you belong to a racial or other minority group (black, Hispanic, gay, long-haired adolescent, etc.), you are considered suspicious in the eyes of many police officers; in some countries in South America, if you do not share the military governments' ideology, the police may terrorize you. (See von Wallenberg Pachaly, Chapter 11, this volume, for case examples of victims of such terror.) As a further illustration of splitting and projective identification, I offer the following example of a group of South American mayors living with the menaces created by police brutality.

In the mid-1960s, I was a cotrainer helping to lead a workshop in the United States for mayors from a South American country. At home, they were facing secret police threats during a military dictatorship. They formed one group of 14 participants.The mayors flew from South America to the U.S. training site, arrived at a motel, and remained there almost sequestered for the week-long training. My cotrainer was an American who did not understand their language. Two interpreters spoke their language to the participants in an audible voice, and whispered in English words for us trainers through an audio system. My cotrainer relied mainly on this simultaneous translation, and our differences in power, language, and style created tensions between us trainers.

The overloaded schedule, the isolation with few leisure activities and the "culture shock" proved to be too difficult for our trainees. The references to their group as an opportunity to learn about leadership were occasionally responded to with "Don't forget we are experienced leaders in our communities!" We trainers had not been briefed on the political situation in the mayors' home country, with the secret police persecuting the opposition. The translators and audio equipment created an artificial emphasis on verbal communications, contributing to an underestimation of the more significant nonverbal cues. The participants were confused, irritated, and also extremely distrustful of each other (was there a dictatorship's "snitch" among them?). They formed a typical paranoid culture in search of their hidden enemies. Hence they doubted everything—us trainers, the interpreters, and the audio system's reliability. They behaved as if they were "in flight," not verbalizing their real feelings, and instead giving nonverbal hints of their intense mistrust. The difficulties in overcoming the fight–flight group dynamics were enormous. The mayors were unable to function as a "work group."

Participants, trainers, and other personnel were all lodged in the same motel. Our meeting room was also there. The fourth night of the experience, we heard unusual noises coming from that room and went there. The mayors were looking for possible hidden microphones in the room. They believed that the translation equipment could be connected to recording gadgets, which could become available to the secret police in their country.

Living with the everyday traumatic threats of a violent military dictatorship, the mayors had transferred their fearful mistrust of their authorities to us trainers, casting us in the role of persecutors. The police activities were then the topics of everyday talk in their home country, where people often disappeared or were sent to jail; if they came back, they reported the tortures utilized by interrogators (mock executions or prisoners suspended from a bar by the backs of their knees and by their tied wrists). The government had created a net of spies to inform on their neighbors, easily accusing them of "conspiring against the safety or political stability of the country." The country was threatened by an anti-Communist campaign comparable to the McCarthy era in the United States, when the House Committee on Un-American Activities terrorized the entire country. Telephones were bugged to gather information against alleged conspirators. The military dictatorship had to dash to pieces the administrative/political network of the previous, legitimate government. This government was too leftist during the Cold War for those who supported the military coup. Because the legitimate government's enemies had to tear down the established control of the country, their attacks were decisive and final. Hence the mayors suffered from a chronic, hidden dread of being annihilated by police brutality.

After their enactment in which they searched for hidden microphones, they avoided examining their anxieties. Details of how and why they were so fearful were not talked about. The transferences to the trainers, the group members, and the group as a whole were displacements of their suspicions and fears of the brutal government police. The right of *habeas corpus* had been suspended, because legally the country was under a state of siege, in an internal war. Hence their seemingly "paranoid" fears were somehow adaptive and appropriate in their home context, but not in the transference. The formidable intensity of their feelings prevented their verbalization; they were instead acted out in the "silence of the night," as the dictatorship's agents acted, during curfew hours.

Like many other victims of trauma and of power abuses, the mayors identified themselves with their aggressors and had a paranoid mentality.

After being caught by us, the trainers, no statements were made by any participant, not even about how or which of the workshop experiences could be brought back home as something they had learned. Unfortunately, they were really retraumatized during this somewhat chaotic experience. Although their traumata were not dramatic, the iatrogenic elements contributing to their retraumatization constituted a significant lesson to extract from our workshop's mistaken design. Because retraumatization can easily happen during work with trauma, this vignette provides an important illustration about the importance of providing the proper setting and structure for resolving trauma and traumatic transference. Another significant lesson offered by this example is the importance of paying attention to nonverbal communications.

VICTIM–PERPETRATOR ROLES AND IDENTIFICATION WITH THE AGGRESSOR

Incest victims sometimes also identify themselves with the aggressors, thus themselves becoming perpetrators and offenders. To understand such a paradoxical development, it is important to keep in mind that projective identification is a reciprocal role reversal. Projective identification is the emotional basis for what I have labeled "the narcissistic contract between incestuous partners" (Ganzarain, 1992b, p. 491). Incest offenders "search for a surrogate source of affection in their own children" in an "act of intergenerational cannibalism, whereby the needs and rights of the younger partner are pushed aside by the exploitative self-centeredness of the offender" (Ganzarain, 1992b, p. 492). The preexisting familial dysfunction is characterized by the mother's emotional unavailability (and a child's consequent deprivation). Hence there is often a confusion of familial roles: The perpetrator is the child's maternal caretaker, while simultaneously demanding reciprocal emotional/sexual attention from that child. By displaying their suffering, because of feeling unloved, offenders elicit compassionate care from their loving children. Their masochistically controlling, guilt-inducing pleas appeal to their victims, who are drawn physically close in the role of comforters. By controlling a child, the abuser feels powerful, yet in so doing he/she simultaneously empowers the victim to exert control over him/her. Believing that he/she occupies a special position in the abused child's life, the abuser reciprocally makes the victim feel "very special." In such a "mutual admiration society," each person gains narcissistic, ambivalent gratifications from the other. As a result, confusion may ensue about who is the provider and who the beneficiary. The so-called "parentified child" (Gelinas, 1983) must lovingly support the older (regressed) partner (Ganzarain, 1992b, p. 492).

The offenders identify themselves with the maternally deprived children while the victims simultaneously identify themselves with the aggressor, feeling narcissistically fused with the offender, whose power they also wish to possess. Violent self-hatred, creating images of themselves as offenders, pleading forgiveness, and fearing punishment complicate the picture later on. Such confusion of identities between victim and offender is the result of the extensive use of projective identification, culminating in the "narcissistic contract": Each party becomes the other, while they struggle for who dominates or controls their relationship.

Buchele and I briefly described the case of a father–daughter pair. The child, whom we called Wilma (Ganzarain & Buchele, 1988), was later—as an adult in group psychotherapy—concerned (as many victims are) about the fear of being like the hated abuser. As an adult, Wilma wished to abuse a child, as her father had. She was attracted to an adolescent male much younger than she was, and as a result perhaps of her guilt about the implied role reversal, she did not want to go on living; she was experiencing depression subsequent to her identification with the aggressor. Her group mates helped her gain insight into herself, and as soon as she was less cruel in judging herself, she was able to put herself in her father's shoes and decreased her condemnation of him. The group's love for Wilma helped her in turn to forgive him. They supported her legitimating the narcissistic exchanges between her and her young lover, to meet her own needs to feel good about herself. But she realized she was repeating her father's typical behaviors.

FURTHER ROLES ELICITED
BY TRAUMATIZED PATIENTS IN GROUPS

The expectations of a group's members are analogous to an implicit, unwritten "job description" of the specific tasks to be performed by them, to meet the group's needs. Each member experiences pressure or "suction" (Redl, 1963) to respond to those expectations by assuming some of the group's functions. Some become "leaders" while others fit in as "followers"; some act as "gatekeepers" and others as "historians"; and so on.

Each individual member receives various nonverbal messages via projective identification, which then "invade" the person, putting internal pressure on him or her to act with a set of behaviors that will in effect constitute the responses to the initial message, originated by the psychopathology of the sender. Thus traumatized patients cast themselves primarily in the role of "victims" of bodily/emotional wounds inflicted upon them. They elicit in their interlocutors feelings of compassion and wishes to "rescue" or to "compensate" them. Group members and therapists alike may be carried away by their "role responsiveness" (Sandler, 1976). These patients defend themselves unconsciously against their possible guilt or responsibility for suffering their trauma, and they expect to be relieved of any guilt; indeed, they often try to blame someone else to protect themselves from their own potentially harsh self-criticisms. Such a plea is often at the core of the victims' initial expectations from the mental health professionals available to help them. Although this is obvious with rape or incest victims, in possible guilt about getting wounded may also be relevant for victims of nonsexual trauma, insofar as they often fantasize that their trauma was some kind of punishment for some previous wrongdoings. Hence in group therapy with traumatized patients, other group members and thera-

pists are often (1) cast in the roles of "witnesses" of these patients' innocence or their "not guilty" pleas; (2) expected to become their supportive
"advocates" in pursuing the indictment of other people (the "real cul-
prits"); or (3) expected to become the patients' "rescuers," magically undo-
ing the painful consequences of the trauma. The patients' defensive attempts lead them to manage their own confusion and guilt by projecting
the blame they inflict upon themselves and then trying to undo it—another
example of projective identification.

As times goes by, victims try unconsciously to induce in those around
them the same feelings of enraged, impotent helplessness that they suffered
during their traumatization. Making others experience the unbearable feelings of pain/anger that the victims could not tolerate is the goal of such a
projective identification. When it is achieved, the senders have succeeded in
getting rid of such painful affects, "dumping" them in the receivers, who
have to face them from then on. The result is a role reversal whereby those
in the therapy group are forced to experience the enraged impotent helplessness the senders felt when traumatized. The therapists may then feel de-
feated, impotent, without effective resources, worn down, and guilty. Other
group members may feel likewise, but they also represent an important res-
ervoir of patience and endurance that may help the group to "contain" and
to elaborate the devaluation of the therapists' and the group's help, which
resulted from the senders' projecting into them the humiliating helplessness
they suffered when they were traumatized. This protracted, unconscious,
nonverbal dialogue is a possible variation of sadomasochism, where the
complementary roles of "winner" versus "loser" and of "dominant" versus
"submissive" are swapped, shifting back and forth during the working
through of the schizo–paranoid anxieties.

Group psychotherapy has the advantage over individual treatment of
being able to utilize the resourceful presence of group members to help the
therapists carry the burden of painful countertransference feelings of humiliated defeat, which are very difficult to contain by the therapist alone.
"Dumping" their unbearable feelings after trauma is the most powerful
weapon in the hands of victims, and one that they all too often use re-
vengefully against the world that hurt them. Thus the gradual sorting out
of these projective identifications can be a very productive aspect of group
therapy (Ashbach & Schermer, 1987).

COUNTERTRANSFERENCE TO THE
GROUP AS A WHOLE

I am using the term "countertransference" in the global sense to describe
all the feelings elicited in a therapist by the patients he or she treats. There

are various countertransference responses to the different transferences in the group. I address here only the countertransference response to the group as a whole.

Two basic roles that groups assign to therapists are those of "treaters" and "members." It is not always easy to discriminate between the feelings generated by being a (special, and hence not so obvious) member of a particular group. Each group has some peculiarities of its own, a special prevailing atmosphere, and a given set of norms. For instance, groups of female incest victims often start promoting an atmosphere of hatred against their male perpetrators; they may develop a norm of ritually dedicating time in every session to ventilating their revengeful rage. One patient often ended such a ritual by swearing "to fix that steer." In an emotional atmosphere like that one, it became impossible for another female member, who was still delusionally in love with her abusive brother, to join the group's curses against their offenders, to the point that she could not continue in this psychotherapy group. (See the case of Vivian, above; see also Ganzarain & Buchele, 1988.)

The following is an example of countertransference in response to such a group formation:

A male cotherapist of a group of female incest victims asked me to supervise him after he found himself several times making the same mistake about announcing his planned absence from a group session. He wished to tell the group about his absence with 2 months' notice, but for week after week he kept forgetting to tell them, until the last minutes of the meeting before his absence. He then remembered to mention his absence only after having closed the session; hence his words were not well heard, since the patients had started to leave the room. Upon his returning to meet these patients after his absence from the group, they gave him a hard time. All the women, he said, including his cotherapist, were furious at him because "he did not care for them." He realized only then that these patients' transferences to him had been highly ambivalent, so that even when they behaved as if they wanted to get rid of him, they were simultaneously fighting against being sexually interested in him. Regarding his countertransference to that ambivalence, he concluded that as a group member he felt he did not belong in such a "for women only" atmosphere, and therefore that he had unconsciously wished to leave the group. In addition, he had split off and overlooked any loving, sexualized feelings between him and these patients, ignoring previous clearly sexualized behaviors of the female group members. His countertransference reactions as a group member had overshadowed his appropriate therapist's responses and obliterated his "knowing better"—his therapeutic ability to raise his head above the turbulent emotional waters, so as to see the whole picture of the ever-present human ambivalence manifested in the group. Perhaps he shared his patients' anxious insecurity about being fully accepted and desired; if that were the case, it would be yet another expression of his identifying with the members.

Notice how therapists' responses in the role of "other group members" replicate what their patients feel, thus becoming an important source of information when therapists examine within themselves their emotional participation in the group (Ganzarain, 1999).

The countertransference reactions to the group in the specifically therapeutic role vary according to the emotional atmosphere prevailing in the group. For example, therapists' internal responses may be different when facing patients furious at them as their "enemies" (the fight–flight BA) than when witnessing patients' struggle with their guilt because they feel they have "destroyed the group" (or are about to do it). They experience then their responsibility for the loss of a good object, which they idealize and pine for (the dependency BA). The paranoid mentality in the first situation casts patients and therapists in antagonistic roles, in an extreme split between good and bad; this was the case when our group of incest victims decided to "fire" my cotherapist and me (see the example involving Betty, taken from Ganzarain & Buchele, 1988). Their sadistic attacks made us feel as if we had lost our capacity to operate as efficient psychotherapists. However, when that same group chose another way to express their anger at males (by attending, as a group, a male strip-tease show), I was able to empathize with their feelings and put them to therapeutic use.

The second situation—that of patients' struggling with their guilt over their "destructiveness"—is well illustrated by this example:

When an outpatient long-term therapy group succeeded in ousting a member after the first eight meetings, they responded with guilt in their ninth session (see Ganzarain, 1992a, for more details). They tried to repair their group functioning, attempting to produce a "very good" session by reporting in detail their sexual problems in order to create an atmosphere of close intimacy, but then they could not go beyond keeping the emotional atmosphere at a level of pseudointimacy through talking about sex while nonverbally giving discreet hints of possible pairings between them. After this ploy failed, two members reported the trauma of their fathers' suicide and their feeling of responsibility for those deaths, which followed their fathers' progressive craziness. The intense activities displayed by this group in that crucial meeting led to their ignoring me and even cutting me off when I twice attempted to say something. After having eliminated a member (whose absence was now being ignored), they were *de facto* eliminating me. (Two sessions before this one, a patient whose father had killed himself had commented that the profession with the highest rate of suicide is psychiatry.)

After being cut off, I felt ignored, almost ousted, like the patient whose dropping out was becoming obvious. I did not have a chance to say anything in the middle of their very rapid exchanges, with each member rushing to speak. Most patients were elated with the "good" session, in which they thought they were creating a "very intimate" atmosphere by talking about sex and death—as if simply by addressing such forbidden topics they had become very close, with love prevailing over hate, and as if they had succeeded in triumphing over their destructive hostility, resorting to the magic of love (the pairing BA). Such a hypomanic atmosphere was being defensively used to avoid dealing with their having violently rejected a patient who was probably dropping out, as well as with eliminating me.

They also substituted for me a patient who acted as if he were a "doctor's assistant"; he depicted himself as a "sex expert," available to help the two younger women of the group with their sexual difficulties. One had described how painful intercourse was for her, because of the intense contraction of the annular muscles at her vagina's entrance, making penetration impossible. Guilt, hostility, and pain were being hypomanically denied, and a pseudoreparatory attempt was promoted to make them feel as if they might magically solve their distressing problems by becoming intimates with each other.

A few minutes before the ending of this meeting, the patients were exploring their vulnerability, and one asked me "formally" a general question: "What makes us so vulnerable?" I interpreted their denial of their guilt for a member's dropping out; their fears that getting emotionally involved with the group would hurt them; and their concerns that I might also commit suicide, which projected into me their depression and their fears of losing their minds. They were denying their anxieties about losing the group and/or me. Such fears/needs of others were making them vulnerable. A patient said, "The group will no longer be available." The woman with vaginismus then began crying out her fear of losing her frustrated husband. At the same time, the children of suicidal fathers were paradoxically happy, stating with laughter their wish to hug everyone (thus repeating their promiscuity).

In order to deal with my countertransference to this group, I had to overcome my guilt and my fear of losing them, as a result of my having undermined their defenses against guilt for destroying the group by eliminating my patients one by one (as in the movie *The 10 Little Indians*), and then doing me in through driving me crazy. I overcame my guilt in calling the bluff of their hypomanic defenses, somehow personified in the two promiscuous patients whose fathers had killed themselves after the failure of "quasi-psychotherapeutic" self-help techniques they had tried (meditation and Alcoholics Anonymous). I had also to accept and to deal with their underlying paranoid fears that the help I was offering them could turn out to be as counterproductive as Alcoholics Anonymous and meditation may have seemed to their fathers. Blaming others is another well-known defense—a paranoid one to externalize or project an individual's unbearable alleged feelings of guilt. They could thus fear what a crazy psychiatrist struggling with his own suicidal tendencies might have to offer them.

Upon the termination of different groups, especially long-term, closed, psychoanalytically focused ones such as the one I have just described, my countertransference to the group as a whole has been significant. Videotaping all their twice-a-week sessions for 42 months and editing them for teaching and writing purposes had made this group an important part of my professional life. I have used those edited videotapes extensively, and now they occupy almost as prominent a place on my bookshelves as the videos of my own children growing up. I feel a similar pride, almost as if these patients had become my own family members.

When ending an open-ended group of female incest victims, I responded to both intense, opposite poles of ambivalence: I felt relief, but I also entertained plans to publish what I had learned during their psychotherapy—as a way of working through my reparatory needs for my frequent irritation with them, and also as an expression of my gratitude for what they had allowed me to learn about them.

THE COURSE OF GROUP PSYCHOTHERAPY WITH TRAUMATIZED PATIENTS

Treatment of an acute trauma may include emergency medical care in addition to brief supportive psychotherapy, which may attempt to produce either "catharsis" or gradual discharge of the pent-up emotions caused by the trauma. Group therapy of long-past trauma utilizes instead a mixture of supportive and exploratory techniques. Exploratory approaches are better tolerated after a substantial time has elapsed following the event. In such cases, the group therapists help patients become aware of how their basic mistrust leads them to avoid dealing with others. Reinforcing transiently the defensive uses of splitting in the initial group meetings helps to locate their persecutors as bad objects outside the group, so that threats of retraumatization are averted. Various transferences may be experienced, focused, and discussed.

As the therapists focus their interventions on the ambivalent group-centered transference, whatever feelings may be exposed become more acceptable, partly because they are addressed to an impersonal, semiabstract entity ("the group") and not to any one member in particular. This quality makes it somewhat less embarrassing to address and to explore "childish" emotions, such as deep mistrust or unlimited neediness. Just as the initial idealization of the psychotherapy group may act as a stabilizing emotional factor, so does the relative "anonymity" of the specific recipient of intense feelings. The initial avoidant, unstable cohesiveness against common enemies may be gradually replaced by the experience of receiving meaningful, nurturant support from the good "mother group." An integrated, ambivalent, positive and negative transference to the group as a whole develops; this facilitates the emergence of a "space of illusion" (Winnicott, 1951/ 1974) where each member can playfully look for a new, real self-identity, beyond being only a resilient survivor of victimization. In the treatment of chronic cases of trauma, it is helpful to reach this stage in long-term therapy. For instance, Betty could thus wish to become a mental health professional, identifying herself with a female group psychotherapist; and Wilma gave herself permission to love a much younger man, working through her hateful yet loving identification with her father, who was her incest offender (Ganzarain & Buchele, 1988).

To provide a further example of the process of working through the ambivalent transference to the mother group, Laura was a victim of parental abandonment: Her father had disappeared when she was 4, and her mother during her adolescence. She was an outpatient whose diagnosis was chronic hypochondriasis and depression. "Working through her help-rejecting complaining attitude allowed her to (gradually) develop a new self-image. From feeling worthless and being content with a menial, back-up part-time job when and if called to replace a missing worker for a few hours, she moved into learning skills in a field of medical technology. She became an E.E.G. technician, thus 're-versing roles' regarding her hypochondriacal anxieties by having her clients anxiously worried about their brain functions, a training tailor-made for her dealing with her own fears of losing her mind by projecting them onto her clients" (Ganzarain, 1989, pp. 163–164). She was angrily resentful and chronically envious of "doctors' power," as she was of her parents' central influence on her life. She acted out her envious attacks on me in different ways.

Upon the cancellation of a session when she had been in the group for 2 years, Laura regressed first to a state of confusion and later to a schizoid withdrawal and "turning away." She did not bother then to explore reality (i.e., she did not ask the receptionist about her group appointment). She reacted instead to the absence of her group as if she were again facing an "empty house" (the traumatic loss of her mother)—in a repetition, within a full transference neurosis, of her previous experience of being deserted. Laura was then flooded with anxiety, which prevented her transiently from using her memory to recall that my secretary had called her to cancel the session. She ventilated her anger and envy of doctors in our next group meeting. She started mastering the experience of abandonment by turning the tables: She imagined reversing the situation by threatening me with losing the group, because of being fired by my angry patients.

Laura used role reversal in another way by taking care of her mother, who was now in a nursing home. The principle of role reversal also influenced her choice of a new, specialized line of work. She learned new behaviors to deal with other persons and with her own anxieties. She replaced the repetition of failure with the repetition of mastery. Her repeated transference distortions, commented upon by several group members, added emotional impact to her insights. Her affects made her insights more believable. Finally, she began making up for all her anger against her father by searching for him, which indicated her (newly acquired) willingness to establish good relations—a favorable predisposition that again reflected her significant internal changes.

I now quote from more extensively from the publication in which I first described Laura (Ganzarain, 1989, pp. 166–168):

The narcissistic envy caused by the effective interventions formulated by the therapist is lessened in group psychotherapy by the effective interpretations by peers or fellow members. The group also offers opportunities for role reversals, such as when a patient can discover and point out in a group peer the same conflicts that have been previously interpreted to him. It allows each group patient to feel helpful and needed by the fellow members. Every one may benefit too, from the transient "co-therapist-like" newly acquired capacity to love, help and to do reparation. . . .

Working through is the essential characteristic of psychoanalytic group therapy that separates and distinguishes it from other group psychotherapy modalities. The other types promote abreactions of briefer duration than working and learning, the two main elements of working through. Separation anxiety is an important aspect of working through. It stimulates a progression to resolve the depressive position or a regression to schizo–paranoid and manic defenses. If the depressive position is successfully solved, the capacity for reparation allows the patient's loving concern to prevail over hate for [his or her] objects.

Laura's case illustrates how she developed her capacity for reparation by taking care of her aging mother. For many years previously, she had hypochondriacally raged against her doctors' carelessness as a displacement of her painful fury against both parents, who one after the other had abandoned her. She also made doctors feel, by projective identification, her own impotent helplessness to change her condition.

DISCUSSION

It is important, by way of integration, to examine the differences among the psychoanalytic theories underlying Hopper's, Lonergan's, and my own views about group dynamics in working with traumatized patients.

British analysts from what is called the "independent tradition" (i.e., analysts who disagree with Melanie Klein) think that their techniques can avoid dealing with envy and annihilation fears, and that such phenomena are intensified as artifacts of Klein's technical approach. When Hopper quotes Turquet on large groups, he ignores the latter's statements that participation in a large group is like a "transient experience of depersonalization" (Turquet, 1975/1994, p. 80), and that the absence of feedback there creates feelings of loss of maternal protection. Thus, in my view, Turquet's observations are misrepresented by Hopper's selectively quoting Turquet to the effect that regression in large groups results from bombardment of stimuli, while omitting that Turquet also wrote about the large-group participants' experience of loss and abandonment. And we know that traumatized patients experience their acute emotional wounds as a loss of maternal protection, or as being abandoned to their own impotent helplessness.

Lonergan's "pre-group dynamics" accurately describe the initial phase of any group, while members test the waters to verify whether their paranoid fears should be taken seriously. Lonergan utilizes the notion of defensive splitting of the objects to differentiate between the "supportive/good" pre-group and subsequent group phases, as well as between the "good" therapist (seeming to encourage patients to gratify their narcissistic needs) and the potentially threatening group members. The therapist, in Lonergan's formulation, thus protects the group from retraumatization and offers them an emotional shelter. By contrast, directly bringing up the patients' paranoid fears runs the risk of provoking them to reexperience their trauma too soon, triggering a "self-fulfilling prophecy" that ends up bringing about such a feared repetition. Retraumatization, however, is much more than simply a consequence of the approach used. Lonergan's is an example of the psychoanalytic principle of dealing first with the surface of defense mechanisms, before focusing on their depths—on their source, on what makes them indispensable. The questions of timing or sequence (e.g., when to shift from one focus to the following one) are not easily resolved. Because the experience of transference is dictated at an unconscious level by the repetition compulsion, there is unavoidable pressure in traumatized patients' minds to relive their wounding experiences. Furthermore, it appears that such patients may develop a neurophysiological addiction to trauma (van der Kolk, 1989), which makes them look for such repetition in order to get a "hit" of a new release of endorphins (the morphine-like neurotransmitters) and a subsequent "high." Hence the likelihood of retraumatization will always, and perhaps inevitably, hamper work with trauma patients, above and beyond our preferred techniques. Thus, in my opinion, neither Lonergan's approach (supportive and self-psychological) nor mine (interpreting the defenses) will always work. These patients' transference will always be an enactment of their trauma. In cases of incest trauma, casting the offenders as the split "bad guys" is not always easy for their victims, since their abusers were also often loved as their caregivers; hence they will confuse and transfer both roles to their therapists, and the distance/difference between the two halves of the split will always be narrow!

Lonergan's technique, like Kohut's, uses a supportive, "run-around" approach to postpone working with aggression. By contrast, my more confrontative technique interprets the negative transference early on as the main strategy to relieve the initial persecutory anxieties, casting the therapist and other group members sooner than Lonergan's technique does in the role of potential persecutors. Kohutian and Kleinian techniques differ essentially on when and whether to deal with aggression and the negative transference. Lonergan's advice may be appropriate with trauma patients early in treatment, when it is necessary to postpone dealing with their intense fears. However, dealing with the psychotic anxieties through interpretation focuses on the total picture of psychic reality, on primitive defenses against such fears of annihilation, instead of minimizing and denying the power of such anxieties. Lonergan's approach introduces instead a temporary split between the "good" therapist and the potentially "bad" group, whose "badness" may be put to test without great risks, given the reliable protection provided by the "good" treater.

In a certain respect, Klein's and Kohut's theories are both object-relations-oriented (Ashbach & Schermer, 1987; Bacal & Newman, 1990). Kohut "developed the view of the *tragic* man, while Klein elaborated on S. Freud's *guilty* image of man" (Ganzarain, 1989, p. 16). Kohut (1977, p. 132) stated: "I identify these by speaking of Guilty Man if the aims are directed toward the activity of his drives and of Tragic Man if the aims are toward the fulfillment of the self." Klein's concern for the object emphasized the maturational ideal of outgrowing the boundary confusion between self and objects, so that each one is distinguished and the differences between them are acknowledged. Self psychology states instead that throughout life we need to sustain the merger of self and object, and to avoid full awareness of their differences, because realizing the existence of these differences becomes a narcissistic injury that provokes tension and envy.

The reasons for the popularity of self psychology among mental health professionals deserve to be explored, since there are now significant indications that many psychotherapists are themselves victims of trauma and significant narcissistic injury. It is important to know that during childhood many psychotherapists were often forced by their overdemanding mothers to become their "parentified" confidants, reversing the generational roles (Miller, 1981); thus they were victimized, trapped by their mothers' self-centeredness (cf. Kohut's [1979] case of "Mr. Z"). They suffered an emotionally incestuous exploitation by their mothers, who triggered serious narcissistic disturbances in their offspring. The self-psychological view of "tragic man" appeals to those who were victimized. Kohut (1968, p. 103) introduced his notion of narcissistic transferences in writing about an analytic candidate "humiliated" by his training analyst, who offered him a crown "as a confrontation, sarcastically mocking his need to be seen as a king." Analytic candidates, who often feel "emotionally battered," welcome Kohut's empathy for humanity's tragic condition, possibly including their own during analytic training (Ganzarain, 1989). Therapists with a history of emotional battering may become good therapists only after integrating their images of "good" and "bad" primary objects, and after learning to accept that they can hate a love object without losing it.

By way perhaps of reconciling Kleinian and Kohutian perspectives in the group setting, Battegay (1983) prefers analytic self-experience groups to treat narcissistic problems, because "it is more possible in a group to recognize narcissistic disturbances than in individual analysis" (p. 209). Groups may alternatively serve as confronting mirrors or as soothing selfobjects for narcissistic personalities. But groups will not let members avoid facing their psychotic anxieties or their alternating feelings of grandiosity and self-depreciation, always doubting their own selves while hiding these doubts.

My own view is that Lonergan's approach is to be recommended when therapists are initiating group treatment of acute cases of trauma, whereas my "Kleinian–Bionian" technique or Battegay's approach may be indicated for the group treatment of nonacute, previously traumatized patients whose "emotional scars" are chronic personality disorders, often of a narcissistic nature. However, I always try to see whether any of the particular trauma patients I am working with can open up to exploring their deepest fears at an early stage, since some seem to do so more readily than others.

SUMMARY

This chapter has described several typical dynamics and roles that unfold during the treatment of traumatized patients in psychotherapy groups, including transference–countertransference reactions. Trauma has been defined in a general way, followed by clinical illustrations from groups with several types of trauma: incest, parental abandonment, abuse in psychiatric hospitals, and police brutality. Every traumatic experience actualizes the basic human fears concerning the annihilation of the self and the loss of maternal protection. Such schizo–paranoid and depressive anxieties trigger primitive defense mechanisms. Clusters of these defenses and fears are the foundations of the three group BAs described by Bion (1961), as well as of the characteristic transference paradigms in the psychotherapy of traumatized patients: fear of repeating the trauma and of the ensuing depressive, lonely hopelessness. Turquet (1974) seems to have defined well a fourth BA of "oneness" as typical of large groups, whereas Hopper (1997) describes one of "incohesion" in small groups, which may be easily confused with the unintegrated or split small group of the fight–flight BA.

Typical roles observable during group psychotherapy of trauma are illustrated, such as "victims," "persecutors," "identical twins," "doctor's assistants," "omnipotent rescuers," "witnesses," and "advocates." The projection by patients of their angry and impotent yet guilt-ridden helplessness into other group members and therapists is described as an important countertransference issue; I emphasize that the presence of enduring group members helps the therapists to carry the burden of "containing" these difficult-to-tolerate emotions. Other expressions of countertransference are also examined, particularly those in response to the deep mistrust within the fight–flight BA and to the unbearable guilt for wishes to destroy the group, the therapists, or both. Techniques that attempt to avoid or soothe the pain and anger of trauma are summarized, such as the one proposed by Lonergan; these are compared with those that aim at bringing such feelings to the foreground in order to work them through. The proneness to and dangers of retraumatization are acknowledged as always present, requiring constant reevaluation of psychotherapy strategies so that therapists can help these patients more effectively. Incest victims, who are sometimes abused by their psychotherapists, are dramatic and tragic illustrations of the tendency to repeat the trauma.

REFERENCES

Ashbach, C., & Schermer, V. L. (1987). *Object relations, the self, and the group.* London: Routledge.

Anzieu, D. (1975). *The group and the unconscious.* London: Routledge.

Bacal, H. A., & Newman, K. (1990). *Theories of object relations: Bridges to self psychology.* New York: Columbia University Press.

Battegay, R. (1983). The value of analytic self-experience groups in the training of psychotherapists. *International Journal of Group Psychotherapy, 33*(2), 199–213.

Bion, W. R. (1961). *Experiences in groups.* London: Tavistock.

Bion, W. R. (1962). *Learning from experience.* London: Heinemann.

Freud, S. (1955). Group psychology and the analysis of the ego. In J. Strachey (Ed. and Trans.), *The standard edition of the complete psychological works of Sigmund Freud* (Vol. 18, pp. 65–144). London: Hogarth. (Original work published 1921)

Ganzarain, R. (1989). *Object relations group psychotherapy.* Madison, CT: International Universities Press.

Ganzarain, R. (1991). The "bad" mother-group. In S. Tuttman (Ed.), *Psychoanalytic group theory and practice* (American Group Psychotherapy Association Monograph No. 7, pp. 157–173). Madison, CT: International Universities Press.

Ganzarain, R. (1992a). Introduction to object relations group psychotherapy. *International Journal of Group Psychotherapy, 42*(2), 205–223.

Ganzarain, R. (1992b). Narcissistic/borderline personality disorders in cases of incest. *Group Analysis, 25,* 491–494.

Ganzarain, R. (1992c). Effects of projective identification on therapists and groupmates. *Group Analysis, 25,* 15–18.

Ganzarain, R. (1999). *Counter-projective identification (C-P. I.) and bi-logic.* Paper presented at the panel in honor of Matte-Blanco at the 41st International Psychoanalysis Association Congress, Santiago, Chile.

Ganzarain, R., & Buchele, B. (1988). *Fugitives of incest.* Madison, CT: International Universities Press.

Ganzarain, R., & Buchele, B. (1993). Group psychotherapy of patients with a history of incest. In H. Kaplan & B. Sadock (Eds.), *Comprehensive group psychotherapy* (3rd ed., pp. 551–525). Baltimore: Williams & Wilkins.

Gelinas, D. J. (1983). The persisting negative effects of incest. *Psychiatry, 46,* 312–332.

Hearst, L. (1981). The emergence of the mother group. *Group Analysis, 14,* 25–33.

Hopper, E. (1997). Traumatic experience in the unconscious life of groups: A fourth basic assumption. *Group Analysis, 30,* 439–470.

Klein, M. (1952). Notes on some schizoid mechanisms. In M. Klein, P. Heimann, S. Isaacs, &. J. Riviere (Eds.), *Developments in psychoanalysis* (pp. 292–320). London: Hogarth Press. (Original work published 1946)

Kohut, H. (1968). The psychoanalytic treatment of narcissistic personality disorders. *Psychoanalytic Study of the Child, 23,* 86–113.

Kohut, H. (1977). *The restoration of the self.* New York: International Universities Press.

Kohut, H. (1979). The two analyses of Mr. Z. *International Journal of Psycho-Analysis, 60,* 3–27.

Laplanche, J., & Pontalis, J. B. (1973). *The language of psychoanalysis.* New York: Norton.

Lonergan, E. C. (1989). Treating wounded self-esteem. In *Group intervention: How to begin and maintain groups in medical and psychiatric settings* (pp. 147–169). Northvale, NJ: Aronson.

Miller, A. (1981). *Prisoners of childhood.* New York: Basic Books.

Redl, F. (1963). Psychoanalysis and group psychotherapy: A developmental point of view. *American Journal of Orthopsychiatry, 33,* 135–147.

Sandler, J. (1976). Countertransference and role responsiveness. *International Review of Psychoanalysis, 3,* 43–47.

Schafer, R. (1997). Vicissitudes of remembering in the countertransference. *International Journal of Psycho-Analysis, 78,* 1151–1163.

Turquet, P. (1974). Leadership: The individual and the group. In G. S. Gibbard & R. D. Mann (Eds.), *Analysis of groups* (pp. 349–371). San Francisco: Jossey-Bass.

Turquet, P. (1994). Threats to the identity in the large groups. In L. Kreeger (Ed.), *The large group: Dynamics and therapy* (pp. 87–144). London: Karnac Books. (Original work published 1975)

van der Kolk, B. A. (1989). The compulsion to repeat the trauma: Reenactment, revictimization and masochism. *Psychiatric Clinics of North America, 12,* 389–430.

Winnicott, D. W. (1974). Transitional objects and transitional Phenomena. In D. Winnicott, *Playing and reality* (pp. 1–50). Harmondsworth, England: Penguin Books. (Original work published 1951)

5

—◄o►—

Hazardous Terrain:
Countertransference Reactions
in Trauma Groups

MAGGIE ZIEGLER
MAUREEN MCEVOY

From Maggie's field journal: It's the first night of group. Eight terrified women sit rigidly on the edges of their chairs staring at the car-
pet, wondering how they will find the strength to talk about what they
have been through, desperate for connection yet certain that they will
be abandoned and betrayed again. I don't like these beginnings. I'm
tense, already creating a wall to protect myself from stories of the terrible things people do to each other, from allowing in the depth of the
woundedness, from having to look in the face (again) the world I live
in and to struggle to make meaning (again) of what I see. I'm protecting myself from a grief so deep I wonder if it can be tolerated. Did this
tightness show tonight, or did I look as relaxed and confident as
Maureen?

From Maureen's field journal: The first hours of group, when I'm
seen as dangerous, are hard for me. Particularly those moments when
I'm handed the perpetrator role. It's like a cup of cold water. It happened tonight, when I was describing how we'll be using containment
skills throughout the group, and Judy made a face of disgust. At that
moment I was the offender in her eyes, trying to conceal and deny the
awful pain. I flushed and wanted to argue with her, to tell her I was a
safe, competent therapist. I wanted to shuck off the slime I felt I'd just
been covered in.

As these descriptions of the opening moments of a trauma group for adult survivors of childhood abuse illustrate, the dance between vicarious traumatization and countertransference begins immediately, as does the dance between the cotherapists. In the first entry—an example of the impact of trauma work on a therapist—Maggie feared she would be overwhelmed by the impending confrontation with violence and pain. In the second entry—an example of countertransference—Maureen found herself vulnerable to transferences that cast her in the perpetrator role. Both of us were in danger of losing the compassionate objectivity essential to trauma work. In the first example, Maggie might have found herself subtly encouraging silence to protect her fragility, and in the second example, Maureen was at risk of overfunctioning to prove her "goodness."

Trauma survivor groups are full of such pitfalls. This complex terrain requires a therapist to identify, understand, and manage complex relational dynamics. She must monitor her responses to the traumatic stories and presentations of the group members, as well as her responses to the group as a whole, group dynamics, and her cotherapist.[1] Although theoretical and clinical grounding in trauma psychology, and strong group facilitation skills, are critical to successful group outcomes, it is essential for each therapist to have a map that supports her in the intricate work of making visible her inner and often conflicted responses to this work. A map (theory) normalizes and contains the difficult task of challenging defense structures and professional egos. Route-finding skills (method) enable her to explore her reactivity and then to respond appropriately.

The map is provided by the concepts of countertransference and vicarious trauma. This chapter adopts a totalistic definition of "countertransference" (Kernberg, 1965; Racker, 1957) that includes all of the trauma therapist's responses to the client, the client's story, and the client's behavior, as well as the conscious and unconscious defenses mobilized by the therapist to protect her from these reactions (Pearlman & Saakvitne, 1995; Wilson & Lindy, 1994).

In the totalistic tradition, countertransference is an important diagnostic tool (Kernberg, 1965). This perspective suggests that a therapist's internal responses are not inherently negative or positive, nor do they constitute a statement about her competency. They are a source of essential knowledge for the therapist about herself, the group, and its members. Rather than being a burden, countertransference can be appreciated as a primary source of insight and compassion into the victim's past experience and present reality. Thus countertransference responses are route-finding markers that can be used to guide therapeutic interventions in a grounded and timely way.

McCann and Pearlman (1990) have noted that countertransference concepts do not encompass the specific impact of traumatic material on the therapist, and have developed the concept of "vicarious trauma" to address the inner alterations of meaning resulting from this exposure. Pearlman and Saakvitne (1995) describe vicarious traumatization as "the transformation of the inner experience of the therapist that comes about as a result of empathic engagement with the client's trauma material" (p. 31). Other authors have conceptualized the therapist's response to trauma as "contact victimization" (Courtois, 1988), "empathic strain" (Wilson & Lindy, 1994), "secondary posttraumatic stress disorder," and "compassion fatigue" (Figley, 1995).

Although therapists have been conducting groups for adult trauma survivors for many years, the literature exploring therapist responses to such groups is surprisingly sparse. The few publications with a primary focus on countertransference issues in trauma group work include descriptions of these issues with persons facing terminal illnesses (Bernstein & Klein, 1995; Gabriel, 1991; Benioff & Vinogradov, 1993), adult children of alcoholics (Vannicelli, 1991), Vietnam veterans (Frick & Bogart, 1982; Walker & Nash, 1981; Parson, 1984), adult children of Holocaust survivors (Fogelman & Savran, 1980), and survivors of childhood sexual abuse (Abney, Anderson-Yang, & Paulson, 1992; Courtois, 1988; Ganzarain & Buchele, 1986; Pearlman & Saakvitne, 1995).

Consequently, group therapists mainly travel this relatively unexplored terrain with maps pertaining to either individual trauma or general psychodynamic group therapy. Neither map exactly fits. It is critical to understand how trauma histories alter the usual group processes, in order to remain grounded in the inevitable flurry of transference, countertransference, and vicarious traumatization reactions. Although understanding the countertransferential traps does not keep them from occurring (Chu, 1988), identifying sources of therapist reactivity is an important first step. Before the therapist can utilize her countertransference responses in trauma group therapy, she must be able to tolerate, manage, and resolve her own cognitions and affects. This processing connects what is happening in her own heart and mind, and enables her to facilitate connection effectively in the group. She is more likely to intervene in ways that promote immediacy (Ormont, 1993) and to demonstrate "willingness and capability to accompany the patient into his past without losing sight of the present" (Kernberg, 1965, p. 53). She is also able to identify unacknowledged individual and group themes and to address them safely. She is able to contain and hold the trauma survivor's disowned parts of self and to make timely interventions that assist the survivor in reclaiming these parts. These examples of countertransference-based interventions enhance the connections of the group members to themselves, each other, and the cotherapists. The hard work that therapists and group members engage in to face themselves, albeit in different ways, leads to a shared joy in the deep connections that occur in successful trauma group work—the connections that are at the heart of trauma recovery.

This chapter examines the link between countertransference and group processes. It focuses on the necessity for therapists to strengthen their capacities for awareness, containment, integration, and presence; these tasks, of course, are also central for trauma survivors. In addition, the cotherapy relationship is viewed as playing a significant role in addressing and resolving therapist reactivity.

Central to our own route-finding efforts are our "field journals." A field journal, as described by Agger and Jensen (1994), is a journal that is used to monitor and process reactions during psychotherapeutic work in the field. Agger and Jensen used such journals while working under conditions of state terrorism in Chile, and Ziegler (1996) kept one while working near a war zone in Croatia. The field journal allows an exploration of both self and the encountered reality, honoring the front-line trenches therapists find themselves in. "In this way, we became our own informants" (Agger & Jensen, 1994, p. 267). Throughout this chapter we share entries from our own field journals (the majority of these entries are descriptions of a recent group); we hope that our self-disclosure encourages other therapists' inner exploration and, most importantly, gives permission to make mistakes. We have learned that our willingness to question our own fears and defenses, risk exposure, and gently confront each other enables us to maintain clarity with ourselves, each other, and the group.

> We realized we needed to continue our field journals through the writing of this chapter. Every time we became blocked, discouraged, or uncertain of where we were heading, we came back to the journal. We would sit together with papers all over the room and say, "Okay, just write for 10 minutes about how we are feeling right in this moment about the topic, about ourselves, about each other." Then we would read it aloud and without feedback to each other. After this, we would say, "Okay, 10 more minutes." We kept doing this until we understood that the blocks had to do with fear. We were afraid of the merging of voices that this chapter required. Our voices had to come closer than in the groups, where our voices dance back and forth, and we were anxious about the impact on our relationship. In the end, we created a balance, using the field journals to portray our individual voices and dialogue for the dance between us.

The group referred to in many of our journal entries and other descriptions was a time-limited 16-week group for severely traumatized women. The women in the group shared complex and chronic childhood trauma experiences, and many had been revictimized in adulthood. Group participants were aware of this project and gave signed consent for personal and group material to be disguised and adapted for this chapter.

THE UNIQUE TERRAIN OF TRAUMA GROUPS

Countertransference issues emerge in unique ways in trauma groups. In individual psychotherapy with trauma survivors, the privacy of the office creates a contained environment for rebuilding safety and trust. The therapist concentrates her energy on one person, tailoring interventions to fit the client's uniqueness, and taking the time required to work safely through the client's transference reactions. The trauma group therapist has to build safety and trust in an exposed environment in which she often has little information about each person's history, traumatic exposure, or response to trauma. She observes at first hand the difficulties in building connection, yet cannot respond to each individual. Often trapped in the past and terrified of the future, group members are frequently numb, dissociated, and absent, desperately avoiding contact with what they crave the most: connection to their own selves and to others. Alternatively, they are flooded with affect, hyperaroused, and hostile. They may use dissociation or self-injurious behaviors as a means of coping with restimulated memories. The therapist faces not only all the transference and countertransference issues of individual trauma therapy, but transferences specific to groups, such as family-of-origin simulations (Courtois, 1988) and victim, offender, and rescuer dynamics (van der Kolk, 1993). Managing all of these complex symptoms and dynamics can raise the therapist's anxiety and mobilize her defenses, compromising her usual thoughtful stance. In the following entry, Maureen described how we defended against our own helplessness with one group member by participating in the re-creation of a family-of-origin dynamic.

> *Maureen:* Carol came faithfully every session but barely participated. When I watched Maggie attempting to draw her out, I saw Carol cringe. I worried that Carol saw Maggie as a dangerous intruder, and I argued that we should allow her to maintain safety by not drawing attention to her. Maggie, feeling frustrated and helpless by her ineffective attempts to make contact, agreed. Then Carol showed me the rash she developed every week just before group, and I finally got it. Between the perpetrator role (Maggie) and the noninvolved bystander role (me), we had participated in the re-creation of a frightened and lonely childhood. She had to develop a rash to get our attention. Consequently, we accessed new patience and compassion to gently but persistently challenge her isolation.

Another unique aspect of trauma groups is their connection to support, self-help, and advocacy organizations. Vietnam veterans' rap groups and women's groups of the 1970s used groups as a means to make public, through shared disclosure, what had been private. This continuing emphasis on breaking trauma-induced isolation puts the therapist in a different position from her position in either individual trauma psychotherapy or a non-trauma-oriented group. Although this community building is often exhilarating and refreshing, it also brings challenges. Many sets of eyes watch to see whether the therapist is willing to stand with them against violence and injustice. Therapists must take a position of ethical non-neutrality (Benedek, 1984; Agger & Jensen, 1994). Yet acknowledging social injustice may bring feelings of powerlessness, despair, responsibility, and fear. Therapists may unconsciously deny social issues in order to protect their world view. Conversely, an overfocus on political discussions can result in intellectualizations and displacements that may serve to protect therapists, as Fischman and Ross (1990) have noted in their group work with torture survivors. As group members develop community and the therapists' role diminishes, therapists may find themselves feeling excluded, irrelevant, and unimportant.

The fragility of trauma survivors results in slower development of group relationships than in non-trauma-oriented groups. Parson (1984) suggests that combat veterans, weakened by symptoms of posttraumatic stress disorder, lack the ability to explore transference and projective identifications through direct confrontation. In incest survivor groups, support and dependency come first, and confrontation much later (Herman & Schatzow, 1984). Fogelman and Savran (1980) have described a process of experimenting with the amount of confrontation they can use in brief group therapy with adult children of Holocaust survivors. Therapists may chafe at the need to use an oblique and extremely gentle approach to transference issues. They may become vulnerable to accepting client transferences of despair and hopelessness and may begin to doubt that change is possible.

All trauma therapists engage to some extent with the complicated social systems in which survivors often become enmeshed. Sponsoring agencies or workplaces, individual therapists, criminal justice systems, and other professionals and institutions involved in the client's care may become sources of indirect (Racker, 1957) or systemic countertransferences. The following entry, in which Maggie wondered how a woman not yet ready for group work got admitted, illustrates these influences on the group therapist.

Maggie: It looks like countertransference responses are at play long before the group began. Were we unconsciously responding to the anxiety of the referring therapist, who appeared desperate to have Frances in the group? Did we feel obligated to the referring agency, who was also sponsoring the group? Did we accept her into the group because of our painful awareness of the lack of other supportive community resources? Were we taken in by Frances's own desperation to join, which led her to present herself as much more able to tolerate a group environment than she turned out to be? Were our hearts overruling our judgment because of the violent nature of the trauma and the bleakness of her current life? Why am I saying "we" when I did the screening interview? Somehow I want to share responsibility, but it was my judgment call.

THE CHALLENGE OF HOLDING

The central task of the trauma group therapist is creating a safe "holding environment" (Winnicott, 1966) in which group members can recover from traumatic injury and regain a connection to life. Group therapists must tolerate and contain negative projections (Hannah, 1984), painful affects, and disturbed schemata. They must hold the collective anxiety, and provide a stable environment in which group members can gently release their tortured pasts.

Trauma survivors and therapists alike must struggle to stay in the present, despite the tendencies of psychotherapy groups to live elsewhere. Ormont (1995) describes how groups prefer to focus on the past, the future, or life outside the group, and suggests that positive group outcomes are dependent on the successful climate of an in-the-moment immediacy. In trauma groups, restimulated memories intensify the need to live elsewhere.

To maintain immediacy or presence, a therapist needs a neutral observing ego that can simply witness without "judging, evaluating or acting" (Ormont, 1995, p. 490). Attention that is impartial, nonjudgmental, and curious opens the mind, "not by attempting to change anything but by observing the mind, emotions and body the way they are. With bare attention we move from automatic identification with our fear or frustration to a vantage point from which the fear or frustration is attended to with the same dispassionate interest as anything else" (Epstein, 1995, p. 111). When the therapist can embrace her countertransference reactions with a gentle, observing mind, she can separate the strands of her reactivity and increase her capacity for holding and presence.

Creating presence in short-term groups and in the early stages of long-term psychodynamic groups is done through gentle, repetitive requests that group members examine their experience in the present moment. It is a slow process, and therapists may easily feel impatient, angry, bored, helpless, and powerless in the face of group members' tentative movements and hasty retreats. When therapists refrain from resolving their feelings through fixing, overprotecting, fusion, avoidance, or denial, they allow survivors the gift of accepting themselves as they are in any given moment. Trauma survivors develop observing egos when therapists are able to hold this nonreactive, bare attention themselves. This is not easy when therapists are "bombarded with so many stories at once" (Fogelman & Savran, 1980, p. 102) and asked to witness the painful sequelae of trauma.

Maggie: Sometimes I'm afraid of the dark side, afraid that I'll collapse and be useless. I don't want to acknowledge the depth of my own despair. I keep to myself the times I can only see destruction and devastation, the times I prefer depression to the grief and despair underneath. Then life's joy is trapped below a plain of misery, and it's impossible to be a purveyor of hope to the despairing, impossible to bring meaning to the meaningless. There is nowhere to go but back to bare attention, to being with the darkness, just letting it be. When I do this, spaciousness grows around the dark. Then I can bear the pain and don't have to convince unhappy group members to be happy.

Maureen: After group I putter. It's the only night of the week that I'm likely to go to bed after my partner. Instead of sleeping, I roam around doing a little of this, a little of that. On smart nights I sit and draw or write in the field journal. When I don't, I sleep fitfully, my dreams attempting to consolidate the unbelievable and the unimaginable. So why do I resist splashing paint or words on paper when I know it will help? My resistance is just like our clients'—the fear of feeling my own pain.

In the following example, Maggie described how a fixation on a group member's story led her to an awareness of unresolved vicarious trauma. If she had not identified this state, she might have been at risk of becoming overly fascinated with the group member or distancing from her.

Maggie: I couldn't get Bernadette's story out of my head. A lifetime of battering: her father, her brothers, her uncle, her husband who kept her isolated on a remote island. This is a terrible story, but I heard a lot of terrible stories tonight and couldn't understand why I was stuck on this one. Only when I raised this with Maureen on the drive home did I realize that it brought back a flood of memories of my years working in a women's shelter—unprocessed memories, because I didn't know at that time what to do with the intensity of my reactions. And here they have emerged, raw and staring me in the face 20 years later.

Trauma therapists must stay present in the face of the massive losses of refugees, the death anxieties of AIDS patients, the wounded attachments of abused children, or the shattered beliefs of sexual assault survivors. Particularly difficult is managing the losses, spoken or not, that can multiply until the therapists' hearts and minds ache with the effort of holding and understanding. In an attempt to manage their own anxiety and unresolved losses, therapists may minimize the losses, limit identification and expression, and prematurely encourage action. When death and mortality are present, group therapists may feel helpless and act to protect themselves. Bernstein and Klein (1995) suggest that therapists may cope in group work with AIDS patients by resorting to omnipotence, engaging in untimely interventions, becoming depressed, or merging with group members. Therapists may also silence the topic of death, and the group members may adapt to contain the therapists' anxiety. Conversely, Gabriel (1991) describes how the chronic mourning that accompanies group work with AIDS patients can lead therapists to focus on death and dying rather than on living. In group work with refugees from Bosnia, Maggie struggled not only to contain the losses, but to understand her responsibility for what she heard.

> *Maggie:* The losses were so extreme: family members dead or disappeared, homes burnt, and communities broken. Loss of future, of personal dignity, of identity. Loss of meaning—an inability to comprehend what had happened, to understand how the neighbors, lifelong friends, could suddenly turn on them. My presence supported naming these losses, the telling of stories, and a tentative rebuilding of community, but this was not enough. It was excruciating to contain all the despair, anger, and sorrow I felt. At the last group, I asked them what they needed from me. Out of a long silence, Amira spoke: "Tell our stories." I promised that I would, and the public advocacy and education I became involved in provided meaning and community that balanced my grief.

The therapist must also hold what group members abdicate through dissociation. When group space is experienced as unsafe, participants can dissociate, either individually or collectively. Saakvitne (1995) describes how trauma survivors can dissociate from painful affect, memory, self, and each other, and suggests that this retreat can evoke feelings of loss, abandonment, insecurity, powerlessness, and incompetence in a therapist. The therapist may be at risk of violating boundaries in an attempt to seek connection, or of fleeing the present moment herself. The intensity of what has been left behind can be overwhelming. In the following example, Maureen described working with Canadian aboriginal people who had experienced several generations of forced removal from their culture and families at an early age into residential schools, which enforced a harsh assimilation into the dominant culture.

> *Maureen:* My worst fears are coming true as I sit in this aboriginal talking circle. I look around the room—the woman holding the talking stick is speaking in a flat monotone, brown eyes never rising from the floor as she lists one horrible experience of physical and sexual violence after another. I know that eye contact is not as important in this culture as it is in mine (European-based), yet I also know I'm seeing

dissociation among the dozen men and women in the circle. Energetically, it's as if the center of the circle is a dissociative vortex, sucking people's life energy and vitality. I'm the only one present in the room, and I can feel my anxiety rising. I feel crushed under the weight of their lost childhoods and shattered futures. I notice an urge to run into the nearby woods and automatically take a deep breath to calm myself. I startle the woman next to me, and I mime that she should breathe too. Gradually the breath moves around the circle.

When therapists experience intense reactions in trauma groups that pull them out of the present moment, they must investigate whether they are responding to traumatic content, personal unresolved issues, or individual or collective transference. In the following, a group member's complaint triggered Maureen's childhood fears.

Maureen: These moments when the energy of the group abruptly shifts always come as such a surprise. Tonight it happened near the end of group. I'm relatively at ease and engaged; then Elaine complains about our straying from tonight's agenda. It's like a plate crashing to the floor. Red alert time. Now, I'm blanking out, so all I know to do is to keep my pen moving and hope. . . . I'm realizing these moments are connected to my childhood experiences of tempers flaring and events suddenly spiraling out of control—when plates did crash to the floor. When I could feel safe one moment and then utterly at risk the next; and how, even now, my limbic system responds to any quick change with the same intensity.

After Maureen made this connection to her own childhood experience, she wondered whether Elaine carried a similar terror of unexpected change, and whether she was absorbing Elaine's fear. At the next session she invited Elaine to explore her distress at the group's shift in focus, and Elaine was able to share her anxiety. For the first time, Elaine felt that someone understood her fear. After this intervention, Elaine began to take more risks in the group.

OVERIDENTIFICATION AND AVOIDANCE

Wilson and Lindy (1994) suggest that most countertransference reactions in trauma therapists fall into the two broad categories of overidentification and avoidance. The overidentified therapist is at risk for empathic enmeshment, leading to loss of boundaries, overinvolvement, and reciprocal dependency (Wilson & Lindy, 1994). Saddock (1993) sees overidentification as the biggest danger in groups with rape survivors and battered women, and Frick and Bogart (1982) caution against overidentification with group themes in group work with Vietnam veterans. In groups, overidentification can result in inappropriate self-disclosure, inability to set clear directions, problems with time limits, and unnecessary availability between group sessions for individual group members (Abney et al., 1992; McEvoy, 1990; Vannicelli, 1991). Overidentification can lead to a reluctance to delve more deeply into a survivor's experience for fear of stimulating additional hurt (Courtois, 1988; Danieli, 1988). The urge to rescue and reparent (Ganzarain & Buchele, 1986; Courtois, 1988; Danieli, 1988) is illustrated in the following entry.

> *Maureen:* A big challenge for me is to manage my awareness of the group members as injured little girls. When they tell stories about the awful things they experienced, I don't hear them as adults, but as the little girls they once were. So tonight when Sally pulled out that skipping rope from her bag and described what her father did with it . . . I just can't stop seeing a little girl tied up and tortured. I'm at risk for treating her like a little girl, not a woman who has survived. She needs to be empowered, not infantilized.

Both individual and group therapists may defend themselves by conspiring with trauma clients to avoid discussing difficult subjects (Benedek, 1984; Courtois, 1988; Danieli, 1988; Fischman & Ross, 1990; Haley, 1974). Therapists may use denial, minimization, depression, dissociation, and distancing to maintain a silent collusion with group members, avoiding themes such as death, loss, anger, or responsibility. For example, Fogelman and Savran (1980) suggest that group leaders, shocked by stories of the Holocaust, may allow group members to change the topic. Therapists may resort to a rigid professional stance or use a theoretical approach not appropriate for trauma survivors, such as focusing on Oedipal conflicts with Holocaust survivors. Finally, therapists may strive for false harmony or stress that life victimizes everyone. In the following example, Maggie explored her desire to distance herself from a group member's neediness.

> *Maggie:* Gail irritates me, and immediately I feel guilty for saying that. I want to cover it up by naming her many strengths and gifts to the group. Gail talks too much, and when I intervene she retracts into an old hurt place like a turtle in a shell and keeps talking how she takes up too much space. Part of me agrees with the harshness of her self-judgment. A large part of me, at the moment, if I'm honest. Does my judgment show? Did I cause the retreat? The depth of her need to be seen and heard irritates me, because it stirs up my own unmet needs. I want her to just get a grip and toughen up as I've done. But I'm not as tough as I pretend, and my shell covers a depleted emptiness. When I acknowledge my unmet needs and the sense of invisibility that sometimes lodges deep inside me, I bring home the projection. When I stop running from myself, I stop running from Gail. I see Gail's desperate longing for connection.

Because Maggie was no longer motivated by avoidance, she was now free to consider potential interventions. She might directly approach Gail and the group members, or she might make a statement about her own immediate experience to encourage present reality. Or she might choose simply to hold Gail's longing until she felt Gail was ready to claim it for herself.

Therapists who are also survivors have particular struggles in the areas of overidentification and avoidance. Overidentification is a particular risk for most incest survivor therapists (Briere, 1992); Vietnam veteran therapists (Catherall & Lane, 1992); and therapists wounded by the same system of political repression that has traumatized their clients (Comas-Diaz & Padilla, 1990). Hartman and Jackson (1994), in a discussion of individual therapy with rape survivors, describe how a survivor therapist was both burdened and stimulated by the enmeshment with her client, and fantasized how they could write an article together. Survivor therapists may also have strong defenses that they employ in groups. For example, incest survivor therapists may have entrenched global defenses, such as dissociation, denial, projection, projective identification, and repression (Pearlman & Saakvitne, 1995). Cotherapy is strongly recommended for survivor therapists as a means of managing vulnerabilities (Catherall & Lane, 1992; Pearlman & Saakvitne, 1995; Vannicelli, 1991).

It is important to acknowledge that therapists who are also survivors bring many strengths to group work. They can offer victims a profound empathy and unflinching clarity. For example, Danieli's (1988) research into therapist reactions to Holocaust survivors revealed that nonsurvivor therapists were more likely to use muted language than survivor therapists who were more likely to use words like "murder."

MANAGING ANGER

Trauma groups inevitably stir up anger in both participants and therapists. Therapists who have difficulty tolerating either their own aggressive urges or anger in others may engage in stifling behaviors. They may join together with group members to keep aggression and rage safely focused on perpetrators—a common dynamic for women leading women's groups. When therapists are unable to cope with group members' projected anger, they may feel victimized (Abney et al., 1992) and may respond with a critical or condemning attitude, feeling hostile toward group members they experience as not appreciating their desire to help. Courtois (1997) suggests that outright displays of anger toward group members are unusual, but that therapists may engage in distancing behaviors such as not preparing for a group session, rushing in at the last minute, avoiding group members during breaks, neglecting follow-up phone calls, or being remote during sessions. Conversely, therapists outraged by accounts of violence may assume that their anger is shared by group members and may prematurely encourage its expression. If therapists are uncomfortable acknowledging their own capacities for violence, they may not be able to tolerate the "perpetrator cloak" that group members so often drape over their shoulders. Haley (1974) highlights the necessity for therapists to examine their own sadistic impulses, especially when working with survivors who are also perpetrators.

In the following example, Maggie attempted to manage her anger by triangulating in the group members' individual therapists. She was displacing her helpless rage at the perpetrators onto other caregivers; this dynamic is similar to how survivors displace rage into revenge fantasies against inept rescuers (Herman, 1992).

> *Maggie:* I'm angry at the women's individual therapists, full of judgments about their competence. Don't they understand the basics of traumatic containment, of symptom management? I realize I'd rather think about how other therapists have failed to "fix" their clients than bend my mind around acts of perpetration and neglect. I'd rather blame my colleagues than really see the source of the shame and pain I witnessed tonight. But in this scenario I allow the individual therapist to stand in for the perpetrator, the group member to be the helpless victim, and myself to alternate between the roles of helpless bystander and rescuer. I need to find a way to open my heart to what really happened to the women, letting go of finding a convenient scapegoat.

In the next example, Maureen facilitated a group for women who had been sexually exploited by mental health professionals, and struggled to maintain her observing ego and contain rage.

> *Maureen:* The women had been sharing drawings of their self-images, and I was completely unprepared for what I saw. Their pictures represented extremes of isolation, disconnection, and distorted perception. They were unable to talk about the drawings, but their eyes and bodies mutually beseeched me to understand. I remember the feeling of blood rising up to my skin, my heartbeat increasing and my hands clenching. I wanted to rant about the people who had done this to them. But I knew I would be the only beneficiary of such a display, as I was feeling the rage that they were not yet able to feel. I'd be allowed to be a good guy, allowed to keep a safe distance from the knowledge of what my colleagues had done. Instead, I had to find a way to hold my own rage, clearly speak to the inappropriateness of these "helpers," and yet leave them room to struggle with their self-blame and traumatic bonding. I had to learn to sit with their distrust of me.

Frick and Bogart's (1982) description of managing their anger in their group work with Vietnam veterans is useful: "Our interventions consisted of . . . admitting our anger when appropriate but containing, holding and hiding our more acute feelings of anger and checking our own impulses to withdraw from or abandon the group" (p. 439).

RESPONDING TO SAMENESS AND DIFFERENCE

Trauma groups have a homogenizing tendency, focusing on commonality rather than difference. Collectively, the group members form a strong enough ego; they need each other in defined ways to keep the group identity intact (Hannah, 1984; Parson, 1984; van der Kolk, 1993). Therapists must identify how their countertransference responses influence group development around sameness and difference. The therapist may rely excessively on "group-as-a-whole" interpretations as a means of avoiding further explorations, which might uncover differences and potential conflicts among members (Alford, 1995; van der Kolk, 1993; Vannicelli, 1991), or of avoiding their own disturbing reactions to an individual group member. Cotherapists may find themselves reinforcing sameness beyond the developmental needs of the group, reducing their own anxiety by creating "order and wholeness out of chaos and fragmentation" (Alford, 1995, p. 131).

We found ourselves one night describing the group to themselves as parts of a whole, stating that each of their symptoms together formed the complete constellation of posttraumatic stress reactions. Obviously we were striving to normalize symptoms, but when we discussed this intervention, it became clear that our timing was off. The need to emphasize the togetherness of the group was ours, an unspoken alliance between us. Our intervention made it easier for us to sit with the array of feelings in the room, and we didn't have to confront or ask the group members to confront their differences and individual responses.

The therapists may also collude with the group as a whole's desire to avoid certain themes, issues, feelings, and conflicts. The therapists do not address what is present but unspoken—for example, the building resentment toward a frequently tardy group participant, or the fear the group members feel about their experiences. In the following example, the group as a whole was more prepared than we were to tackle a difficult theme.

In our recent group, the theme was terror. The fear was ever-present, palpable in the room. Although we constantly addressed the fear, we found ourselves sidestepping a request to devote the evening to specifically discussing fear and anxiety. Unfortunately, in this instance, we modeled that when confronted with an overpowering emotion, avoid it. Why? Later we realized that we were defending ourselves for different reasons. Maggie connected with fear of being overwhelmed by their stories, which produced such terror. Maureen was afraid she'd feel helpless to mitigate it in any meaningful way.

The therapists may become overly protective of the group as a whole, seeing the group members as fragile victims. This is a particularly common pitfall for beginning group therapists.

Maggie: In my first trauma group 20 years ago, with women abused in relationships, the women wanted to talk about sexuality. They said they didn't know anything about healthy sexuality, and some of them had experienced marital rape. My cofacilitator suggested we introduce some discussion of lesbianism into this evening. I thought this would be "too much," that it would raise the women's anxiety even higher, that there was already plenty to cover. I, a heterosexual woman, certainly did not consider myself homophobic, but my cofacilitator, a lesbian, pushed me to address the source of MY anxiety. Consequently we included lesbianism, and it was the most astonishing of all the group sessions. Two of the eight women said they had stayed so long with violent husbands because of their shame about their sexual desire for other women. Another woman revealed a never-told secret about a brief sexual encounter with a girlfriend. A fourth woman confessed to a curiosity about lesbianism that went back to her childhood. That evening, the one I had argued so vigorously against, was a turning point in the group's ability for connection and honesty.

This example also stresses the importance of sensitively addressing difference, even in short-term groups. Even therapists committed to exploration of difference can be surprised at their reluctance to raise these issues if they become caught in the group's desire for sameness. Group participants (members and cotherapists) may be of varied gender, class, sexual orientation, and cultural backgrounds. Gonsalves, Torres, Fischman, Ross, and Vargas (1993) note that when cultural, lingual, and social differences are not addressed, disclosures may be avoided.

Group members will frequently attempt to draw therapists they identify as similar to themselves into their alliance. Therapists with differences may be shunted aside. Therapists who fear abandonment may allow themselves to be drawn into the alliance, while therapists who fear engulfment may protect themselves through self-disclosures that establish their differences.

COTHERAPY IN TRAUMA GROUPS

Much of the non-trauma-oriented cotherapy literature debates the benefits of cofacilitation, but literature describing group work with various trauma populations assumes coleadership (Bernstein & Klein, 1995; Courtois,

1988; Frick & Bogart, 1982; Gabriel, 1991; Ganzarain & Buchele, 1986; Herman, 1992; Herman & Schatzow, 1984; Pearlman & Saakvitne, 1995; Vannicelli, 1991; Walker & Nash, 1981). The dynamics in trauma groups are simply too complex for one therapist to manage alone, but cotherapists must make a significant commitment to their relationship if they expect it to support meaningful therapeutic gains. They must also be willing to address the insecurities that arise from exposing their work to both a colleague and group members.

Successful cotherapy depends on open communication to resolve disagreements and on the ability to accommodate each other's differences (Dick, Lessler, & Whiteside, 1980; McGee & Schuman, 1970; Paulson, Burroughs & Gelb, 1976; Pearlman & Saakvitne, 1995; Roller & Nelson, 1993; Yalom, 1985). Also important are a complementary balance of skills, the capacity to share decision-making power equally, relative noncompetitiveness, and compatibility in orientation (Roller & Nelson, 1993).

Pearlman and Saakvitne (1995) warn therapists to be wary of creating a shared defense or of rescuing each other, particularly from an angry or needy client. In the following example, the two of us were caught in a shared parental countertransference to a member of the group who presented as much younger than her chronological age.

Wendy had a tenuous hold on adulthood. She had trouble containing her internal child states, and her childlike vulnerability put her at risk in the world. We worried about her ability to keep herself safe, and in our worrying we became protective. Wendy found visualization and meditation frightening, and to help her feel safe, we eliminated the meditations with which we usually end the evening. After several sessions, we realized that the unity of this parental countertransference had been so strong that we were willing to sacrifice activities the rest of the group found soothing and containing. Once we recognized we had accepted her transference invitation to be the all-caring parents she never had, we could step back. We reinstituted the activities we had dropped, and worked with Wendy to create a strategy that would enable her to manage her own distress during these times.

Yalom (1985) says that most cotherapists unintentionally split roles. One therapist may be more supportive and the other more confrontative of group members; one may focus on the group as a whole while the other may focus more on individual members. Although he celebrates the differences in cotherapists, he cautions that group members frequently drive a wedge into the cotherapy relationship and exploit any existing tensions. Describing cotherapy in incest survivor groups, Courtois (1988) suggests that cotherapists should "function as a team to guard against being split into good and bad parents but their individuality should come through as they engage with the group and its members" (p. 266). The following dialogue illustrates a strong countertransference response by Maggie, a desire to protect by Maureen, and an exploration of our different styles.

MAGGIE: When Tina said you were the head and I was the heart, I felt instant shame. My face flushed and my heart raced. All I could think about was how I was never smart enough for my father. I was aware enough to notice the group members staring at me, and I remember blurting out how this comment had touched some childhood pain. This was the best I could manage, to let Tina see that she was not the cause of my discomfort.

MAUREEN: I didn't react to Tina calling me the head of the group. I knew she had a strong transference to me because of my authority that started in the screening interview. I was a stand-in for her intellectualizing father, who discounted her ideas, and she wanted me to validate her thinking.

MAGGIE: I appreciated that you weren't caught like me, and I admired how you saw a teachable moment and leapt in, tying my response to an earlier focus on shame reactions.

MAUREEN: I felt stung, though, because after the group you said maybe you believed that I don't have a heart. I didn't respond because it felt so different from our usual interactions. You didn't say, "Of course you have a heart and of course I have a head, but how did we get to this pattern?"

MAGGIE: I don't know why I said that. Perhaps I don't want you to have a heart. Perhaps I want you to be the head so I can have the heart role, an ego attachment to being spiritual and open-hearted. So maybe I'm saying, "Sorry, that role is taken." But on the other hand, I felt deskilled and invisible, because I also have an identification with being smart and articulate.

MAUREEN: Maybe I make it too easy for you. I think I just assume the head role at times because spontaneous teaching moments come naturally to me. You've also been talking about how overextended you are, and I'm trying to help you out.

MAGGIE: If you are going to seize the teaching moment, I'm going to grab the process moment to balance things out. This is a rescue, too, because I take away from you by doing that, and I'm not honoring your process skills.

MAUREEN: I'm also aware that I buffered you from Tina's comment. I saw that you were having a strong reaction, and I looked for a way to call their attention away from you, and so I focused on shame reactions in general. I wanted to give you a bit of time to catch your breath. This touches that place where cotherapists can be a tight unit, taking care of each other rather than maintaining a focus on the group.

MAGGIE: It never occurred to me before that you might have been protecting me. I see now that we both missed an opportunity to go deeper and draw out Tina's transference to us. I had been blaming myself.

MAUREEN: How come it's your fault that we don't go deeper? How come you get assigned responsibility for this?

MAGGIE: If I'm the heart, then it's my job.

MAUREEN: I'm also responsible. Perhaps I'm responding to the group's little scolding that we got sidetracked into process the week before. Maybe that's why I responded to Tina the way I did.

We realized that each of us had played a part in how the group member's comment was handled. Acknowledging our motivations and different styles resulted in a decision both to honor our differences and to encourage each other to stretch.

CONCLUSION

A rigorous exploration of countertransference and vicarious trauma is essential to the trauma group therapist. This sometimes painful confrontation with self needs the support of a cotherapist, colleagues, and supervisors who share the therapist's theoretical map. External support creates containment for the therapist and encourages the development of a caring and objective internal observer. This enables the therapist to be curious about her motivation and compassionate about her mistakes; it illuminates both her resourcefulness and her Achilles heel.

The complex dynamics of trauma groups require master juggling. Juggling demands a concentration that is never automatic; it requires balance, strength, and consistency. Facilitating trauma groups is akin to juggling random objects of differing size and shape that the participants have tossed. Here improvisation is overlaid on training, technique, and understanding. But a therapist will inevitably drop balls, and trouble only sets in when the therapist is unable or unwilling to admit it. Empathic failures serve as route-finding clues unless therapists are unwilling to risk exposure and refuse to examine their conscious and unconscious defenses.

It is essential for therapists to increase their capacities for awareness, containment, presence, and integration. Awareness can be encouraged in therapists' personal lives through meditation, visualization, yoga, journal keeping, art, other creative activities, and personal psychotherapy. Containment abilities can be built through self-care efforts and a balanced life that includes time spent in activities unrelated to work. It is also helpful to engage in advocacy or political action around the causes of violence and catastrophe. Therapists should beware, however, that pursuing any of these activities may simply replicate coping strategies of compartmentalization and separation.

Therapists' compassionate and aware attention to their internal world deepens and integrates the entirety of their experience. No one lives in continuous moment-to-moment awareness, and therapists need patience as we struggle to return to the present. The necessity for therapists to deepen their own integration cannot be overstressed. Herman (1992) reminds us that when therapists foster integration in themselves and in the survivors they work with, they deepen their own integrity. Therapists who can be present while unflinchingly exploring the reality of trauma can help group members reclaim their futures.

> Comments from group members on the final night told us we'd had some success. During our sessions Debra had trouble with the idea that it can be helpful to be curious about painful feelings. "Every week I would go home," she said, "and think that Maggie and Maureen didn't know what they were talking about. I thought it was a really stupid idea that I should be interested in flashbacks when I just wanted help in getting away from them. But somehow I've gotten more interested in these feelings and, at the same time, it's helped me take a big leap into the present."
>
> Wendy described the transformation that came from listening to women exploring their feelings: "I watched everyone sharing painful feelings, without someone trying to fix it and they seemed stronger for it. It gave me the courage to go on and I began to think I could bear my own feelings." Later, after the group was over, she sent a note: "I'm doing things I never imagined being able to do."

NOTE

1. For the sake of simplicity, we use feminine pronouns throughout this chapter to refer to a therapist.

REFERENCES

Abney, V. D., Anderson-Yang, J., & Paulson, M. J. (1992). Transference and countertransference issues unique to long-term group psychotherapy of adult women molested as children. *Journal of Interpersonal Violence, 7*(4), 559–569.

Agger, I., & Jensen, S. (1994). Determinant factors for countertransference reactions under state terrorism. In J. Wilson & J. Lindy (Eds.), *Countertransference in the treatment of PTSD* (pp. 263–287). New York: Guilford Press.

Alford, F. (1995). The group as a whole or acting out the missing leader? *International Journal of Group Psychotherapy, 45*(2), 125–412.

Benedek, E. (1984). The silent scream: Countertransference reactions to victims. *American Journal of Social Psychiatry, 4*(3), 49–52.

Benioff, L., & Vinogradov, S. (1993). Group psychotherapy with cancer patients and the terminally ill. In H. I. Kaplan & B. J. Sadock (Eds.), *Comprehensive group psychotherapy* (3rd ed., pp. 477–489). Baltimore: Williams & Wilkins.

Bernstein G., & Klein, R. (1995). Countertransference issues in group psychotherapy with HIV-positive and AIDS patients. *International Journal of Group Psychotherapy, 45*(1), 91–100.

Briere, J. (1992). *Child abuse trauma: Theory and treatment of the lasting effects.* Newbury Park, CA: Sage.

Catherall, D., & Lane, C. (1992). Warrior vets. *Journal of Traumatic Stress, 5*(1), 19–36.

Chu, J. (1988). Ten traps for therapists in the treatment of trauma survivors. *Dissociation, 1*(4), 24–31.

Comas-Diaz, L., & Padilla, A. (1990). Countertransference in working with victims of political repression. *American Journal of Orthopsychiatry, 60,* 125–135.

Courtois, C. (1988). *Healing the incest wound: Adult survivors in therapy.* New York: Norton.

Courtois, C. (1997). Healing the incest wound: A treatment update with attention to recovered memory issues. *American Journal of Psychotherapy, 51*(4), 464–510.

Danieli, Y. (1988). Confronting the unimaginable: Psychotherapists' reactions to victims of the Nazi Holocaust. In J. Wilson, Z. Harel, & B. Kahana (Eds.), *Human adaptation to extreme stress* (pp. 219–238). New York: Plenum Press.

Dick, R., Lessler, K., & Whiteside, J. (1980). A developmental framework for cotherapy. *International Journal of Group Psychotherapy, 30,* 273–285.

Epstein, M. (1995). *Thoughts without a thinker: Psychotherapy from a Buddhist perspective.* New York: Basic Books.

Figley, C. (1995). *Compassion fatigue: Coping with secondary traumatic stress disorder in those who treat the traumatized.* New York: Brunner/Mazel.

Fischman, Y., & Ross, J. (1990). Group treatment of exiled survivors of torture. *American Journal of Orthopsychiatry, 60,* 135–142.

Fogelman, E., & Savran, B. (1980). Brief group therapy with offspring of Holocaust survivors: Leaders' reactions. *American Journal of Orthopsychiatry, 50*(1), 96–108.

Frick, R., & Bogart, L. (1982). Transference and countertransference in group therapy with Vietnam veterans. *Bulletin of the Menninger Clinic, 46*(5), 429–444.

Gabriel, M. A. (1991). Group therapists' countertransference reactions to multiple deaths from AIDS. *Clinical Social Work Journal, 19*(3), 279–292.

Ganzarain, R., & Buchele, B. (1986). Countertransference when incest is the problem. *International Journal of Group Psychotherapy, 36*(4), 549–566.

Gonsalves, C., Torres, T., Fischman, Y., Ross, J., & Vargas, M. (1993). The theory of torture and the treatment of survivors: An intervention model. *Journal of Traumatic Stress, 6*(3), 351–365.

Haley, S. (1974). When the patient reports atrocities. *Archives of General Psychiatry, 30,* 191–196.

Hannah, S. (1984) Countertransference in in-patient psychotherapy: Implications for technique. *International Journal of Group Psychotherapy, 34*(2), 257–272.

Hartman, C., & Jackson, H. (1994). Rape and the phenomenon of countertransference. In J. Wilson & J. Lindy (Eds.), *Countertransference in the treatment of PTSD* (pp. 206–244). New York: Guilford Press.

Herman, J. (1992). *Trauma and recovery.* New York: Basic Books.

Herman, J., & Schatzow, E. (1984). Time-limited group therapy for women with a history of incest. *International Journal of Group Psychotherapy, 34*(4), 605–616.

Kernberg, O. (1965). Notes on countertransference. *Journal of the American Psychoanalytic Association, 13,* 38–56.

McCann, I. L., & Pearlman, L. A. (1990). Vicarious traumatization: A framework for understanding the psychological effects of working with victims. *Journal of Traumatic Stress, 3*(1), 131–149.

McEvoy, M. (1990) Repairing personal boundaries: Group therapy with survivors of sexual abuse. In T. A. Laidlaw & C. Malmo (Eds.), *Healing voices: Feminist approaches to therapy with women* (pp. 62–79). San Francisco: Jossey-Bass.

McGee, T., & Schuman, B. (1970). The nature of the co-therapy relationship. *International Journal of Group Psychotherapy, 20,* 25–36.

Ormont, L. R. (1993). Resolving resistances to immediacy in the group setting. *International Journal of Group Psychotherapy, 43*(4), 399–418.

Ormont, L. R. (1995). Cultivating the observing ego in the group setting. *International Journal of Group Psychotherapy, 45*(4), 489–506.

Parson, E. R. (1984). The role of psychodynamic group therapy in the treatment of the combat veteran. In H. Schwartz (Ed.), *Psychotherapy of the combat veteran* (pp. 153–220). New York: Spectrum.

Paulson, I., Burroughs, J., & Gelb, C. (1976). Cotherapy: What is the crux of the relationship? *International Journal of Group Psychotherapy, 26,* 213–224.

Pearlman, L. A., & Saakvitne, K. W. (1995). *Trauma and the therapist: Countertransference and vicarious traumatization in psychotherapy with incest survivors.* New York: Norton.

Racker, H. (1957). The meaning and uses of countertransference. *Psychoanalytic Quarterly, 56,* 303–357.

Roller, B., & Nelson, V. (1993). Cotherapy. In H. I. Kaplan & B. J. Sadock (Eds.), *Comprehensive group psychotherapy* (3rd ed., pp. 304–314). Baltimore: Williams & Wilkins.

Saakvitne, K. (1995). Therapists' responses to dissociative clients: Countertransference and vicarious traumatization. In L. Cohen, J. Berzoff, & M. Elin (Eds.), *Dissociative identity disorder* (pp. 467–492). Northvale, NJ: Aronson.

Saddock, V. (1993). Group psychotherapy with rape victims and battered women. In H. I. Kaplan & B. J. Sadock (Eds.), *Comprehensive group psychotherapy* (3rd ed., pp. 525–531). Baltimore: Williams & Wilkins.

van der Kolk, B. (1993). Group psychotherapy with posttraumatic stress disorder. In H. I. Kaplan & B. J. Sadock (Eds.), *Comprehensive group psychotherapy* (3rd ed., pp. 550–560). Baltimore: Williams & Wilkins.

Vannicelli, M. (1991). Dilemmas and countertransference considerations in group psychotherapy with adult children of alcoholics. *International Journal of Group Psychotherapy, 41*(3), 295–312.

Walker, J., & Nash, J. (1981). Group therapy in the treatment of Vietnam combat veterans. *International Journal of Group Psychotherapy, 31*(3), 379–389.

Wilson, J., & Lindy, J. (Eds.). (1994). *Countertransference in the treatment of PTSD.* New York: Guilford Press.

Winnicott, D. (1965). *The maturational processes and the facilitating environment.* New York: International Universities Press.

Yalom, I. (1985). *The theory and practice of group psychotherapy* (3rd ed.). New York: Basic Books.

Ziegler, M. (1996). At the edge of a cliff: Excerpts from a therapist's journal. *Treating Abuse Today, 5*(6)–6(1), 31–37.

PART II

—◄o►—

SPECIAL POPULATIONS
AND TRAUMA GROUPS

6

◄❪O❫►

Group Psychotherapy for the Symptoms of Posttraumatic Stress Disorder

DAVID READ JOHNSON
HADAR LUBIN

Posttraumatic stress disorder (PTSD) is only one of many sequelae of traumatic experience. Trauma has a progressive impact on a person's physical, psychological, social, and spiritual domains, leading to a wide variety of medical, psychiatric, interpersonal, and cultural disorders (Browne & Finkelhor, 1986; Herman, 1992; Kilpatrick, Veronen, & Resick, 1982; Waites, 1993). The modality of group therapy has usually been applied to interpersonal and social problems associated with traumatic experience, due to their salience in the group setting. As a result, group therapy has often been recommended as an adjunctive treatment following primary treatment for symptoms, which is usually conducted in an individual setting. This chapter illustrates how group therapy can have a direct impact on the symptoms of PTSD, and discusses the potential importance of group therapy in trauma treatment.

THE RELEVANCE OF GROUP THERAPY
TO THE TRAUMATIC EXPERIENCE

The group environment is very relevant for traumatized individuals, due to the experience of isolation and separation from communal supports that

141

characterizes trauma. The group serves as a symbolic societal witness to each victim's experience, as it is retold and relived in the group process. Fundamental societal functions—securing safety, sharing affective distress, determining basic attributions of responsibility, and welcoming each victim back into the group—are replayed within the group interaction (van der Kolk, 1987). The successful group experience provides a corrective emotional experience of a victim's "homecoming," in which inevitable dynamics of self-blaming, loss of credibility, and silencing of the victim will be evoked and then worked through (Catherall, 1989; Johnson et al., 1997). The group's intrinsic multiplicity of perspective will highlight differentiated perceptions of each member's traumatic experience; these perceptions will give members the important opportunity to integrate their unique histories into a revised sense of self without feeling cut off, misunderstood, or rejected by others.

It is therefore not surprising that many clinical reports of group therapy with trauma victims indicate that the primary purpose of the treatment is to improve interpersonal and social adjustment. Themes of universality, interpersonal learning, instillation of hope, and existential factors are often addressed (Yalom, 1975). The need for a strongly cohesive group is repeatedly emphasized. Indeed, most clinicians agree that the treatment of PTSD should begin in a highly homogeneous treatment environment, in which clients experience the safety and security afforded by exposure to others who have had highly similar experiences (Bloom, 1997; Herman, 1992; Marmar, Foy, Kagan, & Pynoos, 1993; Parson, 1985; Scurfield, 1993). Feelings of isolation, mistrust, and shame among trauma victims may be more readily overcome in the early stages of treatment within homogeneous environments (Parson, 1985). Learning that one is not alone or crazy appears to be of prime importance in the recovery process, and is facilitated by a high degree of similarity among members. Significant differences in experience among members may place too great a strain on individual members' capacities for accommodation, and may thus lead to a high dropout rate (Parson, 1985). Homogeneity helps keep the focus on the trauma, encourages more detailed recall, authorizes the feedback provided by other group members, and minimizes the "we–they" split that often cripples a treatment group (Scurfield, 1993).

Despite these advantages, several authors have described negative aspects of highly homogeneous groups. Clients may become overly attached to their identities as victims, delaying their adaptation to the normal world (Brende, 1983; van der Kolk, 1987). Collusive group interactions may occur in order to protect individual members from being singled out, and these may prevent members from taking responsibility or acknowledging certain realities (Parson, 1985). Appreciating member differences and engaging in appropriate interpersonal conflicts are important steps toward greater individuation. A group consisting of similarly victimized clients may become too insular, unintentionally increasing the alienation of the clients from their families and from society at large (Johnson, Feldman, Southwick, & Charney, 1994; van der Kolk, 1987). Helping victims differentiate their own experiences from those of others without feeling intense shame or fear may be more likely to occur in heterogeneous groups.

In view of these considerations, a number of authors have proposed treatment models that progress from homogeneous to heterogeneous stages. For example, Herman (1992) proposes a three-stage model of safety, remembrance/mourning, and reconnection. She recommends individual work in the first stage, homogeneous groups in the second stage, and heterogeneous groups in the third stage. Another model aims for a gradual increase in members' psychological differentiation and individuation, in which differences among group members are increasingly identified and explored (Parson, 1985). Johnson and colleagues (1994) have identified first- and second-generation models for inpatient PTSD treatment, characterized by homogeneity and heterogeneity, respectively. First-generation programs are sanctuarial environments highly responsive to clients' expressed needs, whereas second-generation programs encourage transactions across various societal and family boundaries, with less emphasis on intermember bonding.

ADDRESSING THE SYMPTOMS OF PTSD

The diagnosis of PTSD has been in constant revision and redefinition for many years, since the symptoms overlap with those of many other diagnoses, including other anxiety disorders as well as mood, dissociative, and psychotic disorders. The current consensually derived and field-tested definition has been established by the American Psychiatric Association's *Diagnostic and Statistical Manual of Mental Disorders*, fourth edition (DSM-IV), published in 1994. Criterion A is the presence of a traumatic event involving actual or possible death or major injury, or danger to one's own or others' physical integrity, and in which the person experiences severe fear, horror, or helplessness. Seventeen primary symptoms of PTSD are divided into three general categories: the reexperiencing cluster, which includes (1) intrusive recollections, (2) distressing dreams, (3) feelings that the event is happening again (e.g., flashbacks), (4) psychological distress in response to reminders of the event, and (5) physiological reactivity in response to reminders of the event; the avoidance cluster, which includes (6) attempts to avoid feelings or thoughts related to the trauma, (7) attempts to avoid situations or activities that arouse recollections of the trauma, (8) amnesia for important aspects of the trauma, (9) greatly lessened interest in significant activities, (10) feelings of being detached from others, (11) a narrow range of affect, and (12) a sense of a foreshortened future; and the hyperarousal cluster, which includes (13) sleep difficulties, (14) irritability, (15) problems with concentration, (16) hypervigilance, and (17) a heightened startle response. The diagnosis of PTSD is confirmed when the person is determined to have at least one reexperiencing symptom, three avoidance symptoms, and two hyperarousal symptoms. To highlight the tremendous range of effects associated with PTSD, the DSM-IV also lists additional symptoms and disorders commonly seen in persons with PTSD. The symptoms include survivor guilt; phobias; problems with affect modulation; impulsive or self-destructive acts; symptoms of dissociation; somatic difficulties; feeling ineffective, shamed, despairing, or hopeless; feeling forever damaged; losing previously held beliefs; hostility; social withdrawal; feeling continually threatened; problems in relationships with others (e.g., marital conflicts); and changes in personality. Associated disorders include agoraphobia, panic disorder, obsessive–compulsive disorder, specific phobia, social phobia, somatization disorder, major depressive disorder, and substance-related disorders.

Generally, reduction of PTSD symptoms has been attempted through individual forms of therapy, whereas group therapy approaches have targeted more general self-esteem and relationship dimensions (Shalev, Bonne, & Eth, 1996; Solomon, Gerrity, & Muff, 1992). Many clinicians have recommended that individual therapy be used in the initial phase of treatment, followed by group therapy (Gil, 1988; Herman, 1992). The PTSD target symptom clusters of reexperiencing, avoidance, and hyperarousal have been reduced by cognitive-behavioral (Foa, Rothbaum, Riggs, & Murdock, 1991; Frank et al., 1988; Resick, Jordan, Girelli, Hutter, & Marhoefer-Dvorak, 1988), exposure-based (Cooper & Clum, 1989; Fairbank & Keane, 1982; Keane, Fairbank, Caddell, & Zimering, 1989), and psychopharmacotherapeutic (Davidson, Kudler, & Smith, 1990; Shestatzky, Greenberg, & Lerer, 1988; van der Kolk et al., 1994) treatments.

Many earlier models of group therapy for trauma populations have embraced a comprehensive model of treatment that addresses the broad complex of symptoms, interpersonal relations, and meaning dimensions of clients' disorders. These therapies have often presumed that clients' symptoms will diminish over time as a result of the support, insight, and interaction provided by the group. This presumption may be supported by theories proposing that symptoms are manifestations of underlying difficulties, or that the ego-bolstering effects of the group will aid the clients in coping with or managing their symptoms. However, in recent years, specialized forms of group therapy have been developed that specifically target the symptoms of PTSD. These approaches are typically time-limited and not comprehensive in scope. Presumably, group therapy that is directly focused on treating the symptoms of PTSD should be more successful in doing so.

The reduction of primary PTSD symptoms should also enhance the clients' efforts at recovery in other areas of their lives.

Since the most researched and most powerful interventions for PTSD symptoms have included cognitive-behavioral and exposure-based components, it is likely that successful group therapies for PTSD symptoms will incorporate aspects of these techniques. Group therapy specifically designed for PTSD therefore seems to require a clear understanding of the ways in which symptoms manifest themselves in the group, and interventions appropriate to and timed with the emergence of these symptoms.

Avoidance Symptoms

Most theories of PTSD identify avoidance as a primary defense against the distressing affects occasioned by traumatic recall, which prevents a normative process of integration and working through of the trauma. Therefore, clients' avoidance strategies must be identified and interfered with (Foa & Kozak, 1986). Clearly, a certain degree of work must have occurred in order for a client to agree to be in treatment for PTSD in the first place. However, the most significant effect of continued avoidance in the group is the delay in revealing the trauma stories. Postponing the revelation of trauma stories is often justified by concerns about flooding group members too early (prior to the achievement of sufficient cohesion in the group), which may result in high dropout rates. However, without sufficient exposure to the trauma material, therapeutic desensitization designed to decrease reexperiencing and hyperarousal symptoms will not be possible. Thus early disclosure is usually recommended. To reduce the risk of premature flooding or of dropouts, measures that enhance early group cohesion are helpful. Foremost among these is a high degree of homogeneity among group members in terms of type and recency of trauma, social status, age, and gender. Second, a highly formalized approach to revelation of traumatic material is required. Structured approaches such as journals, written formats, time limits, and therapist directives tend to contain and focus the traumatic material and to provide external referents that ground clients during traumatic recall.

Another common expression of avoidance in the group occurs when clients turn their attention to issues not directly linked to their traumatic experience, in order to allow a catharsis in displaced form. The therapists must be ready to interfere with such displacements and remind the clients of the relation of the issue to its traumatic etiology. The goal of "keeping on track" or "sticking to the task" is strictly adhered to in these models of group therapy. These considerations clearly imply that the therapists must be more active and directive than may usually be the case in other group therapy approaches.

Reexperiencing Symptoms

Reexperiencing symptoms will be evoked once avoidance is diminished. Often aspects of the group process remind members of their traumatic experiences; reenactments of traumatic material also occur within ostensibly current issues. Most theories of trauma treatment indicate that traumatic schemata and associated affects such as fear or anger (i.e., reexperiencing) must be activated before they can be mediated or revised through therapeutic interventions. The basic principle is that the best times for interventions designed to help members with reexperiencing symptoms are the times when these symptoms occur. Members therefore should be informed about the likelihood of these occurrences, as well as the need to communicate to the group when they arise. Therapists need to be on the alert for members who may be reexperiencing but not speaking about it, including forms of dissociating. Various methods may be used once reexperiencing symptoms occur in the group, such as grounding exercises, confrontation with discrepant information, corrective interactions, and written exercises. The therapeutic task is to facilitate the clients' reality testing of their experience of danger (reexperienced from the trauma) in the relative safety of the therapeutic situation.

Hyperarousal Symptoms

Hyperarousal symptoms are also likely to occur once avoidant strategies are diminished. As noted above, these symptoms may include irritability, panic and physiological arousal, and lack of attention/concentration. Again, the principle is that the therapy should anticipate symptoms and address them directly in the group via specific methods. Techniques for hyperarousal symptoms include relaxation techniques, cognitive assertions, certain types of distraction, and interpersonal support. These symptoms are likely to occur as group members experience a directed exposure component in the therapy, such as speaking in detail about their traumata, or reading from their journals. Often training in relaxation or affect management precedes such exposure, so that clients can successfully navigate the rush of affect generated (Keane et al., 1989). Generally the intention is to help the clients persevere through their arousal state until it subsides, rather than to abort it midway by avoidant strategies such as leaving the room. For desensitization to occur, it is essential that a client experience both the rise and fall of arousal, so that incorrect ideas such as "I will not live through this" or "I am in danger" can be effectively mediated.

Attention to the likely emergence of PTSD symptoms in the group is critical to group therapies designed to have an impact on these symptoms. Lack of preparation will inevitably lead to these symptoms' interfering with or completely blocking potential therapeutic work of other members. Because the enlistment of group members' healthy egos in such preparation is likely to be helpful, more structured, educational components are often integrated into group therapy formats with such goals. Open, interactive formats are more likely to evoke powerful demonstrations of symptoms without sufficient preparation of group members in techniques designed to handle them. Too often, a productive interaction is stopped dead in its tracks when a member becomes flooded with traumatic memories and the group watches in awkward silence. When the member leaves the room out of embarrassment, the integrity of and confidence in the group therapy enterprise are severely compromised, even when a therapist labels the moment as respecting the client's trauma or giving the client space. In models of group therapy aimed at symptom relief, these moments are opportunities for action, not silence.

TWO MODELS OF GROUP
THERAPY FOR PTSD

There have been few models of group therapy specifically designed to focus on PTSD symptoms. Early PTSD treatments involved support groups of survivors, such as rap groups for Vietnam veterans, which were intended to meet the survivors' basic needs for sanctuary, acknowledgment, and reassurance (Allen & Bloom, 1994; Shatan, 1973). Psychodynamic group therapies provide more generalized treatments designed to help restore individuals' sense of self, integrity, and integration, and to increase their understanding of relations with others (Alexander, Neimeyer, Follete, Moore, & Harter, 1989; Carver, Stalker, Stewart, & Abraham, 1989; Hall, Mullee, & Thompson, 1995; Hazzard, Rogers, & Angert, 1993; Herman & Schatzow, 1984; Neimeyer, Harter, & Alexander, 1991; Roth, Dye, & Lebowitz, 1988). Studies of these groups have reported modest gains in general psychological health variables, such as self-esteem, depression, anxiety, and social isolation. Few have reported specific improvements in core PTSD symptoms. Intensive group-based inpatient programs for Vietnam veterans have shown little impact on PTSD symptoms in this population, though Frueh, Turner, Beidel, Mirabella, and Jones (1996) indicate some potential for a cognitive-behavioral intervention based on trauma management (Fontana & Rosenheck, 1997; Johnson et al., 1996). Evidence for greater efficacy has come from studies of outpatient groups with female survivors of rape and incest. For example, Zlotnick and colleagues (1997) implemented a psychoeducational group intervention aimed at symptom mastery, based on Linehan's (1993) and Herman's (1992) concepts of safety and skill building. Results indicated significant reductions in PTSD symptoms, though 29% dropped out before completing treatment.

Two models of specialized group therapy for PTSD in particular are worthy of greater attention. These are reviewed here in greater detail.

Cognitive Processing Therapy

Patricia Resick and her colleagues have developed a model of therapy for PTSD called "cognitive processing therapy" (CPT), which has been applied to rape victims in both individual and group contexts (Resick et al., 1988; Resick & Schnicke, 1993). CPT is a unique blend of exposure therapy, information-processing therapy, and group support. Memories of traumatic experience are elicited, emotion is generated, and then faulty cognitions and "stuck points" (see below) are identified.

CPT is based on the information-processing notion that symptoms arise from conflicts between one's prior (i.e., normative) schemata and the traumatic schemata. In order to alter symptomatology, first the memory of the traumatic event must be activated, usually through some form of exposure therapy. Then the conflicts between schemata must be allowed to be experienced and processed. "Stuck points" are areas of incomplete processing that must receive particular focus, over and above faulty cognitions of the event; identifying these is of critical importance in CPT. Unlike some forms of cognitive therapy, CPT allows for more complete emotional expression in order to counter the strong avoidant defenses that tend to decrease access to the traumatic schemata.

Structure and Content of Group Sessions

The group format includes 12 sessions of 90 minutes. Table 6.1 lists the themes of these group sessions. Each group usually consists of four to nine members, with two cotherapists. First, clients are provided with a cognitive information-processing explanation of rape reactions in an educational format. Then clients are asked to write about their traumata and to review them repeatedly, as an exposure component. Next, stuck points are identified and confronted via a list of 12 challenging questions, with which the therapists and clients examine the trauma narratives. The purpose of this exercise is to raise questions in the clients about the validity of their views about their traumata. At this point, the therapists introduce a list of seven faulty thinking patterns and ask the clients to find examples of them in their narratives. Here is the text of one client's analysis of her own faulty thinking patterns (Resick & Schnicke, 1993, pp. 78–79):

1. Drawing conclusions when evidence is lacking or even contradictory. Example: All men are untrustworthy.
2. Exaggerating or minimizing the meaning of an event: You blow things

TABLE 6.1. Session Themes for CPT

Session 1: Introduction and Education Phase
Session 2: The Meaning of the Event
Session 3: Identification of Thoughts and Feelings
Session 4: Remembering the Rape
Session 5: Identification of Stuck Points
Session 6: Challenging Questions
Session 7: Faulty Thinking Patterns
Session 8: Safety Issues
Session 9: Trust Issues
Session 10: Power and Control Issues
Session 11: Esteem Issues
Session 12: Intimacy Issues, the Meaning of the Event, and Closure

Note. From Resick and Schnicke (1993).

way out of proportion or shrink their importance inappropriately. Example: Since I was not beat up, my rape is not as serious or bad as others I've heard about.

3. Disregarding important aspects of a situation. Example: Since I did not fight much, it must mean I wanted it.

4. Oversimplifying events or beliefs as good/bad, right/wrong. Example: It was wrong of me not to report the rape to the police.

5. Overgeneralizing from a single incident: You view a negative event as a never-ending pattern of defeat, or you apply an association you made of the rapist to a whole group. Examples: Now that I have been raped, I believe I will be raped again; or All (race, personal characteristics) men are rapists.

6. Mind reading: You assume that people are thinking negatively of you when there is not definite evidence for this. Example: Since my friends and family have not brought up the rape, they must think it's my fault or blame me in some way.

7. Emotional reasoning: You reason from how you feel. Example: Because I feel scared when I am near a man, it must mean that [the man intends] to rape me.

The final phase of therapy addresses how the rape has affected five main areas: safety, trust, power, esteem, and intimacy (McCann & Pearlman, 1990). Extensive homework assignments are given each week and reviewed in the next week's session. The clients practice analyzing their own thought patterns, identifying faulty thinking about these themes both for beliefs about the self and for beliefs about others. Here is how a therapist handled one client's faulty thinking during the "Safety Issues" session (Resick & Schnicke, 1993, pp. 90–92):

The client was accosted by a stranger while sitting in her car in a parking lot as she waited for her husband. The assailant forced his way in at gunpoint, covered her eyes, drove her around, and then raped her. . . . Now she felt she could not go out in her car alone at night. On her worksheet, she said that her emotion was fear (90%) and that her automatic thought about going out alone was that "Something might happen," which she believed completely (100%). She said the evidence was that she had been raped, and that this was logical. Her alternative was to stay home, because if she was raped again it would kill her. The therapist noted that she, like many clients, initially was so entrenched in her beliefs that [she could not] look at them any other way. The therapist focused on the probability of being raped again, and said to the client: "Okay, for you, that means that if everything stayed the same and these events occurred at the same rate, and you went out tonight, you might have a 1 in 1,000 chance of being raped, and a 999 out of 1,000 chance of not being raped. Does it make sense to you that you walk around being terrified all of the time? The rapist owned three hours of your life and we can't change that. Do you want him to own the rest of your life and to dictate what you can and cannot do?" The therapist also pointed out that the client probably had a greater chance of being in a car accident, yet she did not avoid driving at other times. The client agreed with these statements and began to rethink her beliefs by revising her worksheet with the therapist's help. She now wrote that she had "confused a low probability for a high probability event," and that her faulty thinking pattern was "jumping to conclusions and either/or thinking." She re-rated her fear as 40%. The next week she reported that she had gone out one evening and was not as fearful.

Resick's model requires that the therapists keep the group on task. This is accomplished by sticking to a highly defined structure and interfering immediately with clients' tangential maneuvers; by not allowing dominant individuals to keep shy members quiet; and by addressing the need to complete homework assignments. Due to this emphasis on performance, clients with an incest history, or clients who are suicidal or psychotic, are not usually deemed appropriate for a CPT group. The reason clients with an incest history are not included is that it is usually very difficult for them to concentrate solely on the adulthood rape. Since many victims of adult rape have a childhood incest or abuse history, this would appear to limit the applicability of CPT. Conceivably CPT could be adapted specifically for the childhood incest population, though no reports of such an adaptation have yet been published.

CPT can be delivered in either individual or group modalities, though the core therapeutic intervention, true to its cognitive-behavioral orientation, is not intrinsically group-based. Resick notes that the group format has the advantages of providing opportunities for support and validation, social pressure to complete the homework assignments, and the additional credibility of feedback from other rape survivors. Disadvantages of the group format, however, include the greater chances of getting off track because of dominant or personality-disordered members, as well as less therapist time per member. In addition, group members are not allowed to read their detailed rape accounts out loud in the group, to prevent unnecessary secondary traumatization.

Empirical Support

The CPT model has been tested in several empirical studies and has shown consistently positive effects on clients' PTSD symptoms (Resick et al., 1988; Resick & Schnicke, 1993). One study sample (Resick et al., 1988) consisted of 36 women with an average age of 32 years; they were generally college-educated, and 92% were European Americans. They had been raped from one to over five times, and on average their most recent rape had occurred 8 years earlier. Subjects were given a comprehensive evaluation prior to inclusion in the study, and were evaluated at termination and at 3-month and 6-month follow-up visits. Dropout rate was 12%.

Figure 6.1 shows the main results for each of the PTSD symptom clusters, as measured by the PTSD Symptom Scale (PSS; Foa, Riggs, Dancu, & Rothbaum, 1993). Significant reductions occurred in all three clusters by termination, and these were sustained through the 6-month follow-up. At admission, 34 of the 36 women met criteria for PTSD; at the 6-month follow-up, only 2 of 29 women met PTSD criteria. Significant reductions in symptoms of depression and general psychopathology also occurred.

These results clearly indicate that CPT is a promising intervention for victims of rape with PTSD. The efficacy of the group method was equivalent to that of individual sessions, providing evidence of the greater efficiency of the group therapy format in treating these clients.

Interactive Psychoeducational Group Therapy

"Interactive psychoeducational group therapy" (IPGT) is a 16-week form of group therapy we have designed for traumatized individuals with PTSD (Lubin & Johnson, 1997a; Lubin, Loris, Burt, & Johnson, 1998). IPGT is therefore a more concentrated, time-limited intervention than ongoing group psychotherapy approaches (e.g., Cole & Barney, 1987; Goodman & Nowalk-Scibelli, 1985; Herman, 1992; Herman & Schatzow, 1984). IPGT can conceivably be utilized either before, during, or after a course of long-term individual supportive psychotherapy. Many clients find it beneficial to discuss issues raised by the group in their ongoing individual therapy. Like CPT, IPGT is a structured approach involving lectures, cognitive restructuring, exposure to traumatic memories, and homework. In contrast to CPT, the IPGT model emphasizes the interpersonal learning available in the

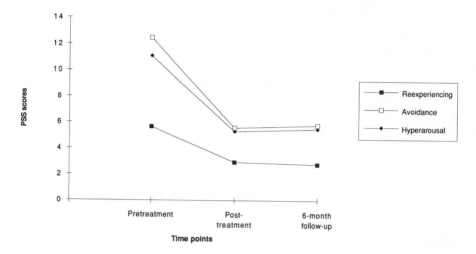

FIGURE 6.1. Reduction of PTSD symptoms in CPT ($n = 36$). Data from Resick & Schnicke (1993).

group format more than that gained from homework assignments. In addition, IPGT tends to focus more than CPT does on the clients' unimpaired traits not associated with the trauma, in comparison with traumatic schemata related to themes of fear, danger, and safety. In part, these differences are due to the fact that IPGT was designed to treat women who have been multiply traumatized by both adulthood and childhood abuses.

The goals of IPGT are (1) to educate clients about how their traumatic experience has affected their lives, and to provoke a reorganization of their ideas and feelings about themselves; (2) to facilitate a differentiation between clients' illness and their unimpaired characteristics; and thereby (3) to reduce PTSD symptoms. These goals are achieved through a process of active engagement among both clients and therapists. Clients are seen as "students of recovery" and are encouraged to utilize personal resources that are not inherently impaired by their trauma, such as their intellect, courage, perseverance, and humanity. The group therapists not only are witnesses to the traumatic stories, but seek to make an active connection with each victim, countering the isolation and helplessness that characterized the moment of trauma. It is essential that the here-and-now relationships established among the clients and the therapists challenge the clients' rigid interpersonal boundaries and distrust of others.

In general, it is best for clients to have achieved a basic sense of safety and cognitive distance from their experience prior to participation in IPGT. Though this is usually achieved through individual therapy, many IPGT clients have achieved these through natural support systems. Since the purpose of this form of group therapy is to target PTSD symptoms rather than interpersonal support or universality, it is best suited for clients in the early stages of recovery, when symptom reduction is a high priority.

The Concept of Differentiation

The IPGT model of PTSD symptom formation is based on the idea that what underlies the faulty cognitions that support avoidant thinking and behaviors is a lack of differentiation. A "differentiated" response consists of making partial distinctions among feelings, ideas, or events, such that one simultaneously acknowledges both similarities and differences. It is this simultaneity that results in the experience of the *autonomy* of a thought or object. The relative complexity of this position is challenged by desires to simplify the experience, so that one only experiences the similarities between two entities (leading to a state of overidentification or merging) or only the differences (leading to a state of isolation or disassociation). Indeed, many of the faulty thinking patterns mentioned by Resick (e.g., exaggeration or minimization, disregarding information, oversimplifying, overgeneralizing, mind reading) are examples of a failure to differentiate a response to the environment. The lack of differentiation, we believe, manifests itself in both the symptoms and the disordered relationships commonly seen in clients with PTSD. It is the driving force behind the tendency to overgeneralize found among clients with PTSD, through which elements of the past trauma infiltrate the experience of the present. Yet if differentiation (e.g., viewing a rape as only one incident and not one's destiny) provides a certain amount of relief from distress, then why do clients with PTSD seem to have difficulty achieving it, or even resist it?

We propose that the inability to differentiate must be directly linked to alterations occurring during the traumatic event, most particularly fear. Certainly a traumatic moment is characterized by a victim's struggle to maintain personal integrity and autonomy in the face of an overwhelming pressure to accommodate to a perpetrator or other external force. Perhaps it is because this struggle is lost and one's sense of self is intruded upon, one's personal boundaries shattered, that the fear of this moment is linked to the state of autonomy itself. Later, in intimate interactions with others, victims attempt to protect themselves by either being one with them or being completely separate from them, for then the victims cannot be singled out. To behave or think independently appears to run a great risk—to lose again what one lost, or to be the only one who has had this particular misfortune.

Thus the dynamics of pseudocohesion in trauma groups (discussed above) are likely to be propelled by fears of differentiating. It is often at times when a distinction among members' experiences is being made that traumatic schemata are evoked and enacted in the group via projective responses to other members or to the therapists. At these times, a direct attempt by anyone else to empathize with the clients regarding their traumatic experience will often be resisted—not to assert their isolation, but to invalidate the capacity of the other to comment on or characterize them. Fortunately, though keeping a group highly homogeneous will diminish the frequency and intensity of major distinctions among members, it is not possible to eliminate differences in the group altogether because of any group's inherent multiplicity. Therefore the therapists will have numerous opportunities to work on differentiation during the course of treatment, and indeed many of the interventions in the IPGT model are intended to address these moments. Treatment attempts to identify and then differentiate the traumatic schemata from the victims' cognitions, affective responses, and behavioral states. When this differentiation is achieved, the clients are able to liberate more resources to deal with their symptoms/illness, and then to direct these resources toward their future lives.

In IPGT, the process of differentiating self from the trauma/illness is accomplished in three basic ways. First, the therapists specifically highlight differences among members' experience, trauma histories, or social contexts. A treatment group consisting of members with different types of trauma histories will facilitate this process, but, again, no matter how well matched group members are, significant differences will exist that can be identified. Paradoxically, the recognition of diversity in perspective or experience of their traumata highlights the members' similarities within the general human condition rather than within the victim role. The acknowledgment of members' differences serves to depathologize their interactions and allows them to acknowledge their unique vulnerabilities and strengths, rather than to generalize their traumatic experiences even further. The acknowledgment of heterogeneity within the clients' traumatic events replicates the diversity they confront in natural social contexts (e.g., workplace, community, society), providing them with opportunities to practice accommodation. The irrational cognition "People cannot understand me unless they have experienced exactly what I have experienced" is dislodged by the achievement of understanding and support in the midst of a diverse social context.

Second, the therapists actively uncover the unique human strengths that still lie within the clients and can be revitalized for the pursuit of recovery. Many victims feel that the trauma has stripped them of everything except their symptoms (Herman, 1992). Universal human attributes and characteristics such as intellect, resourcefulness, humor, and creativity, although affected by the trauma, are usually preserved. The individuals' capacity to be creative, to care for others, and to contribute to society can be rediscovered within the safe interpersonal setting of the group (Bloom, 1997). The result is that unique aspects of their personalities, rather than their traumatic experiences, serve to define them as individuals in the group therapy interaction. It is the conflict between these positive characteristics and the traumatic schemata that Resick posits as the cause of symptoms and "stuck points." In addition to pointing out the inaccuracy of the traumatic schemata, the therapists will strengthen the clients' awareness of the usefulness of their previous schemata.

Third, and perhaps most importantly, the therapists directly confront the overgeneralized responses of clients during reenactments of traumatic material within the group interaction. As we describe below, during each session members bring their own experience to bear on the topics being presented; inevitably, one or more members will be sufficiently engaged to begin to reexperience elements of their traumatic schemata, and to reveal these through their interactions with the group and the therapists. In much the same way that CPT therapists counter the traumatic schemata with discrepant information, IPGT therapists engage with the clients and, through exercises of real-life discovery (e.g., inquiring of each other member of the group about their perceptions of a client), confront the clients with information incompatible with their traumatic schemata. This process puts pressure on the clients to differentiate their responses in the moment.

Structure and Content of Group Sessions

The overall structure of IPGT is described below (the themes of specific sessions are outlined in Table 6.2). We have not found a need to modify this structure despite variations in clinical settings, group size, or clients' level of functioning. The content of the specific lectures has been modified when IPGT has been applied to client populations other than multiply traumatized women, such as substance abusers, sexually abused males, or veterans.[1]

Phase 1. The task of Phase 1 (which lasts 6 weeks) is to explore the effects of the trauma on each individual's self-image, such as shame, doubts about self-worth, and identity confusion. The educational lectures during this phase are centered on the issues of shame, emotional depletion, the inability to trust, and the disturbances in feminine identity. During this phase, each client reviews her traumatic events with the group and receives feedback and support from group members and the therapists. These issues are traced to their origin, which often coincides with the onset of the abuse or the traumatic event. This phase involves direct therapeutic exposure of traumatic material within the supportive group setting.

Phase 2. The task of Phase 2 (which also lasts 6 weeks) is to explore the effects of the trauma on each individual's interpersonal relationships and related difficulties with trust, intimacy, dependency, and sexuality. The group setting provides a naturalistic environment in which each individual's

TABLE 6.2. Session Themes for IPGT

Phase 1: The Self
Session 1: Disclosure of the Trauma
Session 2: Shame and Identity
Session 3: The Void and Emptiness
Session 4: Putting It Right
Session 5: From Rage to Forgiveness
Session 6: Femininity: My Ally or Enemy?

Phase 2: Interpersonal Relations
Session 7: Separating from the Trauma
Session 8: Overcoming Your Isolation
Session 9: Controlling Your Anger
Session 10: Knowing Your Symptoms
Session 11: Befriending Your Body
Session 12: Finding Meaning in Your Life

Phase 3: The World
Session 13: Altering Your Relationship to the World
Session 14: Mourning Your Losses
Session 15: Achieving Transformation
Session 16: Graduation Ceremony

Note. Adapted from Lubin and Johnson (1997b).

constellation of interpersonal beliefs and style is revealed. The lectures during this phase are centered on identifying maladaptive coping strategies and defense mechanisms. Difficulties in relating to others are attributed to the continued application of originally adaptive posttrauma defenses that no longer meet the needs of current relationships. Clients are encouraged to experiment with the freedom inherent in the spontaneous interactions with each other, in contrast to the constraints imposed on them by their rigid traumatic schemata.

Phase 3. The task of Phase 3 (which lasts 4 weeks) is to explore the ways of finding meaning in one's life despite the trauma, and to begin to reconnect with the social world. In this phase, adaptive coping strategies are explored and practiced both within and outside the group through the use of homework assignments. Methods of empowerment are used to facilitate acceptance and generate meaning. For example, at the end of the 16 weeks, a special graduation ceremony is held demarcating the completion of the program. Each client is asked to invite people from her support network to serve as witnesses to her graduation. At the ceremony, each client communicates publicly the impact of her traumatic experience on her life and relationships through a creative project she has designed.

Session Structure. Each 90-minute session begins with a brief psychoeducational minilecture (about 10 minutes), followed by an interactive discussion; the session then ends with a brief, educationally oriented wrap-up. Booklets containing the series of lectures are given out at each phase, and homework for each session is assigned. The therapist giving the lecture utilizes a blackboard to highlight essential points in the lecture. The board and its contents function as an emotional distancing device, allowing group members to explore the traumatic material more safely. Open discussion follows as each member is asked to relate to the presented material. Eventually, some clients will engage more intensely, based on their particular traumata or defenses. They will tend to express elements of their traumatic schemata in their responses. The therapists, as well as other group members who feel empowered by their newly acquired knowledge, may confront these clients' schemata in a supportive way. These enactments then become the primary material for the work of differentiation and processing in the group, rather than the homework assignments used in CPT. Toward the end of the session, the therapist who gave the lecture returns to the board and gives the brief wrap-up; this again provides emotional distancing, and permits closure without an abrupt termination of the discussion. Often group members will remain in the room and continue to talk with one another after the therapists depart. As in CPT, social contact among members between sessions is allowed, as long as it can be discussed in group.

Addressing Symptoms

Avoidance. IPGT addresses avoidance symptoms by including early disclosure of the trauma stories, by making constant references to them during the group, and by providing a special public ceremony at the end of the program. IPGT addresses the traumatic events very early and directly in the treatment. Experience has shown that once the traumatic events have been reported openly in at least some detail, group members feel significantly more relieved and motivated to continue. Suffice it to say that perhaps the only thing on clients' minds when they arrive at the first group meeting is how they will have the courage to speak about what happened to them. Waiting even until the second session risks a decision to drop out. The importance of addressing the impact of the trauma on each aspect of clients' lives is constantly reiterated, and avoidant responses are consistently confronted. The structuring of the group and its psychoeducational format provide the necessary safety for such early disclosure. Similarly, the public ceremony at the end of treatment actively facilitates open disclosure of the trauma to people outside the treatment group. As noted above, the ceremony is structured so that each client presents some creative representation of her journey of recovery (e.g., poems, artwork, narrative, dance, role play) to an audience of family members and invited guests from the community. The clients' sense of shame and isolation is directly challenged, and empowerment and support are offered instead (Johnson, Feldman, Lubin, & Southwick, 1995; Lubin & Johnson, 1998). The clients' revelation of their traumatic experiences in a public arena serves as a metaphor of mutuality rather than privacy; the ceremony thereby breaks the clients' private hold on their traumatic events. The creative process serves metaphorically as an act of differentiating the trauma from the self-representation.

The following clinical example describes how one client's avoidance symptoms were dealt with in a group.

Ruth is 22 years old. At the age of 12, a year after her parents divorced, she was sexually assaulted by her father during a summer visitation. She felt guilty about the divorce and believed that she deserved the abuse. She committed herself to silence and did not reveal the assault. At 18, she presented at a local emergency room with severe PTSD symptoms, but still did not reveal the details of her trauma.

During Phase 1, Ruth was quiet but attentive to the verbal or nonverbal exchange among group members. As the more verbal members expressed their fear and vulnerability, she acknowledged her difficulties in expressing her feelings and said that she could definitely not share what had happened to her. The group nevertheless encouraged her to begin telling her story. Some group members recalled when they could not speak about their traumata, and yet emphasized how relieved they now felt by being able to express their pain more openly. Ruth said she felt envious of the courage of those group members who were capable of sharing their traumata. The therapist congratulated her for making her struggle clearer to the group, which would allow the group to help her overcome her fears. Ruth learned that others felt similar to her, even though their traumata were distinctly different. She realized that her silence was one way she had protected her parents from the pain of the divorce. The group pointed out to her that she needed protection from her parents, not the reverse. This insight finally allowed her to tell the group about the sexual abuse during her visitations with her father. She reexperienced intense shame as she spoke about it in the group, and it became obvious to everyone that she had blamed herself for the abuse.

During Phase 2, Ruth reported that she was able to tell her boyfriend about some aspects of her traumatic experience. She was surprised to find him a sympathetic and supportive listener, and admitted to the group that she had some doubts about the validity of her perception. The therapist asked whether she doubted the authenticity of the group's support. She nodded her head in affirmation. Here her reality testing in the present was impaired by the infiltration of a traumatic schema—namely, that no one would have believed her if she had told them about her father's abuse. The therapist directed her to ask the group in order to verify her suspicion. Ruth asked one member of the group whether she really meant what she had said, and received a warm and caring response that countered her suspicion: The member broke into tears and said, "Yes." The group members were excited about Ruth's newfound courage and more open approach. She subsequently became an active and supportive group member. She revealed to the group that she had written a play about her ordeal, but that until her experience in this group, she had been unable to name any of the characters.

During Phase 3, Ruth appeared brighter and significantly more verbal. She continued to struggle with her tendency to avoid and withdraw, but was increasingly open to feedback from the other group members, who helped her remain present and connected. At the graduation ceremony, with her mother and boyfriend as witnesses, she revealed her traumatic story publicly through the play she had written. The characters of her play were portrayed by different group members, and Ruth functioned as the narrator. Her story was thus revealed for the first time to her mother, who was filled with tears of pain and pride. In comparison with her initial presentation, Ruth's relationship to her trauma seemed to have changed: She no longer carried the burden alone.

Reexperiencing. Reexperiencing symptoms are addressed though corrective enactments of traumatic schemata when these emerge from group members. Interpersonal enactments in the group are evoked by members' engagement with the themes of the session, in which they extend their traumatic schemata into here-and-now interactions with group members or the therapists. During these moments of enhanced emotional arousal and vulnerability, previously protected emotions are often expressed. As each victim's traumatic schema is extended to include the therapists or group members, the boundaries between past and present are weakened. For example, a therapist may be experienced as an ineffectual bystander who looks on while the victim is being harmed. Paradoxically, in this moment the client allows the group into her privately held world. It is at this precise moment that the client's traumatic schema is most available for alteration. Therapists or other group members can identify that a traumatic schema is activated, and can then ask the client to test this schema by asking group members questions about their reactions or perceptions in the moment. For example, the thought "No one here can understand me" can be tested by asking other members to relate their understanding of the client; the feeling "I have nothing to offer anyone" can be confronted by having members identify positive qualities they have seen in the client. Through these corrective enactments, the group can alter a client's traumatic schema by making distinctions between the person and the trauma, between the present and the past, and between the narrow darkness of the traumatic event and the breadth of possibility available to the client in the future.

Another case example illustrates how a client's reexperiencing symptoms were addressed in a group.

Jean had been sexually abused by her grandfather for many years during her childhood. The sexual abuse was violent and accompanied by denigrating and humiliating remarks. Jean stared at the ceiling while the abuse took place, which helped her reduce the overwhelming feelings of emotional and physical pain. The therapist noticed in the group that whenever Jean felt emotionally vulnerable or whenever group members challenged her withdrawal, she would talk softly and stare. The therapist asked Jean to describe how she felt when she stared, and her response was "I just feel pain." In this enactment, Jean's traumatic schema of being abused overlapped with the therapist's putting her on the spot, evoking her staring behavior. The therapist then pointed out to Jean that she had stared at the ceiling when she was abused as a child, and asked her whether the shame she had felt then was linked with the vulnerable feelings she was experiencing now. Jean continued to stare and became tearful. The therapist pointed out to Jean that she was safe now, and encouraged her to establish eye contact with each member of the group. With visible difficulty, she proceeded to establish eye contact with each group member who made supportive and caring remarks to her. In this way she was faced with a differentiation between the time of the abuse and the present—a time when it was now safe to look at others without rejection or humiliation.

Hyperarousal. Hyperarousal symptoms are addressed through the use of cognitive distancing methods and group support. IPGT utilizes cognitive distancing techniques in an educational format to support members' intellectual understanding of PTSD as an illness separate from a victim's motivations, personality, or history. Formal instruction about trauma and recovery helps establish a boundary between the illness and the self. The use of the blackboard to present essential material for each session creates an impersonal element framing the group session at its beginning and end. In addition, during the open interaction—as emotions run high and traumatic schemata threaten to pull everyone in—the board remains an impassive and unalterable reminder of the "facts," which can be referred to by therapists or clients to ground the discussion. The homework assignments provide another arena where the intellectual and reflective aspects of clients are evoked after the group, in their own homes. Reference to these assignments during the group can also serve as a grounding tool to ease the level of arousal. Finally, the atmosphere of real support provided by the group, including verbal praise, caring embraces, and holding hands, allows the process of arousal to be lived through and detoxified.

A third clinical example shows how a client's hyperarousal symptoms were alleviated in a group.

Lisa had been raped by her brother and his teenage friends when she was 8 years old. During the assault she was humiliated and was asked to walk naked in front of the boys as they commented on her body. She was overwhelmed with fear and shame. She primarily felt that she was to blame for the incident, and also felt that her body had let her down. Over the years she did not reveal the assault to anyone, as she felt responsible for it and worried that she would be again humiliated. She suffered from multiple episodes of depression and engaged in quite severe self-mutilation. Even indirect reminders of the trauma evoked intense states of hyperarousal, which led her to avoid many social situations.

During Phase 2, as the group reviewed the topic "Befriending Your Body," Lisa became visibly anxious and agitated. When the therapist asked what she was experiencing, she reported intense shame over her body, similar to the shame she had experienced during her abuse. She said she was afraid she was going to lose control if she couldn't distract herself, and then asked to leave, "before I blow up or cut myself." She became tearful, exclaiming loudly, "I hate my body. It's disgusting!" Lisa was clearly very aroused, and refused to make eye contact with the group members. The therapist instructed her to look directly at each group member and to ask each one whether she felt any disgust toward her right now. With great effort, Lisa asked each group member this question, and received very warm and supportive responses. Some pointed out to her that it was her brother and his friends who had let her down and should be shamed. Lisa smiled with appreciation, but she continued to be visibly agitated. During the wrap-up, the therapist used Lisa's behavior in the group to illustrate on the board how victims of sexual assault sometimes perceive their bodies as their enemies. Lisa contributed several items to the list on the board of methods of punishing the body. The therapist asked her to explain each one, which she did articulately, pointing to the board. Speaking about her self-mutilation in an intellectual framework helped her to gain some control over her feelings, which led to a significant reduction in her anxiety. The therapist predicted to Lisa that she might feel shame later that night at home and might feel urges to cut herself. Lisa was then asked to contribute to a list of support behaviors that might help her not cut herself. The following week she reported that she had not cut herself; instead, she had told her husband about her revelation in the group.

Clinical Challenges

The structured nature of IPGT provides a significant source of safety and control that allows members to attend to the therapeutic process. However, two situations in particular may arise that may threaten the effectiveness of a group. First, clients may become highly aroused during the trauma reenactments, and those with strong dissociative tendencies may be unable to maintain their attention to the therapeutic process and therapist interventions. In such a case, a therapist must maintain close contact with a client to make sure that she is not dissociating; if she is, the therapist waits until she returns and then repeats the intervention. Second, certain clients (particularly those with significant narcissistic features) may respond to the emergence of traumatic memories by attacking the structure, leadership, or rules of the group, and by appearing uninterested in exploring the traumatic material. In this case, the therapists should directly identify the link between the clients' angry response and their traumatic experience, providing them sufficient attention to ameliorate the fears of abandonment that were aroused by the approach to the trauma.

Empirical Support

The IPGT model was tested on a sample of 33 women in five groups, who were aged 18 to 65 and had been victims or witnesses of trauma in childhood and/or adulthood (Lubin et al., 1998). Those who were in acute crisis, were actively abusing substances, or were currently psychotic or suicidal were excluded. Four subjects (12%) dropped out before completing treatment. The groups were led by two cotherapists who were blind to the quantitative assessment data collected by research assistants. Trained clinician interviewers administered the study measures to subjects at baseline, at 1-month intervals during treatment, at termination, and at a 6-month follow-up. This evaluation included a review of trauma history and an assessment of PTSD and general psychiatric symptomatology. Conclusions from this study are limited by the absence of treatment comparison groups.

The sample was on average 41 years old; 86% of the subjects were European Americans, and most were college-educated. The subjects had experienced from two to five traumas from childhood through adulthood, including accidents, physical and sexual abuse, rape, and witnessing murder or suicide. On average, their last trauma had occurred 14 years earlier. The majority of the sample (66%) were victims of trauma or violence perpetrated within the family setting.

The subjects were particularly symptomatic and suffering from several comorbid diagnoses. On average, each subject met criteria for three DSM-

III-R diagnoses, and about half had been hospitalized and/or had attempted suicide. The average Global Assessment of Functioning score was 55. Only 38% were employed full-time. Over three-fourths of the sample satisfied criteria for disorders of extreme stress. Subjects had been in outpatient psychotherapy for an average of 7 years.

Subjects demonstrated significant reductions in their PTSD symptoms, as measured by the Clinician-Administered PTSD Scale (CAPS; Blake et al., 1990) on all subscales and total symptomatology (26 of 29 subjects improved). These reductions were evident within the first month of treatment, and subjects continued to show improvement at termination and through the 6-month follow-up (see Figure 6.2). Subjects also showed significant reductions in depressive and dissociative symptoms. General psychopathology diminished to a lesser extent.

This preliminary study suggests that IPGT was consistently effective across five cohorts of women, primarily in reducing core PTSD symptoms, and secondarily in diminishing the levels of other types of psychiatric distress. These gains were largely retained at a 6-month follow-up. The fact that improvement was more prominent among PTSD symptoms than among general psychiatric symptoms is strongly suggestive of a specific treatment effect. Gains were equally evident among subjects varying in age, type and recency of trauma, type of perpetrator, education, and marital status, suggesting that the treatment may have applicability to a wide range of trauma populations.

These results are particularly encouraging, given the severity of ill-

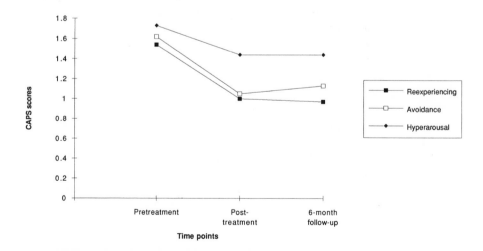

FIGURE 6.2. Reduction of PTSD symptoms in IPGT ($n = 29$). Data from Lubin, Loris, Burt, and Johnson (1998).

ness (e.g., extent of trauma, prior hospitalizations, high comorbidity) and treatment resistance (e.g., years of prior treatment) evident in this sample. Many women reported that significant improvements had occurred in their relationships with their spouses and family members, which persisted at follow-up. The IPGT model, like CPT, appears to have promise as a group-based intervention designed to ameliorate the core PTSD symptoms.

Application

The IPGT model has been implemented with various populations with a comorbid diagnosis of PTSD, including male veterans, female substance abusers, persons with chronic mental illness, sexually abused males, and individuals with personality disorders. Approximately 60 groups have been run over the course of 7 years. The model is designed to benefit from the inclusion of clients with heterogeneous traumas. Qualitative evaluations of results indicate similar positive outcomes among these populations.

COUNTERTRANSFERENCE ISSUES

In CPT and cognitive-behavioral treatments in general, client transference/ projective responses and accompanying therapist countertransference responses are not viewed as essential to the healing action of the therapy, but rather as potentially interfering factors that may diminish treatment effects. As such, intense transference is avoided where possible through attention to the structure and task. In contrast, IPGT anticipates the projection of traumatic schemata onto the group and the therapists, and utilizes such transferences as means of engaging with and then altering these traumatic schemata. Nevertheless, engaging intimately with traumatized clients can be highly stressful for therapists; it can even lead to countertransference reactions best described as "vicarious traumatization" (Pearlman & Saakvitne, 1995; Wilson & Lindy, 1994).

In our experience, transference configurations in trauma groups tend to align themselves along four positions in what might be called the central trauma scenario: "victim," "perpetrator," "bystander," and "collaborator." These positions constitute the core object relations of the traumatic schema, and may shift rapidly among participants. As the client is reengaged in the traumatic schema, often but not always as victim, external representations of the other roles are sought in the therapists or group members. Thus it is common for a therapist to be accused of just standing by and observing a client's pain (bystander), of colluding with family members or society by not believing the client's story (collaborator), or even of putting undue pressure on the client out of sadistic pleasure (perpetrator). Paradoxically, at these challenging moments a therapist can be made to feel like a victim being mistreated by a client/perpetrator. To the extent that these projections find their mark and are supported by defensive efforts of the others to reject them, the here-and-now interactions among group members will become distorted along the lines of the traumatic schema—triggering similar projections among other group members, and thus leading to a rapid descent into regressive group dynamics and inattention to the therapeutic tasks. It is therefore essential for the group therapists to anticipate the evocation of such projective object relations, to be comfortable (i.e., not defensive) with being enrolled in these ways, and to be prepared to utilize these occasions as opportunities to engage clients in moderating interactions. In the IPGT model, as has been described above, a therapist will embrace a projection, but then attempt to introduce discrepant information from the current situation to disrupt the traumatic schema.

As has been discussed in other chapters of this book, treating trauma victims with PTSD is a challenging task, for one must be able to fall back into the darkness of their terror and then be able to return with them. Countertransferential responses that overemphasize rationality and reassurance tend to minimize the truth of clients' experience and support denial and avoidance, whereas countertransference responses that highlight the excitement, heroism, and drama of the event tend to encapsulate clients as "trauma survivors" and to partition their experience of the world (Wilson & Lindy, 1994). In this aspect, we have found that skills developed during training in psychodynamic forms of therapy can be of significant benefit when applied in cognitive-behavioral models of group therapy that target PTSD symptoms (Pearlman & Saakvitne, 1995).

SUMMARY

The field of group therapy for trauma victims with PTSD is a complex and rapidly developing one. Group therapy can serve as a primary treatment for PTSD symptoms when the group format is specifically designed toward that end. Two models of group therapy have been described that hold promise as means of decreasing PTSD symptomatology. Both are time-limited interventions that should be considered as part of a comprehensive treatment for the sequelae of trauma, which may also include long-term individual or group therapy, rehabilitative and creative therapies, and encouragement of public testimony and social advocacy. The essential feature of these treatments is their attention to the symptom pictures of individuals in the context of their psychosocial functioning, as well as a relentless pursuit of distorted traumatic schemata and confrontation of faulty cognitions (CPT) or lack of differentiation (IPGT).

NOTE

1. Because of our original focus on work with multiply traumatized women in IPGT, we use feminine pronouns in this discussion to refer to an IPGT client.

REFERENCES

Alexander, P., Neimeyer, R., Follete, V., Moore, M., & Harter, S. (1989). A comparison of group therapy treatment of women sexually abused as children. *Journal of Consulting and Clinical Psychology, 57*(4), 479–483.

Allen, S., & Bloom, S. (1994). Group and family treatment of posttraumatic stress disorder. *Psychiatric Clinics of North America, 17*, 425–437.

American Psychiatric Association. (1994). *Diagnostic and statistical manual of mental disorders* (4th ed.). Washington, DC: Author.

Blake, D. D., Weathers, F. W., Nagy, L. M., Kaloupek, D., Klauminzer, G., Charney, D., & Keane, T. (1990). A clinician rating scale for assessing current and lifetime PTSD: The CAPS-1. *The Behavior Therapist, 13*, 187–188.

Bloom, S. (1997). *Creating sanctuary.* New York: Routledge.

Brende, J. (1983). The psychodynamic view of character pathology in Vietnam combat veterans. *Bulletin of the Menninger Clinic, 47*, 193–216.

Browne, A., & Finkelhor, D. (1986). Impact of child sexual abuse: A review of the research. *Psychological Bulletin, 99*, 66–77.

Carver, C., Stalker, C., Stewart, E., & Abraham, B. (1989). The impact of group therapy for adult survivors of childhood sexual abuse. *Canadian Journal of Psychiatry, 34*, 753–758.

Catherall, D. (1989). Differentiating intervention strategies for primary and secondary trauma in post-traumatic stress disorder: The example of Vietnam veterans. *Journal of Traumatic Stress, 2*, 289–304.

Cole, C., & Barney, E. (1987). Safeguards and the therapeutic window: A group treatment strategy for adult incest survivors. *American Journal of Orthopsychiatry, 57*, 601–609.

Cooper, N. A., & Clum, G. A. (1989). Imaginal flooding as a supplementary treatment for posttraumatic stress disorder in combat veterans: A controlled study. *Behavior Therapy, 20*, 381–391.

Davidson, J., Kudler, H., & Smith, R. (1990). Treatment of post traumatic stress disorder with amitriptyline and placebo. *Archives of General Psychiatry, 47*, 259–266.

Fairbank, J., & Keane, T. (1982). Flooding for combat-related stress disorder: Assessment of anxiety reduction across traumatic memories. *Behavior Therapy, 13*, 499–510.

Foa, E. B., & Kozak, M. J. (1986). The emotional processing of fear: Exposure to corrective information. *Psychological Bulletin, 99*, 20–35.

Foa, E. B., Riggs, D. S., Dancu, C., & Rothbaum, B. O. (1993). Reliability and validity of a brief instrument assessing posttraumatic stress disorder. *Journal of Traumatic Stress, 6*, 459–474.

Foa, E. B., Rothbaum, B. O., Riggs, D. S., & Murdock, T. B. (1991). Treatment of post-traumatic stress disorder in rape victims: A comparison between a cognitive-behavioral procedure and counseling. *Journal of Consulting and Clinical Psychology, 59,* 715–723.

Fontana, A., & Rosenheck, R. (1997). Effectiveness and cost of inpatient treatment for posttraumatic stress disorder. *American Journal of Psychiatry, 154,* 758–765.

Frank, E., Anderson, B., Steward, B. D., Dancu, C., Hughes, C., & West, D. (1988). Efficacy of cognitive-behavioral therapy and systematic desensitization in the treatment of rape trauma. *Behavior Therapy, 19,* 403–420.

Frueh, B., Turner, S., Beidel, D., Mirabella, R., & Jones, W. (1996). Trauma management therapy: A preliminary evaluation of a multicomponent behavioral treatment for chronic combat-related PTSD. *Behaviour Research and Therapy, 34,* 533–543.

Gil, E. (1988). *Treatment of adult survivors of childhood abuse.* Walnut Creek, CA: Launch Press.

Goodman, B., & Nowak-Scibelli, D. (1985). Group treatment for women incestuously abused as children. *International Journal of Group Psychotherapy, 35,* 531–544.

Hall, Z., Mullee, M., & Thompson, C. (1995). A clinical and service evaluation of group therapy for women survivors of childhood sexual abuse. In M. Aveline & D. A. Shapiro (Eds.), *Research foundations for psychotherapy practice* (pp. 263–279). New York: Wiley.

Hazzard, A., Rogers, J. H., & Angert, L. (1993). Factors affecting group therapy outcome for adult sexual abuse survivors. *International Journal of Group Psychotherapy, 43*(4), 453–468.

Herman, J. (1992). *Trauma and recovery.* New York: Basic Books.

Herman, J., & Schatzow, E. (1984). Time limited group psychotherapy for women with a history of incest. *International Journal of Group Psychotherapy, 34,* 605–610.

Johnson, D., Feldman, S., Lubin, H., & Southwick, S. (1995). The use of ritual and ceremony in the treatment of post-traumatic stress disorder. *Journal of Traumatic Stress, 8,* 283–299.

Johnson, D., Feldman, S., Southwick, S., & Charney, D. (1994). The concept of the second generation program in the treatment of post-traumatic stress disorder among Vietnam veterans. *Journal of Traumatic Stress, 7,* 217–236.

Johnson, D., Lubin, H., Rosenheck, R., Fontana, A., Southwick, S., & Charney, D. (1997). Measuring the impact of homecoming on the development of post-traumatic stress disorder: The West Haven Homecoming Stress Scale. *Journal of Traumatic Stress, 10,* 259–278.

Johnson, D., Rosenheck, R., Fontana, A., Lubin, H., Southwick, S., & Charney, D. (1996). Outcome of intensive inpatient for combat-related PTSD. *American Journal of Psychiatry, 153,* 771–777.

Keane, T. M., Fairbank, J. A., Caddell, J. M., & Zimering, R. T. (1989). Implosive (flooding) therapy reduces symptoms of PTSD in Vietnam combat veterans. *Behavior Therapy, 20,* 245–260.

Kilpatrick, D., Veronen, L., & Resick, P. (1982). Psychological sequelae to rape: Assessment and treatment strategies. In D. Dolays & R. Meredith (Eds.), *Behavioral medicine: Assessment and treatment strategies* (pp. 473–497). New York: Plenum Press.

Linehan, M. M. (1993). *Cognitive-behavioral treatment of borderline personality disorder.* New York: Guilford Press.

Lubin, H., & Johnson, D. (1997a). Interactive psychoeducational group therapy for traumatized women. *International Journal of Group Psychotherapy, 47,* 271–290.

Lubin, H., & Johnson, D. (1997b). *Training manual for IPGT.* New Haven, CT: Post Traumatic Stress Center.

Lubin, H., & Johnson, D. (1998). Healing ceremonies. *Family Therapy Networker, 22,* 39–42.

Lubin, H., Loris, M., Burt, J., & Johnson, D. (1998). Efficacy of psychoeducational group therapy in reducing symptoms of posttraumatic stress disorder among multiply-traumatized women. *American Journal of Psychiatry, 155,* 1172–1177.

Marmar, C. R., Foy, D., Kagan, B., & Pynoos, R. (1993). An integrated approach for treating post-traumatic stress. In J. M. Oldham, M. B. Riba, & A. Tasman (Eds.), *American Psychiatric Association review of psychiatry* (Vol. 12, pp. 239–272). Washington, DC: American Psychiatric Press.

McCann, I. L., & Pearlman, L. A. (1990). *Psychological trauma and the adult survivor.* New York: Brunner/Mazel.

Neimeyer, R., Harter, S., & Alexander, P. (1991). Group perceptions as predictors of outcome in the treatment of incest survivors. *Psychology Research, 1*(2), 148–158.

Parson, E. R. (1985). Post-traumatic accelerated cohesion: Its recognition and management in group treatment of Vietnam veterans. *Group, 9,* 10–23.

Pearlman, L., & Saakvitne, K. (1995). *Trauma and the therapist.* New York: Norton.

Resick, P., Jordan, C., Girelli, S., Hutter, C., & Marhoefer-Dvorak, S. (1988). A comparative outcome study of behavioral group therapy for sexual assault victims. *Behavior Therapy, 19,* 385–401.

Resick, P., & Schnicke, M. (1993). *Cognitive processing therapy for rape victims.* Newbury Park, CA: Sage.

Roth, S., Dye, E., & Lebowitz, L. (1988). Group therapy for sexual assault victims. *Psychotherapy, 25,* 82–93.

Scurfield, R. M. (1993). Treatment of post-traumatic stress disorder among Vietnam veterans. In J. P. Wilson & B. Raphael (Eds.), *International handbook of traumatic stress syndromes* (pp. 879–888). New York: Plenum Press.

Shalev, A. Y., Bonne, O., & Eth, S. (1996). Treatment of posttraumatic stress disorder: A review. *Psychosomatic Medicine, 58,* 165–182.

Shatan, C. (1973). The grief of soldiers: Vietnam combat veterans self-help movement. *American Journal of Orthopsychiatry, 43,* 640–653.

Shestatzky, M., Greenberg, D., & Lerer, B. (1988). A controlled trial of phenelzine in post-traumatic stress disorder. *Psychiatry Research, 24,* 149–155.

Solomon, S. D., Gerrity, E. T., & Muff, A. M. (1992). Efficacy of treatment for posttraumatic stress disorder: An empirical review. *Journal of the American Medical Association, 268,* 633–638.

van der Kolk, B. A. (1987). The role of the group in the origin and resolution of the trauma response. In B. A. van der Kolk (Ed.), *Psychological trauma* (pp. 153–171). Washington, DC: American Psychiatric Press.

van der Kolk, B. A., Dreyfuss, D., Michaels, M., Shera, D., Berkowitz, R., Fisler, R., & Saxe, G. (1994). Fluoxetine in posttraumatic stress disorder. *Journal of Clinical Psychiatry, 55,* 517–522.

Waites, E. (1993). *Trauma and survival.* New York: Norton.

Wilson, J. P., & Lindy, J. D. (Eds.). (1994). *Countertransference in the treatment of PTSD.* New York: Guilford Press.

Yalom, I. (1975). *Theory and practice of group psychotherapy* (3rd ed.). New York: Basic Books.

Zlotnick, C., Shea, M. T., Rosen, K., Simpson, E., Mulrenin, K., Begin, A., & Pearlstein, T. (1997). An affect management group for women with posttraumatic stress disorder and histories of childhood sexual abuse. *Journal of Traumatic Stress, 10,* 425–436.

7

◄◦►

Group Psychotherapy for Survivors of Sexual and Physical Abuse

BONNIE J. BUCHELE

SPECIAL ASPECTS OF SEXUAL AND PHYSICAL ABUSE

All trauma involves being overwhelmed by an event beyond the range of normal human experience. Sexual and physical abuse, however, are unique traumatizations because the psychological fear of death or annihilation is coupled with physical activities and/or sensations; thus disturbances that have physical components (e.g., eating disorders, sexual dysfunction, hypochondriasis) are common sequelae. In addition, another human being organizes, implements, and inflicts these traumatic events. The resulting fear of helplessness (i.e., once again being at the mercy of fate) is accompanied by the terror of becoming the focus of intentional and mobilized evil. Achieving mastery—the pillar of recovery from trauma—means trusting others when the mind and the body of each survivor know that in some way trusting another made him or her vulnerable to being hurt. There are no short cuts here: Trust cannot be reestablished by denying the existence of evil in the world or in people, as many of us typically do from time to time. The solutions are developing a belief that good can overcome evil and developing confidence that one can cope with whatever happens. These are Herculean tasks that must be accomplished step by step over time; only then can the survivor feel safe enough to risk trusting again.

Trauma intentionally inflicted by another human being—often a trusted person—is more damaging than trauma associated with a natural disaster (Allen, 1995; Gelinas, 1993). Just as trust is at the center of these traumatizations, so are power dynamics. Whether the actual abuse of power involved misuse of larger physical size, abdication of caretaking responsibility, or both, the survivor's view of and coexistence with power and authority are forever altered. These traumatizations also involve boundary violations, which are experienced as psychological and physical assaults on the self; these often leave the survivor with a fragmented, narcissistically troubled, and poorly defined sense of self. Most frequently, sexual or physical abuse occurs in an atmosphere of privacy, enhancing the subsequent sense of shame, which reinforces the need for secrecy. Public feedback, which would help the victim to know that self-blame is inappropriate, is not available.

Any trauma has a characterological impact, but these traumata may have a more profound effect because of the trust issues involved, as well as their often prolonged and repeated nature, leading to a pervasive interweaving of character with posttraumatic stress disorder (PTSD). The earlier in life the events occur, the more significant their impact on later character development and resolution of subsequent developmental conflict, such as Oedipal conflicts and conflicts associated with achieving the depressive position as posited by Melanie Klein (1946/1975).

In this chapter, I discuss group psychotherapy for survivors of sexual and physical abuse. The types of traumatization reviewed here include incest, child molestation, childhood physical abuse, rape, and spousal abuse. "Incest" as defined here involves three factors: (1) inappropriate sexual activity (2) initiated by a caretaker or caretaker surrogate (3) in the context of an ongoing caretaking relationship. In this definition I am taking a position that sexual abuse of a child by any ongoing caretaker (blood relative or not) is a type of or close to incest, because of the violation of trust within the relationship. "Child molestation" is inappropriate sexual activity initiated with a child by an adult without an ongoing caretaking relationship between those persons. "Physical abuse in childhood" includes harsh beatings, threats of violence, and deprivation (Allen, 1995). "Rape" is forced sexual intercourse between adults. Finally, "spousal abuse" involves battering and/or rape occurring in the context of an ongoing committed relationship between two adults. (All of these definitions are clinical, not legal.) Of note are the facts that these types of trauma are initiated (1) by human beings who (2) often have some kind of relationship with the people they are traumatizing and (3) usually have physical components.

RATIONALE FOR GROUP
PSYCHOTHERAPY FOR ABUSE

Group psychotherapy is particularly suited for treatment of sexual and physical abuse. The psychotherapy group, with its intimate yet public atmosphere, affords opportunities to safely dilute the sense of shame and secrecy by hearing about others' experiences and sharing one's own. A therapist facilitates this process, especially early in the group, by drawing attention to similarities in members' experiences—including fears of being exposed as defective, and fears of retaliation should the silence be broken.

> In a women's group, one member experienced immense relief as she, for the first time, talked about a beating she had received from her husband during a previous marriage. Many months later, she reluctantly revealed that she had won a lawsuit, the terms of which included no public disclosure of the settlement. As other members talked about fear of retaliation from those who had abused them, she discovered that she was repeating a pattern—"keeping the secret," just as she had been ordered to do when beaten by her husband, for fear of retaliation. She had kept the "secret" of the lawsuit in its entirety from the group, not even mentioning it despite its importance in her life, even though the terms of the settlement had been simply that she not disclose the *amount* of the settlement.

The isolation begins to be replaced by a sense of affiliation. As group members speak and interact, work on trust issues begins. This work is dramatically augmented as the transference to the therapist blossoms, so that trust issues can be examined in the context of a relationship with an authority figure. Time and time again, the therapist will be feared and hated as he or she is perceived to abuse power or neglect group members; alternatively, idealization may stubbornly persist for many months as the group protects itself from the thought that the therapist could do harm. Group boundaries, such as timely payment of fees, punctual attendance, confidentiality, and minimal extragroup contacts, will be violated. Only as the therapist firmly encourages exploration of transference distortions and boundary violations are the intense conflicts about authority worked through.

THE ROLES OF DEFENSES

Certain defenses are particularly suited to coping with trauma and greatly influence the transference and group ambience. Although this is not meant to be an exhaustive list, the most frequent are dissociation, splitting, projective identification, denial, acting out, identification with the aggressor, and repression. The primary purpose of all defenses is to lessen the piercing psychological pain that continues after the trauma has ended.

When dissociation is present, a group member experiences a vertical split or rupture of the sense of self, memory/affect, and consciousness; there is a gap in these functions. The painful experiences are deposited in the separate, parallel consciousness, memory, and sense of self. Very often, individuals describe living through the original trauma by "going away" from the actual experience into a fantasy, wallpaper on the wall, a painting, or the like. Dealing with dissociation can be a very difficult task for the group's therapist for several reasons. The dissociation at the time of the trauma can substantially alter the actual psychological experience of traumatization, so that memory is distorted. In addition, when events in group sessions occur that act as triggers for retraumatization (e.g., another group member's traumatic story), dissociation can occur as a protective mechanism *during the session*, thus preventing the group member from taking in the session as it occurs. When this happens, the group therapist must draw attention to it and facilitate the member's return to being consciously in the here and now (Buchele, 1993).

In a mixed-gender long-term psychotherapy group, the theme of one particular session was that the world is a dangerous place, especially because women will betray and neglect others. The therapist began by updating the group on her discussion with a female clerk in the state office for disability benefits, who was threatening to refuse to authorize additional reimbursement for Nancy's group psychotherapy. Another patient empathized with Nancy's distress, and then Nancy grew silent. A different member talked about how she was fearful of attending a class reunion, because she expected her female classmates to ridicule and exclude her as they had in school. A fourth woman, a teacher, reported that her female students had pulled a prank on her and she had fallen as a result. A fifth member told the group how his mother had recently verbally berated him for associating with his father, from whom the mother was divorced. Following the therapist's interpretation that it sounded as if the group felt the world to be a very unsafe place, in part because the women one trusted would neglect, betray, and even attack, Nancy—much of whose experience with her mother had consisted of criticism and rejection—stayed silent. The therapist waited a while to see whether Nancy would resume participation, but she sank deeper in her chair and made eye contact with no one. Other members did not address her. Finally, as soon as there was an opportunity, the therapist asked Nancy directly how she was faring. Cryptically, Nancy answered, "I'm fine." The therapist and members observed that Nancy seemed to have been "going away" (the group's term for dissociating). Nancy denied this, but appeared silently attentive for the remainder of the session. It is likely that the patient experienced the announcement that the woman case manager was thinking about discontinuing payment for her treatment as a stimulus for reexperiencing situations when her mother was critical, depriving, and neglectful. Nancy attempted to ward off the pain by dissociating, but the stimulus grew stronger as other members recounted betrayals by women and the therapist made the interpretation; then Nancy, in response, sank into a deeper dissociative state. Transferentially she experienced the women and female therapist in the group as dangerous, so that Nancy could not engage in dialogue about her symptoms. Being addressed, however, did at least reorient her to the here and now.

The rupture of ego functions (i.e., memory, consciousness, sense of time, management of affect) that is central to dissociation has particular consequences for the trauma survivor. There is little sense of continuity of self because of the huge gaps in memory; the survivor cannot remember what he or she was doing at various times, and therefore worries about past behavior. There is an experience of inability to count on oneself to respond in predictable ways. A sense of being calm and competent can be completely disconnected from the state of being angry. The resulting experience is of oneself as scattered, fragmented, and behaving very differently at times for what seems like no reason. Many survivors, searching for an explanation for this experience, believe they are crazy.

In contrast to dissociation, splitting does not remove painful mental contents from awareness; instead, splitting involves the unconscious act of separating good from bad in order to keep the bad from destroying the good and to protect the good. Here an individual (both oneself and others) cannot be experienced as simultaneously good and bad; people are not perceived as whole but as part-objects, either good or bad. Integration of good and bad within the same person is a developmental achievement that can be delayed in childhood trauma victims or regressed from into splitting as a result of trauma.

Karen had three older brothers and was 13 when her parents divorced. Completely preoccupied with fighting each other, the parents and brothers ignored Karen, who acted out significantly during adolescence. She experienced terrible guilt over her adolescent behaviors, believing herself to be a bad person. Her terror and rage over being abandoned, and her own potential subsequent defenselessness, were defended against by seeing herself as a very bad person—the cause of the family's unhappiness and distress. This then allowed her to preserve a view of her parents as loving and caring. When she was mugged in her early 20s, she initially felt totally to blame and believed the world helpful, but this view quickly shifted to seeing everyone in the world as potentially dangerous and herself as good but helpless.

In the group, she lamented the state of her relationship with one brother, stating that he was insensitive and mean. She then could feel herself to be a well-intended, blameless person. In one group session, fearful that she had not passed an important examination, she reported that she had sabotaged her exam; she stated with conviction that the only thing she was certain about in life was her own badness. As others tried to empathize and remind her of her good attributes, she withdrew into silence. She missed the following session without calling, and then there was an interruption due to the therapist's vacation. Upon returning, she declared that the group was not helping her. In response to some expressed disagreements among members that everyone took things too personally, it appeared that Karen was utilizing splitting in order to preserve a good self-image. She needed to see the group as unhelpful—a feeling enhanced by hurt and anger at the therapist about the interruption.

Projective identification is a defense that is a three-step process: (1) Within the context of an emotionally intimate relationship, the unwanted mental contents are projected into another, and there is a grain of truth in the projection; (2) the recipient absorbs the projection, but alters or personalizes it in so doing; and (3) the projector identifies with the recipient, taking the altered projection back in (Ogden, 1989). Several other authors have described this defense in coping with incest.

A colleague and I (Ganzarain & Buchele, 1988) conceptualize incest victims as assuming alternating sides of reciprocal roles in interactions with family, friends, and treaters. Examples are victim versus abuser, rival versus dependent small child, and seductress versus shameful, ignorant one. Both roles exist as identifications within the patient, but one role must be extruded via projective identification to ward off painful conflict. Davies and Frawley (1994) describe four transference–countertransference paradigms that also rely heavily on projective identification in the clinical situation: the unseen, uninvolved parent and the unseen, neglected child; the sadistic abuser and the helpless, impotently enraged victim; the idealized, omnipotent rescuer and the entitled child; and the seducer and the seduced. In Davies and Frawley's formulations, the countertransference is viewed as the treater's experience of being the recipient of group members' projective identifications (i.e., one side of these transference–countertransference paradigms).

After considerable work in individual therapy on her fears of revealing shameful parts of herself, Jan told the group about an affair she had had, which had resulted in a pregnancy that she aborted. Group members empathized and shared similar experiences, but then the group had a scheduled interruption of several weeks' duration. In the next session, Kathy, with considerable drama, stated that the group's previous session had upset her so much that she had required extra sessions with her individual therapist during the group's break. She was morally opposed to affairs and wondered whether she should even be in a group with people who held such beliefs. Jan verbally attacked Kathy, saying that being criticized for the affair had been her worst fear in telling the group. Furthermore, she said, Kathy was usually critical, and Jan found group sessions tense because of her. Kathy became angry in return, saying that her opinion was always seen as wrong, that Jan thought she was special and always right, and that she (Kathy) should just leave this group.

With great difficulty, the therapist and group contained this angry situation for weeks. Ultimately the therapist said, after everyone had struggled to formulate an understanding, that a legitimate disagreement about the issue of affairs had become a life-and-death matter under the force of several transferences (which the therapist understood to be related to projective identification). Jan was projecting her own critical, rejecting side in identification with her mother into Kathy and then struggling mightily against it. Kathy was projecting her competitive, judgmental, attacking side (based on an identification with a cruel sister) into Jan and fighting for survival. Furthermore, the therapist had made the environment an unsafe one by leaving the group, stimulating a "bad mother" transference related to experiences when members' mothers were neglectful or had abandoned them. Shortly thereafter, Kathy and Jan each softened. Other group members verbalized their feelings about affairs, as well as the therapist's absence during the group's break, and Kathy decided to stay.

Denial is often used extensively in surviving trauma. Life events are viewed in an optimistic light, while painful aspects are banished from awareness. Denial can be very adaptive in coping with life until it is used excessively, in which case perceptions of reality are seriously distorted.

One group member who had been raped in early adulthood proudly informed the rest of the group that she was enjoying the new sport of running and doing it at night. When others voiced concern about her safety, she denied that there was any danger, saying that she "stayed close to home."

Dissociation, splitting, projective identification, and denial are some of the more primitive defenses. The extreme pain caused by the trauma pulls for their use. As such, however, they come with considerable psychological cost to a survivor. With all of them, parts of reality are not seen or are distorted markedly. They prevent the survivor from being aware of certain things or from simultaneously comprehending contradictory aspects of self and others. In addition, quick fluctuations in projective identification, dissociation, and splitting add to an internal sense of instability. Since the view of reality can be so altered, and the internal world so quixotic, the overall level of functioning is decreased (i.e., self-care and decision making can be compromised functions).

A defense closely related to projective identification is identification with the aggressor. Here the victim identifies with or takes in the abusing person, becoming like him or her in order to protect against the fear of further traumatization and to achieve mastery. Many traumatized individuals find the idea that they might be like their abusers and hurt someone else consciously terrifying, shameful, repugnant, and therefore unacceptable. When traumatization is prolonged and repeated, however, utilization of the defense is more likely. A deep sense of shame often accompanies and complicates discovery and exploration of this defense in the group. Members are certain that their peers will hate them. Furthermore, many survivors of physical and sexual abuse find having any anger or aggression abhorrent, because they confuse the healthy expression of aggression with abusive behavior. In fact, for survivors to have the best chance for the most complete recovery, analysis of their own aggression and management of it must occur; however, this aspect of the treatment can easily be omitted. The longed-for self-image of many survivors is one absent of aggression, and a frequent countertransference difficulty is experiencing patients as simultaneously abused and aggressive. The emotions can be so strong that therapists, as well as their patients, manage the painful confusion by taking a unidimensional view that excludes patients' aggressive sides.

As noted elsewhere (Ganzarain & Buchele, 1987), acting out is taking action to express feelings rather than thinking, talking, or reflecting about them. These actions keep the particular emotional conflict out of awareness, but simultaneously are communications about the problem. Examples may be missing sessions rather than verbalizing anger and mistrust of the therapist, or going from one romantic relationship to another instead of exploring the painful conflicts associated with intimacy. The solution to the problems attendant to acting out is working through, which involves several sequential steps in group psychotherapy:

1. Identifying interactions in the group that are instances of acting out.
2. Helping group members verbalize the impulses being acted out in understandable ways.
3. Facilitating each member's application of the newly discovered material to understanding him- or herself better, especially to understanding how the same behaviors appear repeatedly in different contexts.
4. Fostering members' new realizations in reflections of themselves based on new awareness of the repetition of the behaviors.
5. Integrating these fresh awarenesses into the images of self and other, thus leading to character change.

In one heterogeneous, extended psychotherapy group, a number of changes and interruptions occurred within several months. One member terminated in a planned way; another left with short preparatory time; a new member joined; one session was canceled unexpectedly by the therapist; and another session was canceled due to a holiday. Two members with trauma histories angrily attacked the therapist for being insensitive, incompetent, and uncaring, but disagreed when the therapist suggested that they might be feeling abandoned because of the cancellations and a feeling of instability in the group. Amidst all the changes, a third member maintained her stance that she was angry because, despite her being visibly upset, the therapist had insisted on ending the meeting on time. The group was able to work shortly thereafter, but the underlying atmosphere contained elements of an unresolved trust issue. Meanwhile, the therapist learned that the two angriest members were staying in the lobby and talking for an extended time after group sessions. The therapist brought the issue up in the group, as a third member disclosed her feeling of alienation from the group. The therapist wondered aloud whether it might be helpful to discuss in the session what had occurred in the outside contacts, since it was possible that the third member was feeling excluded as one part of her sense of alienation. Both members said that much of their discussions had been about matters other than therapy, but then the member feeling cut off said she had asked one of the other two members (a man) about additional treatment modalities he had utilized, wondering whether they would be helpful for her. The therapist suggested that the cut-off member may have been expressing her feeling of being unattended to and anger about being cut off by, in effect, extending the session with the other two members and exploring other treatments. The cut-off member agreed that she had those needs and might have expressed them that way. The therapist was attempting to move the expression of feelings from taking action to putting them into words; however, she chose to emphasize the adaptive aspect of feeling needy first, with less emphasis on the expression of anger, since the atmosphere of the group was still volatile. She was trying to minimize narcissistic injury and the chance of further explosions of anger.

Repression and dissociation both banish painful experiences from consciousness, but they operate quite differently. Repression eliminates painful events from consciousness so that they are forgotten; a horizontal division of mental contents occurs. Some memories are allowed into consciousness, but painful material is pressed down into the unconscious. Entire traumatic experiences or specific aspects of them are often repressed. It is not unusual for new group members to retrieve previously repressed memories as they enter a trauma group and hear the histories of other members. One challenging task for the group therapist is to attempt to titrate the amount of actual trauma material in group sessions, so that members are not overwhelmed and retraumatized by memories' surfacing as they listen to peers.

In a group of women with trauma histories, Ursula tearfully updated the group on her inability to become pregnant and her upcoming appointment with an infertility specialist. Sobbing, she revealed her fantasy that she would never be able to conceive, as punishment for the venereal disease she had contracted during adolescence. Stories of interrupted pregnancies and childbirths poured forth. One member, in a subsequent individual session, confessed that when she was very young, she had miscarried after receiving a similar diagnosis. She said she thought she had worked the resulting guilt, anxiety, and self-hatred through and had virtually forgotten the experience, but she had found the group session itself very disturbing. Shortly thereafter, her self-destructive behavior resumed with such vengeance that hospitalization was required.

Identification with the aggressor, acting out, and especially repression are somewhat higher-order defenses. They protect against psychic pain in a less costly way. Perception of reality is less distorted, and since rapid internal fluctuations are less prominent, the survivor's sense of self is less fragmented and disrupted by their use. One would hope that in a successful treatment process, the group members become able to utilize higher-level defenses more and primitive ones less.

NEUROBIOLOGY OF TRAUMATIZATION

The experience of traumatization alters brain chemistry and structure. When a trauma is sufficiently long, intense, or frequent, neurophysiological activation (i.e., changes in receptor sensitivity following increased neurotransmitter activity and increased catecholamine activity) leads to sensitization. Responsiveness is quicker and greater and can contribute to affective lability, hypervigilance, increased startle response, and other reactivity associated with PTSD (Bartlett, 1998). Decreased responsiveness to reward related to stress-induced changes in the dopaminergic mesocorticolimbic system may contribute to the depression and anhedonia that accompany PTSD (Allen, 1996). Serotonin dysfunction induced by stress can result in impaired functioning of the behavioral inhibition system, effecting compulsive reenactment of trauma-related behavior patterns, aggressive outbursts, and impulsivity (van der Kolk, 1996). Intense fear also stimulates increased secretion of endogenous opioid peptides, which in turn interferes with the storage of experience and explicit memory; thus traumatic experiences are often not stored as verbal memories, but rather as physical states (i.e., unsymbolized experiences).

It is likely that a return to normal physical brain functioning following trauma is facilitated by turning to a trusted figure for comfort. When the abuse has been inflicted by the very person who would normally be the source of comfort, however—as is the case in incest, childhood physical abuse, and spousal abuse, for instance—this return to normal brain functioning is hampered and the likelihood of permanent change is enhanced.

These recent findings about the neurobiology of trauma have direct treatment implications. Reworking traumatic experiences at a higher cortical level (i.e., creating new associative networks) is one important aspect of healing and can probably best be accomplished within the soothing security of a set of safe, trusting relationships in the group. Decreasing arousal, focusing on the here and now, and promoting self-care are essential to make the environment safe and to facilitate formation of new associative networks; often these steps must precede interpretation, which facilitates the acquisition of understanding and insight. Therefore, it may be necessary to employ parameters that are somewhat nontraditional. For instance, contact with the individual or group therapist via extragroup calls or the addition of individual sessions to decrease arousal, especially in early phases of treatment, may be crucial to promoting these neurobiological changes.

> Anita, a college professor, was a member of a women's group; she had been raped in young adult life by a family friend, but had told no one for decades. As Anita began in the group, she recounted many somatic problems, several of them related to anxiety arousal (i.e., gastrointestinal difficulties, sleep disturbance, suspected cardiac problems). Furthermore, the physical difficulties themselves stimulated anxiety. Much as she had done after the rape, however, she usually discussed her physical stress with no one, including the group. Anita appeared to have a low anxiety threshold, either not realizing she was anxious or taking it for granted as her normal state. Often she could not put her distress into words. In the group, the work consisted of helping her identify when she was anxious, encouraging her to verbalize it, and providing psychoeducation about the neurobiology of the brain relevant to trauma and how it applied to her (especially her hyperarousal and difficulty in containing anxiety). To further these goals, the therapist urged Anita to phone her in two sets of circumstances: (1) whenever she became intolerably anxious between sessions, to facilitate containing; and (2) to report achievements in managing her anxiety (e.g., good results from a doctor's appointment or successful resolution of a particular anxiety-provoking problem), to increase her sense of reward for her efforts.

COUNTERTRANSFERENCE

Diagnosing and managing the countertransference in the treatment of survivors of sexual and physical abuse are crucial. Recent research on memory tells us that both treators and survivors will never know the *exact* truth about what happened, because of normal alteration of memory and the idiosyncratic ways in which traumatic memory is taken into the brain (Brenneis, 1996; Fonagy, 1999; Target, 1998). A therapist can, however, acquire vital information about traumatic experiences and the impact they have had on an individual's object relations via the relationship with the therapist, especially via the countertransference (Scharff & Scharff, 1994). A few of the more problematic, but common, countertransferences are discussed here. Therapist dread of group sessions may be the first indicator that patients are responding to impending interruptions with fear of victimization: The group atmosphere, losing its consistency, is experienced as unpredictable and unsafe, and the therapist is experienced by the patients in the transference as an unreliable, incompetent protector/parent. In turn, the therapist may feel deskilled and incompetent, dreading the experience of interventions that repeatedly have no apparent therapeutic effect.

Although any trauma patient awakens a wish to rescue in a group therapist, this countertransferential response may be more compelling when the trauma has been intentionally inflicted by another human being. The therapist feels the need to make up for the heinous acts of his or her fellow humans and may thus inadvertently interfere with group development. Brabender (1992) posits a model of group development wherein initially group members need to idealize the therapist. Traumatized individuals may also need to idealize the therapist as a defense against the fear of further traumatization. Brabender suggests that in a subsequent phase of group development, the idealization of the group and the therapist must be broken down in order to promote growth. The interaction of the rescuer countertransference with the patients' defensive use of idealization may prolong the idealization phase and stifle group development. In these instances, it would be helpful for the therapist to be vigilant for other countertransferences, such as anger at the survivors and fascination in response to some revelations.

Group therapists can experience intense frustration as they attempt to create a safe "play space" within a very paranoid atmosphere. Extensive use of splitting and projective identification—defenses used in the paranoid–schizoid position, according to Klein (1946/1975), and to which many survivors may need to regress—can lead to an atmosphere filled with wariness and suspicion. In addition, natural development may be impeded because there is little or no play space. Winnicott (1945) described a transitional space created by mother and infant, within which the child learns to fantasize and symbolize. Ogden (1989) has called this phenomenon "play space." When abuse occurs within a family, this space—where ideas can be played with, as well as boundaries between "me" and "not me" explored—is collapsed and destroyed. To begin to rebuild the play space, it is crucial that the group therapist accept the presence of the projections and gently (not defensively) respond by disclaiming them and tenderly beginning to play with ideas and explore boundaries. To the extent that the group therapist is able to be spontaneous and genuine under such tension and stress, the creation of the play space is facilitated; this is a frustrating and demanding task, but, especially in homogeneous groups of traumatized persons, group members can have tremendous difficulty relaxing after their initial relief at being together. Their suspiciousness is heightened in the presence of those who would customarily be thought of as trustworthy figures (i.e., persons in authority and sibling figures).

Managing the paranoid atmosphere, diagnosing the countertransference, monitoring very serious psychopathology of individual members, and experiencing vicarious traumatization (being victimized by listening to another's account of traumatization) can combine to create therapist exhaustion. Sometimes these factors lead to the therapist's experiencing a kind of entitlement, as if he or she deserves special recognition for working so strenuously. For instance, the therapist may feel that he or she should be spared the burden of contacting other treaters of patients in the group, or may expect colleagues to recognize his or her "special" status for working with such a difficult population. The reality aspects of the hard work can blind the therapist to the likelihood that this experience is also a countertransference, mirroring patients' frequent experience of believing that the world owes them many things (including special consideration and status) because they have been deprived so severely and have suffered so much. When this countertransference goes undetected, the group and therapist can collude to avoid analyzing these reactions, and growth is thereby limited.

> Susie, a middle-aged woman suffering from borderline personality disorder and a proclivity for self-mutilation, announced to the group that she was terminating. The group was concerned, and the therapist was worried and anxious. As the subject was explored, the group therapist became aware that several of Susie's other treaters had changed without the group therapist's knowledge; this had occurred because Susie had not reported these events, but also because the therapist realized that she had not maintained contact with the other team members. Tired in her attempts to maintain genuineness and spontaneity in the face of a paranoid, distrustful group ambience, the therapist realized she had felt entitled to recognition for doing such difficult work. She wanted acknowledgment from colleagues for doing this difficult work, and wanted them to initiate contact rather than her taking the responsibility.

Given the disturbed object relations and the intense, primitive transferences and countertransferences that exist in work with this population, the therapist as a real person is very important. Many survivors have an eye-opening first experience within the context of their therapy: a relationship with a safe, collaborative human being who is not perfect (usually idealization is a constructive but tentative first step toward trying to manage the fear inherent in trusting, but it must be worked through or the treatment is incomplete), but whose faults will not lead to retraumatization. Superficial self-disclosure is not ideal or desirable, but being with each patient in an experience-near way (i.e., being emotionally available) is essential. The therapist will be helped tremendously by having a clear theoretical understanding of how he or she is perceived as a transference object, but when the therapist is actually relating to the patient, staying close rather than distant facilitates the therapy. In this way, group psychotherapy of sexually or physically abused patients may be somewhat different from the treatment of other types of problems, where distance is less likely to be perceived as dangerous or abandoning.

TYPES OF GROUPS

Most victims of trauma could benefit from group psychotherapy at some point in their recovery. There are many kinds of group psychotherapy, however, so the question becomes this: What type of group psychotherapy at what point in the healing process is best (Buchele, 1994)? Group psychotherapy commonly varies according to group duration (time-limited vs. extended) and group composition (homogeneous vs. heterogeneous). Time-limited homogeneous (trauma patients only) group psychotherapy can be very helpful as a patient begins to work through trauma issues; breaking the secrecy and isolation in an atmosphere of acceptance is very powerful and can provide the victim with hope that recovery is possible. This type of group is ideally suited to inpatient settings.

Extended group psychotherapy for a homogeneous group of trauma survivors is a second option, but in recent years this has become a somewhat controversial issue. On the positive side of the debate, this type of group psychotherapy is useful because the length of time allows for desired character change through identifying and analyzing patterns of behaving and interacting that emanate from the trauma and occur in many contexts. One common occurrence is that traumatized individuals, especially when the abusive events took place in childhood, often see no relationship between their presenting problems and their trauma histories. Members often realize the connection between their reaction to the trauma and subsequent characterological patterns for the first time as they hear peers unravel the connection in group sessions. In addition, the sine qua non of any therapy (i.e., that the therapeutic setting itself be a safe place) has heightened importance for survivors of sexual and/or physical abuse. Since the abuse often occurred in what should be the safest of places—their homes and intimate relationships—they are skeptical and suspicious about the therapist's promise of a safe atmosphere. Achievable safety may be equated with being in the presence of similarly abused persons; everyone else, including the therapist, may be feared and dealt with in a guarded way. When a history of sexual abuse is present, talking about sexual matters is laden with shame, danger, and fear. Although discussing sex is seldom easily accomplished, making sexual disclosures is especially difficult for sexual abuse survivors—not only because of the terror, but also because there can be an indistinct boundary between speaking and taking action. A homogeneous group that includes sexual abuse survivors may provide greater safety, because other members are known to be managing fear and shame as well.

On the other hand, one liability associated with extended homogeneous group psychotherapy is that acceptance can become a resistance: Group members may fear a loss of identity associated with being traumatized persons if, in treatment, they grow and move beyond their trauma experiences and their perception of their group mates as trauma survivors (Ganzarain & Buchele, 1988). Nicholas and Forrester (1999) postulate that a traumatized individual is insufficiently treated in an extended psychotherapy group of trauma survivors. They state that in order for the treatment to be maximally effective, factors causing and perpetuating abuse must be addressed in interaction with nontraumatized individuals who have been passive when aware of abuse or who have been abusive themselves.

A third liability, seldom mentioned in the literature, is the difficulty of the therapist's role in an extended homogeneous group. The negative transferences are powerful and painful for the therapist. Likewise, the resistances can be very powerful, and it is not unusual for the therapist to feel that he or she is alone, without group allies, in acknowledging these resistances and encouraging exploration. Therefore, consultation and supervision are very important for the therapist of an extended homogeneous group.

For these reasons, it is sometimes advisable for a trauma survivor to become part of a heterogeneous group (i.e., a general psychotherapy group composed of men and women who are trauma patients at later stages of recovery or who have not been traumatized at all). Exposure to a safe, therapeutic environment including nontraumatized individuals can present a victim with new options and can promote hope, growth, and facilitate the working through of various transference distortions that are related to the trauma. The survivor is reminded consistently that his or her identity consists of far more than a traumatized sense of self. In addition, the presence of both genders in a heterogeneous group (extended homogeneous groups are often composed solely of women) affords abuse survivors the opportunity to examine their object worlds and to change interaction behaviors via association with both genders; it is, for instance, far less likely that the men in the group can be viewed without challenge by female incest survivors as "the enemy." Central in this option is a group that can accept and relate to a trauma survivor so that the survivor's sense of being "different" and isolated is not reinforced.

Another factor central to the use of a heterogeneous group by an abused person is the extent of damage related to the trauma (i.e., the severity of the individual's psychopathology). Although one could argue, as Nicholas and Forrester (1999) do, that the most effective treatment for the trauma survivor includes membership in a heterogeneous group, there are instances when this is not the case. When the patient's capacity to trust is so compromised that relationships are experienced in an almost phobic way, or when the abuse has contributed to severe paranoia, the safest atmosphere possible (in the patient's view) may be all that can be risked— and this atmosphere may be perceived to be found only in a homogeneous group. Also, for some individuals whose PTSD is, despite best efforts, so incompletely resolved that the symptoms are easily restimulated and retraumatization occurs easily, their belonging to a heterogeneous group may be too disruptive for the heterogeneous group itself. In these cases, other types of groups can be utilized instead (i.e., a homogeneous group, women's groups, stress reduction groups, or anger management groups).

SUMMARY

Group psychotherapy is typically a treatment of choice for most survivors of sexual and physical abuse. Although recovery from PTSD and even the subsequent character pathology has a good prognosis, the group therapist working with this population can expect some special problems and dilemmas.

When a group is homogeneous, cohesion is easily fostered in early stages. However, the similarity of experience and limited range of options in a survivor group can lead to members' developing a resistance to move beyond having an identity primarily as survivors.

In any group, the serious psychopathology of survivors leads to challenging work, usually because of members' preferred defenses. Dissociation alters memory and, when it occurs in the group, alters group participation; the therapist must interrupt the flow of the group when the group itself does not do so and must attempt to retrieve the distanced member. Vigilance to the presence of this defense demands extra effort from the therapist.

Use of the other more primitive defenses (i.e., denial, splitting, and projective identification) can periodically create a paranoid atmosphere. It is quite a dilemma for the therapist to stay experience-near in order to rebuild a safe "play space" when the ambience is such a suspicious one. Maintaining this balance, however, is important, because taking distance removes the therapist as a real person and impedes the treatment.

With traumatized persons, the countertransference is often intense and kaleidoscopic, but crucial to diagnosis; ultimately, its competent management contributes significantly to a successful outcome. Finally, vicarious traumatization is a hazard of treating sexual and physical abuse survivors. Staying affectively with these patients increases the therapist's vulnerability to this injury. Consultation and at least periodic supervision, as well as therapist self-care, are essential.

Whatever the type of group, working with survivors of sexual and physical abuse can be an exhausting, challenging, and somewhat daunting task for the group therapist. It can also be a source of existential refueling: The strength and resilience of the human spirit, when seen at close range as survivors recover, are inspiring indeed!

REFERENCES

Allen, J. (1995). *Coping with trauma: A guide to self-understanding.* Washington, DC: American Psychiatric Press.

Allen, J. (1996). Neurobiological basis of posttraumatic stress disorder: Implications for patient education and treatment. *Bulletin of the Menninger Clinic, 60*(3), 377–395.

Bartlett, A. (1998). *Neurobiology of early childhood trauma: Attachment style and affect dysregulation in the context of the "dangerous other."* Paper presented at the Fielding Institute, Chicago.

Brabender, V. (1992). The psychological growth of women in a short-term inpatient group. *Group, 16*(3), 131–143.

Brenneis, C. (1996). Memory systems and the psychoanalytic retrieval of memories of trauma. *Journal of the American Psychoanalytic Association, 44*(4), 1165–1188.

Buchele, B. (1993). Group psychotherapy for persons with multiple personality and dissociative disorders. *Bulletin of the Menninger Clinic, 57*(3), 362–370.

Buchele, B. (1994). Innovative uses of psychodynamic group psychotherapy. *Bulletin of the Menninger Clinic, 58*(2), 215–223.

Davies, J., & Frawley, M. (1994). *Treating the adult survivor of childhood sexual abuse: A psychoanalytic perspective.* New York: Basic Books.

Fonagy, P. (1999). Memory and therapeutic action. *International Journal of Psycho-Analysis, 80,* 215–223.

Ganzarain, R., & Buchele, J. (1987). Acting out during group psychotherapy for incest. *International Journal of Group Psychotherapy, 37*(2), 185–200.

Ganzarain, R., & Buchele, J. (1988). *Fugitives of incest: A perspective from psychoanalysis and groups.* Madison, CT: International Universities Press.

Gelinas, D. (1993). Relational patterns in incestuous families, malevolent variations and specific interventions with the adult survivor. In P. T. Paddison (Ed.), *Treatment of adult survivors of incest.* Washington, DC: American Psychiatric Press.

Klein, M. (1975). Notes on some schizoid mechanisms. In M. Klein, *Envy and gratitude and other works, 1946–1963* (pp. 1–24). New York: Delacourt Press. (Original work published 1946)

Nicholas, M., & Forrester, A. (1999). Advantages of heterogeneous therapy groups in the psychotherapy of the traumatically abused: Treating the problem as well as the person. *International Journal of Group Psychotherapy, 49*(3), 323–342.

Ogden, T. (1989). *The primitive edge of experience.* Northvale, NJ: Aronson.

Target, M. (1998). Book review essay: The recovered memories controversy. *International Journal of Psycho-Analysis, 79,* 1015–1028.

van der Kolk, B. (1996). The body keeps the score: Approaches to the psychobiology of posttraumatic stress disorder. In B. A. van der Kolk, A.C. McFarlane, & L. Weisaeth (Eds.), *Traumatic stress: The effects of overwhelming experience on mind, body, and society* (pp. 214–241). New York: Guilford Press.

Winnicott, D. (1945). Primitive emotional development. *International Journal of Psycho-Analysis, 26*(3–4), 137–143.

8

-◄O►-

Group Psychotherapy for Psychological Traumata of Prolonged, Severe, and/or Terminal Illness

MYRNA MARCUS
HAROLD S. BERNARD

The diagnosis of a serious illness is often accompanied by feelings of helplessness and questions about one's ability to influence events related to the illness. A sense of isolation may develop, perhaps accompanied by overwhelming feelings related to a lack of ability to count on one's body, or to believe any longer in the fantasy that one can control one's destiny. Some individuals may organize their defenses in order to present themselves as positive, determined, and in charge. Others may appear to be helpless and bewildered.

Patients with certain illnesses sometimes obtain a complete remission of their symptoms. For others, there can be a lessening of pain; the acute aspects of the illness may be diminished. Many serious illnesses are nevertheless irreversible. Some lie dormant, exhibiting no evidence of their existence, but still lurking in the background. Others carry with them constant reminders that life as it once was is now forever changed.

Even if a serious illness is not diagnosed as terminal, an underlying and usually unexpressed concern with death often exists. Stress can also accompany lifestyle changes, which vary according to type of illness. For example, diabetes necessitates a change in eating habits and constant monitoring of such bodily sensations as dizziness and fatigue. Constant monitoring of the environment and of one's ability to breathe easily becomes part of the life of a patient with advanced asthma. Patients diagnosed with a neurological illness will usually have some interruption in functioning, although this may be reversible and/or slow to progress. Cardiac patients are advised to change their eating habits. Patients with kidney disease become dependent on machines as a lifeline (Roback, 1984; Stewart, Kelly, Robinson, & Callender, 1995).

Despite the differences related to particular illnesses, certain stressors are shared by many of these patients. In addition to the suddenly increased awareness of one's own mortality, there can be concerns about sexual activity, for both psychological and physiological reasons. There may be an overbearing sense of uncertainty about the near future, or even the immediate future. Some individuals may develop feelings of being out of control.

Feelings of helplessness and lack of control over life choices, as well as the dissolution of what was once safe and predictable, are indications of trauma (van der Kolk, 1987). In describing posttraumatic stress disorder, the fourth edition of the *Diagnostic and Statistical Manual of Mental Disorders* (American Psychiatric Association, 1994) emphasizes the significance of unexpected, life-threatening, or seriously harmful experiences for an individual or for family members or other persons close to that individual. The diagnosis of a life-threatening illness is specifically mentioned, as well as the fact that typical responses include fear, helplessness, or horror.

Also indicative of trauma is the sense of being "different" from others, which can be a marker for the beginning of isolation—the beginning of the disruption of affiliative bonds, as described by Lindemann (1944). Group therapy is one method of addressing the traumatic effects of serious illness on patients, family members, and other significant persons in the lives of those directly affected by the illness.

Group interventions for seriously ill individuals can take several forms. The initial group experience for the newly diagnosed and those close to them is often an "education" group. These groups are structured around (1) presenting information to patients and family members about the illness, types of treatments, and ways others have coped with the illness, and (2) responding to questions from those attending. Although in this chapter we refer to these groups as "education" groups, these groups are usually also experienced as very supportive: As individuals experiencing the trauma of diagnosis of a serious illness become more informed in a group setting, they usually have feelings of being supported by others as they receive pertinent information.

Another group experience for the newly diagnosed is a "support" group. Support groups are not insight-oriented groups; they are not designed to interpret interpersonal dynamics or to analyze defenses. Rather, they are groups in which members have the opportunity to experience a safe environment where they can discuss the illness-related issues that have interrupted their lives (Cordoba, Shear, Fobair, & Hall, 1984; Roback, 1984; Spiegel & Yalom, 1978). Van der Kolk (1987) recommends that the initial group experience for traumatized individuals be more supportive than confrontational, at least for a brief period of time. Decreases in anxiety, isolation, and helplessness are goals of these initial groups. "Psychotherapy" groups, which address the intra- and interpersonal dynamics of individuals, may be helpful to some patients and/or their family members as they adjust to the trauma of illness.

Our plan in this chapter is to discuss the different types of groups that can be helpful in providing information, support, and a sense of relief from the traumatic effects of illness. We attend to Yalom's (1995) descriptions of "therapeutic factors" that help to produce change in groups. In addition, we explore critical stages in the span of an illness during which a group may be useful for those affected. We believe that education and support groups are by and large the most effective ways to provide group interventions for greater numbers of those dealing with serious medical illness. Because of this, and because there is a more extensive literature on insight-oriented psychotherapy groups in general, we have chosen to focus primarily on education and support groups in this chapter.

TRAUMATIC REACTIONS TO ILLNESS

Many variables influence the manner in which individuals react to the intrusion of serious illness in their lives. Most frequently mentioned are age, developmental background, previous methods of coping with crises, types of defenses employed, and familial patterns in dealing with stress (Weisman, 1979; Rolland, 1987). A crucial determinant of one's reaction is the availability of supports, as well as the nature and depth of those supports. Thus the effect of the illness on those in one's support network is very important. Also to be considered is the meaning to the individual of his or her work life. For those with a great deal of support and relational ties that will be of help during a difficult period, there may be less need for help from outside their own circles. This chapter addresses possible ways in which different types of group interventions may be helpful for people with relatively little support who suffer the trauma of serious illness.

Following the diagnosis of any serious illness, it is likely that there will be concrete questions regarding the effectiveness of various treatment options, and ways to begin determining the best medical care for the illness. Treatment for some illnesses can involve great financial expense; for some individuals and families, this can lead to questions about the adequacy of their health insurance, and other concerns about how their finances will be affected. In some cultures and religious communities, prohibitions are maintained regarding certain medical treatments. For people in these sub-groups, questions may arise about whether or not particular treatment options will fit within the cultural and/or religious traditions of their belief systems. These and other difficult issues often arise amidst the earlier-described feelings of helplessness and isolation, all of which are accompanied by a great sense of loss.

Another set of reactions may surface after decisions have been made regarding treatment, when the next phase of the illness begins. The previously overwhelming uncertainty has possibly been replaced by a plan that may involve one or more types of treatment, or no immediate treatment until further indicated. Feelings may arise regarding any of the decisions, such as relief that there is a proposed strategy, fear that the choice is incorrect, fear of side effects as a result of the treatment chosen, anger that this interruption has occurred, or some combination of these feelings. As time goes by, feelings may subside, increase, or otherwise change, depending upon the course of the illness and the individual's psychological makeup. Some people may vigilantly monitor any changes in their bodies; others may opt (consciously or unconsciously) not to notice unless the changes are persistent and/or intrusive.

Treatment for prolonged and/or life-threatening illness does not necessarily result in cure. Although a number of illnesses today have a better chance of being cured than in previous years, uncertainty continues to exist for many others, and helplessness for some. In these cases, therefore, treatment is designed with the hope of controlling or ameliorating an individual's symptoms for varying amounts of time.

Chronic illness affects not only the body or the physical being of an individual; there is always an emotional component, sometimes hidden, at other times expressed. In addition, the social aspect must be considered (Vugia, 1991; Weisman, 1979). The professional mental health care provider who is offering the possibility of group intervention as a support to any individual with a serious physical illness must consider both the needs of that individual and, simultaneously, what the individual can tolerate. Many people consider a group of any type as too overwhelming. Instead of being considered anxiety-relieving, a group may be thought of (and actually experienced) as anxiety-producing.

A relatively nonthreatening group designed to reduce anxiety and isolated feelings is the education group. As described above, this is a group that offers information to patients and families about specific topics. Such a group may meet for only one session, or may meet at monthly or other intervals.

Alternatively, the provider may determine that an individual can benefit as a member of a group of people who have recently experienced similar crises in their lives, and who have joined together with the provider (or another professionally trained individual) for group discussions leading to the possible resolution of the helpless feelings often accompanying such diagnoses. In this chapter, as noted earlier, we call that type of group a support group.

Some who have been dealing with the "crisis of the moment" may wish to learn more about dealing with their relationships with others, or may even have some curiosity about exploring unresolved issues from the past. For these people, the provider may suggest an insight-oriented psychotherapy group. It is important for the therapist leading such a group to bear in mind the recent significant and critical events centering around a recent diagnosis; however, the focus of such groups is on interpersonal and intrapsychic issues rather than on the impact of the illness.

It is important to keep in mind that the losses and traumatic reactions previously described are experienced not only by the patient diagnosed with the illness, but by all those who have significant relationships with the patient: spouse or partner, other family members (including children), and friends. Work or school colleagues, neighbors, and others who seem more peripheral to the patient may also be affected. These losses can generate a variety of feelings and behaviors, which in turn affect the individual who is ill. Family life may change—sometimes temporarily, at other times more permanently. The same may be true of the world in which one is employed. Roles may be exchanged; for instance, dependent and independent roles are often reversed. Relationships may shift, and values may be called into question. Conflicts may be seen differently; goals may need to be readjusted (Vugia, 1991; Weisman, 1979). Thus a group may be of value not only to the patient, but also to family members and significant friends of the patient as well.

The following case examples introduce two patients prior to their participation in groups. These patients are described again later in this chapter, to illustrate some of the key principles we wish to communicate.

A 52-year-old male, Mr. C, a high school guidance counselor who could "turn any problem around," began to notice tingling sensations around his mouth. At the same time, he became aware that he was occasionally unable to pronounce certain letters of the alphabet clearly, and that some words he spoke were unintelligible as a result. He ignored these symptoms for months, rationalizing that he had not been getting enough sleep and had been somewhat stressed about his aging parents. Some months later, when his symptoms appeared more frequently, he reluctantly sought medical help. He was diagnosed with amyotrophic lateral sclerosis (ALS), otherwise known as "Lou Gehrig's disease."

Prior to seeing a physician, Mr. C had not told his wife of 26 years about his concerns. He believed that it was important for her to be protected from "unnecessary worries"; in fact, he had always believed that protecting her from many of life's burdens was a part of his role as her husband.

Mrs. H was diagnosed with breast cancer when she was 39, after her gynecologist found a small lump that she had not noticed. The surgeon to whom she was referred recommended a mastectomy followed by 6 weeks of radiation and 1 year of chemotherapy. She did not know why these treatments were selected, nor did she question them. The mastectomy was performed a week later, and radiation therapy began about 3 weeks after her surgery. Her husband believed that if they both had positive attitudes and did not discuss any negative thoughts, she would have a better chance for survival. Her 12-year-old son and her 10-year-old daughter were told that she was being hospitalized for "women's problems"; her radiation was arranged to take place while they were in school, so there would be no chance for the children to question her whereabouts. During the fourth week of radiation therapy, Mrs. H found that she was crying in the most unlikely places and for no identifiable reason. Her family physician suggested that she see a psychiatrist for evaluation. She saw the psychiatrist for several months, and found some relief from the fact that "there was something to do about all this crying."

These two cases illustrate patients at different stages in the courses of illnesses—one at the time of his diagnosis, the other during the period of her treatment. As stated earlier, we return to these case examples later in this chapter, when each patient is reintroduced as a member of a group.

TYPES OF GROUPS

Again, there are three basic models of group intervention for people with prolonged and/or severe illness: education, support, and psychotherapy. In this section we describe each of these models in greater detail.

Education Groups

Groups that have been designed primarily to provide information to patients and/or family members and friends are often referred to as "education" or "information" groups. They are organized around a topic or a set of topics presented in lecture format; the lecture is usually followed by discussion. They may occur on a one-time basis, or may be offered as part of a series, meeting at regular intervals (e.g., monthly). The leader of an education group is usually referred to as the "group facilitator" rather than as the "therapist." In these groups, which are more cognitively oriented than the types of groups described later in this chapter, the facilitator attempts to create a supportive environment in which information can be disseminated.

These groups are not limited in size, nor is their membership restricted by variables that may influence participation in the other types of groups to be described (such as age, phase of illness, or level of functioning). In other words, there is no need for a structured selection process to determine those who are appropriate to include. Education groups are interventions designed to deal with people's traumatic reactions to their lack of control over a serious physical illness, as well as their isolating feelings of being "different." The topics chosen for presentation and discussion are aimed at the key issues of a particular illness, such as pain or symptom control, treatment and side effects, and (at times) insurance coverage. Those who attend education groups have the opportunity to ask questions and to integrate information about various aspects of their illnesses (Cordoba et al., 1984; Spiegelberg, 1980).

As noted earlier, although education groups are not billed as support groups, people who attend often find these groups supportive. For instance, participants often feel less isolated as a result of hearing questions posed by others whose concerns are similar to their own. When such groups are effective for the individuals who attend, there can be a clarification of significant issues, such as uncertainty about the course of the illness, treatment choices, and treatment side effects. A lessening of uncertainty allows for increased feelings of control over decision making (Fobair, Cordoba, Pluth, & Bloom, 1982). Information delivered by presenters as well as by other group members can set into motion several of Yalom's (1995) therapeutic factors: namely, the universality of common dilemmas, including the need to face a common enemy (the illness); the catharsis involved in expressing feelings that have often never been expressed; and the group cohesiveness that often emerges when people with a common struggle get together and share their experiences. Family members and friends often participate in these groups and frequently experience similar positive reactions (Plant et al., 1987), as a further description of Mr. C (the man with ALS) and his wife indicates.

> Despite the efforts of Mr. C's physician, he was unable to convince Mr. C to discuss his concerns with his wife. Mrs. C appeared distraught and confused on the one occasion in which she was included in a visit. Stressing the importance of education about ALS, the physician strongly suggested that the couple attend an informational meeting.
>
> Mr. and Mrs. C attended the meeting, and as they listened to the speaker, watched a videotape, and heard the questions and answers that followed, they experienced validation of their respective feelings and concerns. Following the meeting they were approached informally

by some of the other attendees, who invited them to sit and chat for a while. After a few minutes, the facilitator who had presented the lecture asked whether he could join them.

Mrs. C found herself discussing the fact that her husband was eating very little and had begun to lose weight. She was not only perplexed by this, but concerned that his lack of interest in food was a result of depression about his diagnosis. She found herself telling this "spontaneous support group" about her dilemma, saying that her husband wouldn't talk to her about his illness or let her know how he was feeling emotionally. She reported feeling "all alone," adding that she was afraid to discuss the situation with their children, as she didn't want to worry them unnecessarily.

The people in this informal group, who were both patients and family members, began to talk about themselves. They began to educate Mr. and Mrs. C about the illness from each of their perspectives. The process of telling their stories and educating others was cathartic and supportive for these participants each time they met with new attendees. It also became helpful for Mr. C, who, after listening to the others, revealed with apparent relief how he had become embarrassed about his more frequent mispronunciations and concerned about how they would be perceived by the students with whom he met. He found himself beginning to avoid personal contact with the students, claiming that he had to catch up on his paperwork. He told the group how difficult it was getting to go to work, and how he had become withdrawn at home, as he did not want to trouble his wife with his feelings about his illness.

As Mr. C unburdened his reactions to his illness to the group (which included his wife), he was finally able to begin to understand information that he had previously been told but had not been able to integrate. Both Mr. and Mrs. C reported feeling less isolated and less helpless. They learned that Mr. C's symptoms regarding food might be related to depression, and they were encouraged to report them to his physicians so that it could be determined whether the symptoms were emotional or whether they might have a physiological basis. Although there was some anxiety associated with the question about the etiology of the symptoms, they both reported feeling more in control. They were also relieved to have been open with each other and others, so that they could approach together whatever was to come.

In the case described above, it is easy to imagine that Mr. C might have chosen not to attend the group. And, had he attended what began as an educational, information-imparting experience, he might have chosen to leave as some people initiated conversation with others. It is important not to forget that the prospect of participating in a group is frightening for many individuals, and that facilitators and other group members can best respond to the fear by accepting it rather than by working harder to encourage participation.

As education/information programs are concluded, one may notice small groups of people gathering informally to continue discussions inspired by the large-group meeting. A wise facilitator will make him- or herself available during this time to serve as a consultant, if invited, and to consider offering those gathering the option of returning at a future time for more regular discussions. In this way, those who wish may find opportunities for ongoing support.

Professionals who design education groups should keep in mind that providing information and a question-and-answer discussion period is helpful both for those who actively participate and for those many individuals who merely want to listen and absorb material that they found difficult to understand when it was first told to them. It is also important to maintain a sharp awareness of those who may want time for small-group discussion, and perhaps to suggest that for a brief period of time the large group break down into smaller groups. For example, an ongoing support group reported in the literature (Spiegelberg, 1980) for multiple sclerosis patients was formed following informational discussions about treatments, diets, exercise, and theories about the illness. Patients recruited a psychologist and social worker to be facilitators, who helped the group to structure itself and to begin to discuss feelings about living with multiple sclerosis.

There may be occasions when professionals perceive the need for a supportive group situation, while those for whom they think it would be useful may be mostly fearful of it. Sometimes an education group will attract these patients or family members, as it is usually less threatening to attend an informational meeting. In addition to providing a warm, nonchallenging atmosphere for group exchange, the creation by the facilitator of a comfortable and pleasant physical environment for group sessions can help to allay some of the participants' anxieties.

A group of physicians specializing in hematology began to have increased numbers of patients who were HIV-positive. Some of the patients seemed particularly isolated, as did some of the people who accompanied them to their visits. One of the doctors engaged the services of a social worker and a nurse to design a support group for the HIV patients and their significant others. The group was to take place in the waiting room of the office one evening each week, after office hours had been completed.

The other physicians in the practice agreed to the idea, and each referred some newly diagnosed patients to the group. Many of the patients indicated interest and agreed to attend—some with partners, friends, or parents; others alone. Following office hours on the first evening the group was scheduled, the social worker and nurse prepared the waiting room for a meeting, and then waited. No one came. The following week patients indicated that they would attend the next meeting; each had a reason for not being at the first meeting. Again, however, no one arrived.

When they spoke to their patients, the physicians were unable to ascertain the reasons for the lack of attendance. Those patients who had been referred had all expressed interest in being part of a "discussion group." It was decided to change the format to an education group. Responses from patients were positive, and the program was redesigned, but again no one attended.

The social worker and nurse, who had each repeatedly been able to engage these patients individually, were puzzled. As they spoke more with the patients, one man remarked about how strange it would seem to be having a meeting in the waiting room, noting that he always felt anxious there.

For one last attempt, the education meeting was scheduled a month later to meet in a conference room elsewhere in the building. Seven people attended—three patients and four significant people in their lives. They were appreciative of the program that was presented, and of the refreshment period following. They requested another program in a few weeks, which was attended by some of the same people as well as a few others. Before long, these education sessions became the basis for a slowly forming support group.

The needs of patients and family members regarding information and support are often not clearly defined. It is not always easy to know which type of group will be most helpful to particular people. If the professional maintains an awareness of the basic needs of those who are experiencing illness-related trauma, he or she can attend to the additional specific concerns of the individuals in the group. In these groups, as with all of the groups described in this chapter, the facilitator must consider how he or she will interface with physicians. Physicians can be an important resource for helping to determine the needs of specific patient groups, as well as for making referrals as groups are designed.

Support Groups

Support groups for those affected by a serious or prolonged illness are created to provide a forum for patients and family members to express their feelings about aspects of the illness and ways in which it has changed their lives. Support groups can be designed to serve only patients, only family members and significant others, or all persons affected by an illness. Self-help groups are support groups without a therapist. They often develop when a time-limited support group has ended, or following participation in some education group sessions.

As stated earlier, support groups aim to help decrease feelings of anxiety, helplessness, and isolation. These groups encourage cohesion and interpersonal exploration of current life issues, with very little confrontation involved. Problems unrelated to symptoms of the illness (e.g., marital discord) can be discussed in support groups, although they are not usually explored in great depth (Bernstein & Klein, 1995; Deans, Bennett-Emslie, Weir, Smith, & Kaye, 1988; Hunt, Bond, & Pater, 1990; Spiegel, Bloom, & Yalom, 1981; Spiegel, Kraemer, Bloom, & Gottheil, 1989; Spiegelberg, 1980; Vugia, 1991).

Support groups differ from education groups in that (1) they are limited in terms of size and composition, and (2) topics for discussion typically emerge from the participants rather than having been previously set by the leader. These groups should be led by individuals who have been professionally trained as clinicians; a facilitator/therapist may be a psychologist, a social worker, a nurse, or a psychiatrist. The size of a group can vary from 4 to 14, although it is most effective if the numbers stay within the range of 6 to 10 participants. The facilitator must determine whether the group is to be open-ended or time-limited, and whether the membership will be open or closed. He or she will also decide on the numbers of participants, as well as the numbers of sessions.

Open-ended groups meet at regular intervals at a specific time of day for an indefinite period of sessions (e.g., every other Thursday at 5 P.M. until further notice). Time-limited groups meet regularly for a defined number of sessions (e.g., every other Thursday at 5 P.M. for six sessions). Open-ended groups usually also allow for new members to join at any time; thus the term "open membership." Closed groups dictate that after a certain time (usually by the second or third session) new members will not be welcome.

The composition of the group is also of significance; the therapist must select the members on the basis of a common theme (e.g., the illness itself, or a particular stage or phase of the illness, or an age range). The facilitator also needs to interview potential participants briefly, in order to screen out those who seem inappropriate (e.g., individuals who seem overly narcissistic, acutely paranoid, or actively suicidal). An interview can conceivably be accomplished by telephone, but is much better done in person.

Although it is often easy for professionals to identify people who might benefit from a group experience, it is nevertheless difficult to get groups started. It is wise for those attempting to form support groups to be creative in their approaches in terms of marketing such groups, and flexible (as mentioned earlier in regard to education groups) in terms of being able to change direction so as to attract those who might respond. For example, it may be easier for those who work in a setting where patients are treated (e.g., a hospital, physician's office, physical therapy practice, etc.) to consider offering a group as part of the services offered by that setting.

We have observed that support groups move through different phases of development. These phases occur in all groups of this type, no matter for how brief or extended a time they are offered. In the first stage of such a group, there is marked ambivalence, curiosity, and skepticism. The facilitator must be quite active in outlining objectives, defining confidentiality, establishing respect for differences, helping to maintain the focus, and modeling acceptance. The group then moves into a phase in which the members become competitive with and/or challenging of each other and the therapist. The role of the therapist becomes that of helping the group to set appropriate limits so that it solidifies and moves forward. The next phase involves group members' developing relationships with each other that are supportive and even friendly. The facilitator has a less overt role, as the members will have integrated the earlier structuring. These phases of development are more obvious if the group meets on a regular basis over a period of time. They can be noticed, however, even in a group that meets for just a few sessions, although in such cases the third phase may not have an opportunity to develop fully. In the fourth, or termination, phase, group members are reflective about their experiences and expressive of feelings about ending the group.

Sometimes after a support group is terminated, it may evolve into a self-help group, which is formed by the group members and meets in another location. The therapist may or may not be aware of this occurrence. The following example illustrates the development of such a group:

A group of people who had been widowed following the extended illnesses of their spouses met with one of us (Marcus) as therapist for a few months (10 sessions). Several years later, Marcus encountered the entire group in a restaurant. The members reported that they had been meeting once monthly for all of the intervening years, because they had felt the need for and the gains from the support derived from each other.

Self-help support groups (with no designated leader) can often be helpful, though they are more likely to be helpful if they have some professional guidance at the outset. Such groups often need assistance in screening out potentially destructive members (e.g., overly narcissistic people, delusional people, etc.). Also, they often need help in establishing norms of genuine acceptance and respect. Especially with assistance of this sort, support groups can evolve into well-functioning self-help groups.

The goals of helping to decrease group members' feelings of anxiety, helplessness, and isolation can be achieved through the use of specific techniques by the support group therapist. For example, by framing issues within the context of short-term goals, the therapist can foster feelings of being in control in both patients and family members. This can be useful for people struggling with illness-related trauma, no matter what the prognosis. Whenever possible, too, concrete suggestions can be offered. For example, through group discussions members may become aware of how they and others address concerns with physicians. They may observe that some are timid about asking questions or describing illness- or treatment-related symptoms to their doctors. Other group members and the therapist can often help increase assertiveness in this area (Spiegel et al., 1989). It should be noted that although there may be some insight to be achieved, it is not explored and developed, as it might be in a psychotherapy group.

Another example of employing specific techniques is the use of behavioral strategies to help with anxiety or pain control. Many support group therapists teach participants self-hypnosis, relaxation, and/or deep breathing exercises.

> After one of us (Marcus) offered a 5-minute deep breathing and muscle relaxation exercise to a group of family members of patients with Parkinson's disease, the members requested that the exercise be incorporated into each session. They reported that they were able to use these techniques at various junctures during the week when they felt stressed.

Members often help each other solve problems by exchanging ideas and experiences about similar issues. These exchanges can center around such practical matters as what particular medical supplies have been most helpful and where to purchase them, or deeper issues such as how individuals have dealt with role changes in their families. It has been reported that self-esteem and feelings of competence are increased as participants help others, while feelings of helplessness are diminished (Spiegel et al., 1989; Spiegelberg, 1980).

Such exchanges exploit what Yalom (1995) calls "altruism," one of his therapeutic factors. Although people come into psychotherapy groups for the help they can receive, they often find they can give help to others, and further discover that this has benefits for them. In contrast to this, people often come to support groups with the idea that they might be able to offer help to others, and in the process find that the group has been helpful to them. Many people who find themselves in situations where they are facing a crisis such as prolonged or serious illness have not ever considered participating in group therapy; in fact, the idea of therapy of any kind is alien. For those people who feel frightened by the idea of revealing personal feelings to a group of strangers, it is often less threatening to think of participating in a group by giving rather than receiving help.

> In a support group for breast cancer patients (described later in connection with the case of Mrs. H), a woman who had been treated for breast cancer 15 years prior to the start of the group began attending

so that she could give advice to the other women, since no groups had been available to her when she would have found them helpful. The other members looked to her for information about what they could expect. She soon reported that her husband said she "spoke with a lilt in her voice" after these group sessions, and appeared to be more "in charge of her life." She also reported that she was slowly learning from the other members about related subjects that she hadn't thought about.

Yalom's (1995) therapeutic factor of group cohesiveness highlights the importance of valuing and being valued by one's fellow group members. The resultant unconditional acceptance that can flow between members can lay the groundwork for building trust, so that the goals of reducing anxiety, helplessness, and isolation can be accomplished. One way of achieving cohesion is by encouraging members to attend the group regularly. Cohesiveness can be further encouraged by the therapist's highlighting common themes and areas of concern among participants and identifying common illness-related experiences among group members (Cordoba et al., 1984; Spiegel et al., 1989; Vugia, 1991). The support group thus becomes an arena for adjusting to serious changes and legitimizing the feelings that accompany these changes.

Encouraging participants to express their feelings, particularly feelings about the losses in their lives as a result of the illness, is a major objective for the therapist in a support group. A variety of losses may be discussed, such as physical changes in one's body, loss of hope, and loss of a job or career aspirations. Loss of relationships can be significant, according to Getzel (1994), in that any life-threatening disease or chronic disease may result in the loss of important relationships at precisely the time one needs them most. It is helpful for the therapist to learn about early losses in the lives of group members—not from the perspective of trying to resolve them in the group, as would be the goal in a psychotherapy group, but to learn how feelings were expressed about the losses (if at all).

Although group members will not necessarily experience the same losses, the therapist can identify the common thread of loss among the participants, helping them to make this connection as they become able to express their feelings of sadness, anger, and fear. Genuine relief can be experienced as group members come to develop a sense of belonging, and (ideally) as they come to feel less helpless.

Family members and friends may discuss the effect on them of the losses described by the patients, as well as the effect of the illness on their relationships with the patients (Wellisch, Mosher, & Van Scoy, 1978). For example, members of a family may need to process their feelings about a patient upon whom they depended for most of their needs, when the patient now needs to depend upon them for the most basic life necessities.

It is important for the support group therapist to have a simultaneous awareness of the individuals in the group and of the group as a whole. Differences among the participants often need to be pointed out even while similarities are highlighted. Several authors have emphasized the value of positive reinforcement of individual strengths, as well as acceptance of individual values and needs (Fobair et al., 1982; Vugia, 1991). Respect is generated in a group as the therapist gives permission to the more passive members to remain less involved, and as he or she helps participants accept the different ways in which they express their feelings. An example of this is encouraging individuals who cope by using humor to tolerate those who need to express anger, sadness, or fear, and vice versa. In fact, respect is modeled whenever the therapist encourages participants to express differences and disagreements about their styles of coping with and discussing their illnesses.

Whenever cotherapy is possible, there are a number of reasons to consider it for a support group that focuses on illness-related trauma. One rationale for cotherapy is that the group will be able to meet even in the absence of one of the cotherapists, thus providing consistency for individuals for whom predictability in life has been seriously interrupted. In addition, the cotherapists can be supportive to each other as countertransferential issues arise for them, such as helplessness, depression, or demoralization (Bernstein & Klein, 1995; Getzel, 1994). Furthermore, the intense transference to the therapist that may develop in support groups addressing the trauma of illness can sometimes be diluted when there are cotherapists (Vugia, 1991). The intensity of transference material is primarily determined by how little or much attention is focused on the material by the therapist(s). The cotherapy structure can be helpful when there is a wish to deemphasize transference material. Cotherapy offers the advantage of one therapist's being able to take some distance from the group process temporarily as issues of transference and/or countertransference arise.

Change is mediated by the operation of therapeutic factors. Yalom's (1995) descriptions of these factors have become almost universally accepted as a way of understanding how group therapy works—both ego-supportive therapy (support and education groups) and ego-regressive therapy (psychotherapy groups) (Rutan & Cohen, 1989).

The operation of therapeutic factors varies from group to group because participants' needs differ and therapists work differently. In the following continuation of the case of Mrs. H, we suggest how some of Yalom's therapeutic factors become activated.

Mrs. H, the woman with breast cancer described earlier in this chapter, was referred by her psychiatrist to a support group as an adjunct to her ongoing therapy. She reported to the group that she was attending because her psychiatrist had told her to. She made little eye contact with anyone in the group, expressed almost no affect, and spoke only in response to questions from the other members, which related to her diagnosis and treatment. She was in the midst of her chemotherapy treatments, which caused her to become nauseated even before she walked into the office where the treatments were administered.

The support group was an ongoing, open-ended group for women that met once weekly for 1½ hours. It had been meeting for about 5 years at the time Mrs. H joined. About 10 women who attended regularly had become the "core" members of the group. Many others attended less often, or had come for a while and stopped. New members were always welcome, with new arrivals occurring about once a month. The women ranged in age from 27 to 73; they had different types of breast cancer, different treatments, and different prognoses.

Topics focused on feelings of isolation and helplessness, struggles with assertiveness regarding health care options, ways to discuss their illness with family members, many practical problems, concrete decisions that needed to be made, fear of recurrence, and fear of death. Although the members tried to include Mrs. H, she let it be known by her one-word answers that she was not comfortable with being an active participant. Mrs. H attended the group weekly, maintaining the same posture and affect—and, incidentally, wearing the same sweater and skirt each week.

Several months after the completion of her treatments, Mrs. H appeared at a group meeting in different clothing. She had been unaware that she had dressed in the same clothes each week, and was surprised when the members commented on her new outfit. She now made eye contact with the other women and told them that she felt as if she had awakened from a long nap. She reported that her anxiety level had been so high during the treatments that she "felt like a robot, just going through the motions." She told the members that without them she would not have been able to endure the chemotherapy. Each time she went for a treatment, she would sit there and think of each group member who had been through this treatment; she would think of what the other women said they did during the treatments, or what they thought of. Sometimes she would just sit there with their faces in her mind and think to herself that it would all be over in a few more minutes. The other women were pleased to know that they had been helpful to Mrs. H, even though they had previously been unaware that she had found them supportive.

The treatment experience of Mrs. H illustrates several of Yalom's therapeutic factors. She had attended the group for about 6 months before she returned and told the others of her experiences. During that time, she was identifying with different group members and trying out some of their strategies in her mind to see what would fit for her (Yalom's factor of imitative behavior). As she did this, she was learning that she was not so unique or isolated as she might have thought (Yalom's universality). When she was thinking about how they got through the treatments, and when she told herself that it would be over in a few minutes, she appeared to be able to be hopeful—not hopeful for a cure, necessarily, but hopeful of being able to get through a difficult time (Yalom's instillation of hope). And her internalizing the group (carrying some of the members with her during a tough time) was an example of still another therapeutic factor at work (Yalom's group cohesiveness).

Support groups differ from psychotherapy groups in that the former are not insight-oriented groups; the therapist does not offer interpretations of interpersonal dynamics, nor does he or she analyze defenses. Although the two types of groups are characterized by similar interactive processes, which result in participants' developing feelings toward the therapist and each other, the therapist does not explore this material in depth.

The therapist in a support group usually takes a more active role in the group process—being actively responsive to group participants, offering suggestions, and so on. A more neutral position is typically assumed in psychotherapy groups, particularly those that are more psychodynamically oriented. Psychotherapy groups are addressed more fully in the next section of this chapter.

Support groups are generally nonconfrontive and have flexibility in terms of attendance, between-group boundaries, and expression of feelings (members' touching or hugging each other) (Frost, 1993; Spiegel et al., 1981, 1989). Although support groups are not therapy groups, when such groups are conducted for people who are dealing with trauma resulting from serious or prolonged illness, they can indeed be therapeutic.

Psychotherapy Groups

In contrast to support groups, which are ego-supportive and geared toward helping individuals move on with their lives, psychotherapy groups are aimed at exploring and (ideally) resolving past conflicts. Members are helped to learn about the effects of those conflicts on their current relationships. In contrast to education and support groups, psychotherapy groups attend to the intrapsychic as well as interpersonal needs of group members. Although we believe that the first two types of groups can often meet the needs of those who are experiencing the trauma of newly diagnosed and/or terminal illness, psychotherapy groups can be significantly helpful for those who are motivated to work on themselves as well as to learn how to cope with their illnesses. In some instances, an individual may be seen by a clinician as having deeper internal conflicts, self-esteem issues, or difficult behavior patterns that may be interfering with adjustment to the illness. Dealing with the losses resulting from the illness may exacerbate feelings about earlier losses (including early object losses), which need to be explored if progress is to be made.

Once the initial trauma has been addressed, a patient or family member may be amenable to, and interested in, learning more about the nature of the impact of the illness. In a psychotherapy group, many of the same therapeutic factors that get mobilized in a support group also have their positive impact (e.g., universality, altruism, group cohesiveness, catharsis, etc.). In addition, conflict exploration and resolution can sometimes occur.

One of us (Marcus) received a request to join an ongoing psychodynamic psychotherapy group from a young man who had been diagnosed with colon cancer 2 years earlier. He had already sought individual therapy to enable him to deal with the many changes in his life as a result of the diagnosis, including the loss of his career dreams, the inability to have more children as a result of treatment, and the fear for his future at such a young age (he was 34). He had also attended support groups at his church and at the hospital where he was being treated. After 2 years, however, he found himself dealing with early family conflicts that were interfering with his relationships.

The patient became a member of a group of physically healthy men and women, and remained in the group for 4 years. He experienced universality from a perspective other than his physical illness: The common experiences in this group involved early object loss. There were also experiences in the group of universality related to human dilemmas precipitated by a variety of causes. Universality was not the only factor in this group that helped to create changes in the patient's life; he experienced deep feelings of catharsis and cohesiveness, as well as instillation of hope in terms of his family problems, and he integrated well the existential factor of learning what could not be changed. The group became a place where he also sought support with illness-related issues such as anxiety prior to scheduled examinations, and the other members spoke about the knowledge they acquired from him about the existential qualities of hopefulness (not necessarily hope for an ultimate cure, but hope of being able to get through a difficult time).

An individual who has been a member of a psychotherapy group at the time of a diagnosis or at another significant juncture in the span of an illness does not necessarily have to leave the group. The material that emerges at this point can be explored by group members, and the therapist can help the group adjust to the trauma (which the members may be experiencing as well). On the other hand, if the problem becomes too preoccupying for the group and becomes the primary focus, the therapist must help the member leave and find another venue for the crisis being experienced.

There are many different types of psychotherapy groups, some of which explore the underlying causes of individual difficulties, while others work to effect change without looking deeply into members' psyches. Our focus is on insight-oriented groups, which often but not always involve some encouragement of ego regression; these groups operate on the theory that by fostering regression and encouraging exploration of past conflicts, the therapist will help group members ultimately achieve a higher level of functioning. The primary goal of insight-oriented psychotherapy groups is characterological change, which occurs as members gain increased self-understanding.

Psychotherapy groups, especially insight-oriented ones, help individuals learn about their relationships and actions within the context of the group experience. A group offers the opportunity to learn about one's feelings and experiences regarding intimacy, conflict resolution, and individuation, as well as to learn how one's actions and expressions of thoughts and feelings affect others (Rutan & Stone, 1984). Insight-oriented psychotherapy groups are geared toward members' learning about their own perceptions and distortions as they and their fellow group members each expose shameful aspects of themselves within the group setting. This process encourages characterological change as members repeatedly express their feelings about what has been revealed. When it works, members can achieve forgiveness, resolution, and self-acceptance (Alonso & Swiller, 1993).

Working with transference is an essential component of insight-oriented group psychotherapy. Transference may be directed toward the therapist (representing parents and authority figures) as well as toward other group members (representing siblings, friends, colleagues, and others in one's world). Transference can provoke affective reactions that help members to learn about themselves and how they relate to others. Although transference occurs in all groups, as well as in all interpersonal situations, it is only in insight-oriented psychotherapy groups that it becomes important for the transferences to be explored and understood. Therapists in such psychotherapy groups both encourage and explore transference material, whereas such material is given minimal attention in support groups (Rutan & Cohen, 1989).

It can be quite difficult for individuals to focus on the work in an insight-oriented psychotherapy group when they are in the midst of a life crisis. A psychotherapy group experience moves beyond the immediate issues of isolation and helplessness related to a serious illness. Obviously, when individuals are preoccupied with acute feelings related to illness such as those described earlier in this chapter, they are in no position to do the work that is ultimately the aim of an insight-oriented psychotherapy group.

Countertransference issues are present for every therapist who leads any type of group described in this chapter. Therapists who lead psychotherapy groups for people who have been traumatically affected by a serious or prolonged illness are constantly inundated by loss. Such therapists' existential awareness of their own limited control, of their own helplessness, and of the unpredictability of life can be overwhelming. Therapists must remember that their own feelings may parallel those of the group members, and that they need to be as creative in the alleviation of their own stress as they are in attempting to lower the stress levels of the group members. There are many ways to accomplish this; some of these may be finding a support group of other therapists who lead similar groups, being sure that supervision or consultation is available, and/or having colleagues who are willing to listen when a therapist's stress level needs some reduction.

SUMMARY

In summary, the initial group intervention offered to individuals who have been newly diagnosed and their families is usually an education group. A support group often proves useful both for those who are newly affected by an illness and for those who are entering acute phases of an illness, such as treatment, an increase in symptoms, or recurrence. The critical nature of what is occurring in patients' and families' lives usually precludes beginning insight-oriented psychotherapy at these times. There may be other times during a prolonged illness, however—such as during a long period of remission, or after adjustment to the initial impact of a serious illness—when an individual may want to engage in psychotherapy to explore such issues as unresolved earlier losses and/or unresolved relationship issues that have been exacerbated by the illness.

REFERENCES

Alonso, A., & Swiller, H. (1993). Introduction: The case for group therapy. In A. Alonso & H. Swiller (Eds.), *Group therapy in clinical practice*. Washington, DC: American Psychiatric Press.

American Psychiatric Association. (1994). *Diagnostic and statistical manual of mental disorders* (4th ed.). Washington, DC: Author.

Bernstein, G., & Klein, R. (1995). Countertransference issues in group psychotherapy with HIV-positive and AIDS patients. *International Journal of Group Psychotherapy, 45*(1), 91–100.

Cordoba, C., Shear, M. B., Fobair, P., & Hall, J. (1984). *Cancer support groups.* Oakland, CA: American Cancer Society.

Deans, G., Bennett-Emslie, G. B., Weir, J., Smith, D. C., & Kaye, S. B. (1988). Cancer support groups: Who joins and why? *British Journal of Cancer, 58*, 670–674.

Fobair, P., Cordoba, C., Pluth, C., & Bloom, J. (1982) Considerations for successful groups. In *Cancer rehabilitation: Proceedings, Western States Conference*. Palo Alto, CA: Bull.

Frost, J. C. (1993). Group psychotherapy with HIV-positive and AIDS patients. In A. Alonso & H. Swiller (Eds.), *Group therapy in clinical practice*. Washington, DC: American Psychiatric Press.

Getzel, G. S. (1994). No one is alone: Groups during the AIDS pandemic. In A. Gitterman & L. Shulman (Eds.), *Mutual aid groups, vulnerable populations, and the life cycle* (2nd ed.). New York: Columbia University Press.

Hunt, R. W., Bond, M. J., & Pater, G. (1990). Psychological responses to cancer: A case for cancer support groups. *Community Health Studies, 14,* 35–38.

Lindemann, E. (1944). Symptomatology and management of acute grief. *American Journal of Psychiatry, 101*(2), 141–148.

Plant, H., Richardson, J., Stubbs, L., Lynch, D., Ellwood, J., Slevin, M., & De Haes, H. (1987). Evaluation of a support group for cancer patients and their families and friends. *British Journal of Hospital Medicine,* 317–322.

Roback, H. B. (1984). Introduction: The emergence of disease-management groups. In H. B. Roback (Ed.), *Helping patients and their families cope with medical problems.* San Francisco: Jossey-Bass.

Rolland, J. S. (1987). Chronic illness and the life cycle: A conceptual framework. *Family Process, 26,* 203–221.

Rutan, J. S., & Cohen, A. (1989). Group psychotherapy. In A. Lazare (Ed.), *Outpatient psychiatry.* Baltimore: Williams & Wilkins.

Rutan, J. S., & Stone, W. N. (1984). *Psychodynamic group psychotherapy.* New York: Macmillan.

Spiegel, D., Bloom, J. R., & Yalom, I. (1981). Group support of patients with metastatic cancer: A randomized prospective outcome study. *Archives of General Psychiatry, 38,* 527–533.

Spiegel, D., Kraemer, H. C., Bloom, J., & Gottheil, E. (1989). Effect of psychosocial treatment on survival of patients with metastatic breast cancer. *Lancet, 2,* 888–891.

Spiegel, D., & Yalom, I. (1978). A support group for dying patients. *International Journal of Group Psychotherapy, 28,* 233–245.

Spiegelberg, N. (1980). Support group improves quality of life for MS patients. *Association of Rehabilitation Nursing Journal,* 9–11.

Stewart, A. M., Kelly, B., Robinson, J. D., & Callender, C. O. (1995). The Howard University Hospital transplant and dialysis support group: Twenty years and going strong. *International Journal of Group Psychotherapy, 45*(4), 471–488.

van der Kolk, B. A. (1987). The role of the group in the origin and resolution of the trauma response. In B. A. van der Kolk (Ed.), *Psychological trauma.* Washington, DC: American Psychiatric Press.

Vugia, H. D. (1991). Support groups in oncology: Building hope through the human bond. *Journal of Psychosocial Oncology, 9*(3), 89–107.

Weisman, A. (1979). *Coping with cancer.* New York: McGraw-Hill.

Wellisch, D. K., Mosher, M. G., & Van Scoy, C. (1978). Management of family emotional stress: Family group therapy in a private oncology practice. *International Journal of Group Psychotherapy, 28*(2), 225-231.

Yalom, I. (1995). *The theory and practice of group psychotherapy* (4th ed.). New York: Basic Books.

9

◄◦►

Children of Trauma and Loss: Their Treatment in Group Psychotherapy

JANIS L. KEYSER
KATHY SEELAUS
GLORIA BATKIN KAHN

Jason's father routinely comes home drunk and beats up his mother. The last time, he used kitchen knives to threaten her. Many times during the day now, when Jason's mother goes to look for him, she finds her 5-year-old lying under his bed, eyes wide open.

David's mother does not take him to visit his father in jail. His mother tells him that his father doesn't want to see him. She also tells him he's worthless like his father. David broke two chairs in fourth grade last week by throwing them against the wall.

Nine-year-old Kia's parents are divorced. Kia and her little brother, 4, were formerly living with their mother, who takes drugs. Some nights she wouldn't come home at all, leaving the children by themselves. Her father hadn't shown up for visits for a while, and his whereabouts are currently unknown. Now they have been placed in foster care. Kia, usually well behaved and a good student, has just cut up her favorite poetry book.

A year ago, when Michael was 6, he was a passenger in the car his mother was driving. An accident ensued, and his mother was killed. He is now living with his grandmother, and nobody talks about his mother's death. They "shush" him when he mentions her name. Michael refuses to eat because his tummy hurts; his head hurts, too.

WHAT IS TRAUMA FOR CHILDREN?

Something powerful and hurtful has occurred in the lives of the children described above. Their normal development has been impaired by traumatic events, and there is a real risk of their situations' remaining unchanged or deteriorating unless some intervention occurs.

In our consideration of the nature of trauma in the lives of children as opposed to trauma in the life of adults, one reality is apparent and of the utmost concern: Children are *still growing*, and they need to put their attention and energy into the developmental tasks of growing. This is hard to do at best. When a "curve ball" occurs in a young life, the growing process receives an assault, and development is arrested unless some therapeutic intervention occurs. Something needs to be done.

What is traumatic for children? A basic working definition of "trauma" for children is any experience or event that threatens a child's sense of safety and security to such an extent that it is perceived by the child to be unmanageable. There is a continuum from extreme trauma, "distinctly unusual and deemed abnormal" (Apfel & Simon, 1996, p. 6) in quality and requiring intense intervention, to relatively uncomplicated grief, which by its nature may require minimal intervention in order for satisfactory recovery to occur. A trauma may be acute or chronic. Although all trauma inherently includes a multitude of losses, not all loss is traumatic. In the case of children, though, it is harder to maintain a distinction between trauma and loss. For instance, a child's loss of a parent—whether to death, incarceration, substance misuse, or mental illness—is a traumatic loss.

Some children's view of the world is one of "reasonable stability and sanity," while others may in fact live in a world that in their view is always "predictably violent and cruel" (Apfel & Simon, 1996, p. 6). A trauma creates a sensation of overwhelming arousal, to which children are particularly susceptible. They take in and record the blunt, raw impact of the experience (Young, 1996). Research has indicated that traumatic experiences in childhood can alter brain development and chemistry in such a way that learning and concentration are affected (DeBellis, 1999). With their coping skills and sense of who they are still in the process of development, they end up feeling frighteningly helpless and out of control. They can feel as though their world has been cracked open and turned upside down. Over time, there is a strenuous struggle to make sense of their experiences, to search for meaning or meanings (Garbarino & Kostelny, 1996; Webb, 1991). In the process, there is often a battle with the contradiction between feeling powerless and feeling that the traumatic events were their fault. The self-blame, and the shame that accompanies it, are hard for a child to speak of.

There are many disruptive happenings in the lives of children: poverty, illness, parental drug/alcohol addiction, parental incarceration, or death of a family member. These things are not just aspects of the inner-city environment; they are the "monsters" of the suburbs as well. When further significant traumatic experiences are added to the mix—for instance, murder, separation from family, AIDS, a mass disaster (e.g., the Oklahoma City bombing), or a natural disaster (e.g., a hurricane)—children's sense of the world's order and safety may be shattered (Garbarino & Kostelny, 1996). The boundaries around their safe haven are destroyed as the world becomes much bigger and more fearful. Their response to this crisis is often played out in destructive or violent acting out of the craziness of their inner turmoil, for lack of any other sense of how to handle it (Wolfelt, 1996).

CHILDREN'S RESPONSES TO TRAUMA

For children as well as for adults, grief is a normal reaction to loss. Grief reactions are evident in even very young children as responses to separation from their mothers (Bowlby, 1960). Even when a loss is temporary, a child can respond with intense distress. Webb (1993, pp. 8–10) makes a distinction between "grief" and "mourning," with mourning being dependent upon an understanding of the permanence and irreversibility of the loss. Although young children may be unable to understand these concepts, they experience the grief process, which is accompanied by many thoughts, feelings, and behaviors (Wolfelt, 1983).

Grief is undeniably psychologically, socially, behaviorally, and physically challenging, but it may or may not be traumatic, depending on the circumstances. A traumatic reaction may be experienced after a loss that is sudden, unexpected, and/or violent, or after a loss that disrupts a child's whole life, such as the death of a parent. For children as compared to adults, there is a greater overlap between grief and traumatic loss reactions. A loss that may cause a grief reaction in an adult may precipitate a more profound traumatic reaction in a child. When, just as children are developing a capacity to understand the world, that world is turned upside down by a loss, they can be left feeling threatened, anxious, helpless, guilty, dissociated, and distrustful (Rando, 1993).

Webb (1991) notes six factors that play a part in a child's reaction and that should be part of the assessment process after a child has been through a crisis: age and developmental factors; precrisis adjustment; coping style and ego adjustment; past experience with crisis; Global Assessment of Functioning score (Axis V of the DSM diagnostic system); and the specific meaning of the crisis to the child. This concept of meaning is of particular interest. Janoff-Bulman (1985, 1992) has studied the assault upon the assumptive world that comes with grief and trauma. She emphasizes the differences in this assumptive world for a child versus an adult: The child is more open to new input and more able to accommodate new stimuli. Janoff-Bulman adds that this capacity is a two-edged sword, allowing for both psychological protection and destruction.

While growing up, a child has to have an idealistic understanding of his or her world. Children who have dealt with trauma in the past or who are dealing with ongoing trauma have been robbed of their innocence prematurely. Their suffering has shown them that life is not easy or fair—that it has not conformed to the ideal they had hoped for or that they see their peers still holding as valid. For a while, they cling to and yearn for the lost assumptive world to be restored and for their cherished ideals to be reinstated.

The work of processing grief or trauma can be interrupted by current needs and happenings in a child's life; conversely, psychological development can be interrupted by grief and trauma. A disruption or derailment during a critical period of development results in a more rocky path for the resolution of that particular period of growth. Certain tragedies, such as a child's own life-threatening illness or that of a loved one, can lead to much earlier refinement of death- and trauma-related concepts.

Children can demonstrate amazing resilience, even in the face of trauma, if the key element of social support from significant adults in their environment is in place. A fundamental requirement for the healthy growth of children is the presence of loving, caring adults who are there on a consistent basis for them. Children, due to their dependence, are particularly reliant upon family resources (i.e., parents or guardians) and their extended support network (e.g., teachers, club leaders, members of the clergy) for help and guidance, especially after a traumatic event. In a classic study of children during the London Blitz of World War II (Freud & Dann, 1951), it was demonstrated that children who stayed with their parents in the bombed area fared better than those who were moved to a safe area but separated from their parents. The nurturing that parental presence provided was invaluable in reducing the impact of the traumatic events. The value of a child's healthy attachment to adults in the family and in the extended support network when a traumatic event occurs is to "reframe and transform the event" (Janoff-Bulman, 1992, p. 86)—to help the child obtain a perspective on it that makes it less overwhelming to the child's inner schema, and/or to help the child do the work of revising his or her inner world to obtain a degree of resolution.

In the event that an adult who would have filled this role is missing (due to death, substance abuse, incarceration, etc.), other adults must become reliable sources of support and caring. Many adults, however, are not prepared for this role. When these important people react with panic and despair in response to the child's need, the child's adaptation may be compromised (Garbarino & Kostelny, 1996). In addition, a whole different set of implications results when children are the recipients of "victimization by the very people who are looked to for protection and safety" (Janoff-Bulman, 1992, p. 86). A more hopeful view of this subject comes from studies by Young-Eisendrath (1996), who suggests that in some cases it may take one particular adult in an at-risk child's life to precipitate a turn toward resilience. A counselor, a teacher, or other adult may fill this role by providing valuable mentoring for even a short duration of time. The way in which such an adult is present to the child in offering guidance and support can help the child summon up the strength he or she needs to move through challenging situations.

THE ROLE OF GROUP THERAPY FOR TRAUMATIZED CHILDREN

The group therapy experience provides a setting in which a child's psychic and developmental wounds can receive some healing. Family members are often unable to deal with the trauma constructively, and they give either direct or indirect cues that talking about the painful event is unacceptable. Thus the wounds continue to fester and development is blocked. The group offers a model for the restoration of an ideal—a caring "family" consisting of empathic adults and other children who are accepting and understanding. This "family group" creates for the children a caring circle of people who will walk with them through the suffering, allowing them to verbalize the stories of their experiences.

Children's Response to Group Therapy

Therapeutic support in the group setting can be as helpful for children as for adults facing trauma. Most children find groups to be a natural environment in which to play, grow, and express their physicality. In the Freud and Dann (1951) study of children during the London Blitz, it was found that some of the children who were separated from their parents spontaneously developed a peer group that provided some of the nurturing they needed. Unfortunately, there is a paucity of literature on the subject of group therapy with traumatized children.

Short-Term Trauma-Focused Groups

Children who have experienced trauma benefit from belonging to short-term groups focused on their specific trauma. Children's communication styles and patterns are different from those of adults. Pynoos and Nader (1988) have observed that school-age children often do not make direct statements about their emotional status, so that it is easy to underestimate the strength of their feelings. Since these children may not typically look to words for expression of fears, the therapist uses the children's play, artistic expression, and peer encounters in the group as clues to their inner thoughts, feelings, and fantasies. Schamess (1993) notes, "A capacity for and an interest in verbalizing feelings should be viewed as a desired outcome of treatment, rather than as a prerequisite for participation" (p. 565). He adds,

> Trauma-focused groups work because their psychoeducational structure contains anxiety and reduces the likelihood of regression and decompensation, even in the face of highly stimulating material. Those groups are effective in ameliorating particular aspects of the pain and the dysfunction caused by repeated trauma, and they help prevent retraumatization. (p. 561)

Healing in the Telling of Children's Stories

When children get the opportunity to tell their stories in the group, they can share as much or as little as they choose. They are telling these stories to others within whom there is a place in which the stories can resonate, because these "others" are their peers who have also been traumatized. Each child not only is validated by peers (e.g., "Yeah, I thought I was going crazy, too, when that happened to me"), but gets the chance to hear his or her own story spoken aloud. Paradoxically, by hearing themselves in the company of listening peers, who are being compassionate toward their own experience—validating its reality and the accompanying feelings, thoughts, and sensations—the children also become more objective about it, slowly gaining distance from it. They move beyond that first horror of being helpless children in an out-of-control world, to being bearers of stories, narrators in the midst of peers. This also gives the children the beginning of a sense of control: They determine when and how much they will tell of their tales. They can choose a *Reader's Digest* version, compressed and edited to meet their needs, or they can take one aspect and explore it more fully. They learn over time in the supportive atmosphere of the group that, as Fred Rogers (1979) of public television's *Mister Rogers' Neighborhood* has said, what is mentionable can be manageable. The restoration of self-esteem and mastery is an important outcome.

The therapist starts by accepting that each child's initial story (though it may include many fantasies and misconceptions, from the helper's point of view) is the child's reality at the moment. At least it is where he or she is willing to begin, and a place from which the full story can unfold. Over time, with the help of the therapist and peers, fantasies and misconceptions can begin to fall away. Within the safety of the group, the child begins to process the nuggets within the story—to get to the heart of the trauma and its assault upon the child's world.

For children this process has a different flavor than for adults, in that it can be a huge breakthrough for children even to know they have stories to tell. Children, putting their entire beings into who they are, may not distinguish their experiences from the core of who they are. For example, if they feel shameful about elements of their traumatic events, their shame can become the reality that they accept without question. They may not reason or rationalize any differently, and consequently may not gain any distance from the events to examine them more objectively. Their propensity toward magical thinking, in which they believe the power of their thoughts and wishes can cause things to happen, may further reinforce their feeling. When they share in the group or hear other children share a similar feeling, their view of themselves as the sole containers of that feeling can crack, if even just a little—enough to let in the light of day. That is a start. A connection is made to another; a link is forged; identification with the group has begun. Healing becomes a possibility.

Often children may have the opportunity to reenact their stories in the group. For instance, the therapist's use of group activities to help the children identify bodily states of anger or fear may allow a child to demonstrate how he or she reacted when angry or afraid as a result of the traumatic event. At other times, certain triggers may spontaneously lift to awareness particular feelings or events related to the trauma, offering an impromptu opportunity for a child to play out his or her story in the group. The therapist's guidance in identifying and naming of this reenactment process can help it to be a safe experience for the child. With the support of the group, positive changes and adaptations can be learned.

Through attention to children's stories, they can be reassured that they are not alone and will not be left alone in their grief and trauma. As others are compassionate toward the children, they can learn to be compassionate toward themselves. As the children receive support, they can begin to give support to others. These empowering interactions help the children begin to trust once again, in what has otherwise become a scary world. In the group, the meaning of and the feelings connected to the trauma are recognized on many levels. Thus addressing the trauma within the group creates a curative experience.

The Development of Children's Groups

Grounding in group development theory is necessary for the successful facilitation of a group for traumatized children through its many vicissitudes. It is essential for the therapist to have a model to use as a lens through which to view group process, and to keep in mind that group development theories are based on research with groups of adults. They are not specific to children's groups, nor are they specific to children's traumatic loss groups. Still, they can be helpful in informing the therapist's work with groups of children.

The view that we find particularly useful in working with children's groups is Johnson and Johnson's (1987) life cycle model. This model builds upon Tuckman's (1965) linear-progressive theory. Tuckman's scheme includes (1) "forming" a group through a stage of testing and dependence; (2) "storming" through intragroup conflict and emotional expression; (3) "norming," through which cohesion and commitment is built in the group; and (4) "performing" the group task. In applying Tuckman's model to cooperative learning groups, Johnson and Johnson propose a seven-stage model that includes a terminal phase; they liken the period of a group's existence to a life cycle that includes decline and death. Groups, including those with children, can move rapidly through the first five stages, which are (1) defining and structuring procedures and becoming oriented; (2) conforming to procedures and getting acquainted; (3) recognizing mutuality and building trust; (4) rebelling and differentiating; and (5) committing to and taking ownership for the goals, procedures, and other members. The next stage is (6) functioning maturely and productively. The group may remain in this stage for a number of sessions. The last phase is (7) terminating. The termination phase acknowledges the finiteness of the group and the feelings of separation and loss that can accompany its ending. In a group designed to help children deal with traumatic loss, attention to how this termination phase is handled is particularly important. The more cohesive the group has become, the stronger the emotional attachments will have become. It can be painful to leave the security of the "ideal family" that the group has become for the children over many weeks. Through the therapist's skill and intentionality, this stage provides important learning for the children. It can offer some sense of closure, which may not be possible in regard to many of the losses with which they are dealing.

Through attention to group processes and roles, the therapist can encourage children to stretch into new, positive, healing behaviors. Children may demonstrate a natural proclivity toward certain roles in groups, and the therapist may need to actively "run interference" to a child's repeated enactment of certain roles to the exclusion of others. The therapist may also need to work toward keeping a balance so that no one member contains a particular function or emotion for the entire group, and so that children have the freedom to try on roles that they haven't played before. For instance, a previous harmonizer can be guided to take the risk of being a gatekeeper or an opinion giver. If a child tends to enact the role of parent in the group, the therapist may encourage him or her to try the role of follower or information seeker. Behavioral disruptions in the group can result from a child's denial of his or her pain. Those who bully others, who get the group to laugh at their antics through their clowning, or who hold out from participating by sulking or clinging are children who cannot easily let themselves go on a path of discovery that they know will be painful. Depending on the developmental level of the group, children may or may not benefit from the therapist's attempt to interpret these maladaptive roles to them. For latency-age and younger children, it is often more effective for the therapist to maintain enough structure in the group that the roles do not have a negative impact upon the group process. Through attention to group process and roles, the therapist can prevent scapegoating, sub-grouping, and other potential problems that can proliferate in groupings of children.

In addition, a knowledge of children's developmental stages is important. For example, Piaget's stages of development are helpful. However, as Webb (1993) notes, research on children's conceptualizations of death suggest that children may have a realistic perception of the finality and irreversibility of death at age 9 or 10, which is earlier than would be suggested by Piaget's stage of formal-operational thought. It is important for the therapist to be mindful of individual differences among children in their conceptualizations of death and trauma.

The ways in which successful groups for children are run may vary as a function of the children's age. The value of group psychotherapy for traumatic loss has been demonstrated for preschoolers through adolescents, though each age level brings its own challenges. Preschoolers are less verbal and tend to focus greatly on play materials and activities. Progress is rather slow, and much patience is required on the part of the therapist, but an important grounding in terms of trust building and familiarity can be established for future group and individual work. Groups for latency-age children require the therapist to develop structured plans and utilize varied materials for projects and crafts, honoring their proclivity toward concrete thinking. Groups for preadolescents and adolescents require the therapist to work with resistance issues that come from a more defended stance toward group participation.

In establishing a group, the therapist has to consider many factors. These include demographic issues, such as potential differences between the needs of inner-city children and those of children from suburban neighborhoods. Whether the group is held in a neighborhood school, a local hospital, a psychology clinic, or another location in the community can influence children's participation and perceptions about the group. Consideration should also be given to the duration of the group (i.e., time-limited or ongoing). Younger children can benefit from a shorter series of time-limited groups, with the potential opportunity to participate in a future series, whereas teens may benefit from ongoing groups over months or years.

The Therapist: Role and Person

In order to understand how the group serves to deliver a curative effect, we must first look at the therapist. The therapist is the pivotal person in creating the environment for healing to occur. The therapist needs to have attributes that make him or her, in a way, the ideal parent. These attributes include a genuine love for children and a recognition and respect for their unique personhood, as well as the ability to give and receive affectionate responses. The therapist must be able to tolerate frustration, chaos, and aggression, while possessing his or her own sense of wonder at and hope for the world, even when children's assumptions about it have been shattered. The therapist must understand what it means to play, and must cherish the qualities of joy, creativity, and curiosity that accompany play, while also being able to assert limits. In embracing these contradictions, the therapist becomes the ideal and protecting parent—providing unconditional acceptance of each child, though not always accepting as constructive the ways in which the symptoms of the child's traumatization are acted out in the world. That the children in the group come to depend on the therapist is a healthy and appropriate development, given that they *are* children; this makes such a group different from an adult psychotherapy group (Siepker, Lewis, & Kandaras, 1985).

It is important for the therapist to have the clinical training to pace the therapy to meet each child's needs and to start from the place where the child is. The therapist needs to understand a child's tempo, particularly a traumatized child's tempo. Often these children are highly defended, withdrawn, or hostile; they need time to settle into the group and to trust that this is in reality a safe and a consistently caring place. The therapist needs to be a patient person who can give each child the time to begin to trust and let down the barriers.

Group work with traumatized and bereaved children requires particular openness to the examination of the therapist's own processes, including coming face to face with his or her own childhood experiences of trauma and grief (Schamess, Streider, & Connors, 1997). In fact, without this examination, the therapist's effectiveness is likely to be limited. The children's stories and personalities will inevitably stir feelings within the therapist. It is important to understand this so that the therapist does not "react" out of his or her own needs and feelings. It is essential for the therapist to know him- or herself as much as possible before beginning this challenging work with groups of traumatized children; then it is necessary to remain continually alert to the countertransference reactions that may arise. It is helpful for the therapist to have a cotherapist and/or supervision to help keep a perspective on the process.

A CLINICAL EXAMPLE

The Context and Setting

There is no better way to make real the concepts of group practice that we have been discussing than to illustrate them with an extended clinical example. We give an overview of the 6-week life of a children's traumatic loss group, in order to convey the reality of the experience both for the children and for the group therapists. In pursuing this approach, we identify specific guidelines for the cotherapists and share with the reader their path—sometimes discouraging, and sometimes richly gratifying. It is important to note that not all goes well even for experienced practitioners, who realize that any group represents many unknowns, and who are excited and challenged by that fact. In working with groups of children, our knowledge gained has been great; our progress has often been moderate; and our hopes remain firm.

The group we describe here included seven children, aged 7–9, who had each experienced one or more traumatic losses (e.g., incarceration of a parent, the witnessing of the murder of a sibling, movement among multiple foster homes, or death of a close family member). The sessions were conducted after school in the school library.

The Therapists

The two therapists who led the group brought both similarities and differences to the group experience. One therapist had been the bereavement coordinator at a children's hospital in the city, and in that role had dealt with hundreds of bereaved family members over many years. The other therapist had begun grief work unexpectedly, working with families who had lost an infant to sudden infant death syndrome; she then went on to work with child and adult survivors of trauma (especially homicide), and from there to work with children who had experienced any severe kind of loss. Both therapists felt qualified by experience and supervision for this particular activity; more importantly, they had a personal commitment to the work, especially in this neighborhood, which was known to both of them as bleak and often fearful for children. They had each, however, experienced the hidden richness of survival qualities in these families, and they longed for the community to be able to "turn a corner" and see the possibility of change. In addition, they each genuinely loved children and enjoyed them. Both were mothers; indeed, they were mothers who each had suffered the loss of a child. They had known the heartbreak of untoward death many years ago, and had come to hold in high regard everything about the process of grief work.

Factors Considered in Setting Up the Group

Previous experience led the therapists to recognize certain factors that were very important to consider in setting up the group. These included attention to the selection of group members and the degree of traumatic loss suffered, as well as the recency of each child's loss and its relevancy to the child; the meeting time and setting of the session; and the inclusion of refreshments.

Selection of the Children

Careful screening of the children was of utmost importance. The children needed to be selected most specifically on the basis of a very common trauma, which for this group was bereavement. The therapists decided that the traumatic loss must be recent and/or must still be causing a child significant pain. For example, a child whose grandparent had died several years ago would not be appropriate for the group if he or she were not in current distress. Although there might be some residual feelings of loss, the child might easily be distracted into playing that strayed away from the group task. The therapists would not exclude those children whose suffering resulted in extreme behavioral problems, because they believed that the need of these children was possibly greater. They would either deal with a child's difficult behavior in the group or invite that child to meet with one of the therapists separately from the group.

The Meeting Place and Time

The therapists knew that the group needed to be held at the conclusion of the school day and planned as one of the after-school clubs. During a school day, norms exist that are counterproductive to the purpose of a traumatic loss group. A child in school is programmed to adhere to a "get it right" approach; this is different from the approach needed in trauma-related grief work, where the only "skills" required are openness and acceptance of all feelings, as well as a consistent, respectful availability. Placement of group sessions in the middle of the school day does not allow children to integrate the experience fully, as they may be required to shift gears rapidly to adjust to the demands of the next class, and this leaves them no place to go with affect. Schedules can also be disrupted by fire drills and other demands. In addition, it is more obvious that the children are involved in a "different" activity from that of their classmates.

Finally, the meetings of a children's traumatic loss group need to take place in a space that allows a warm setting for circle time and conversation. A typical classroom is not ideal for these purposes. The school library was chosen for this particular group, since meeting in the library allowed ample space for movement, play, and writing activities.

Refreshments

For children, the inclusion of food in a group experience is a necessity (Schleidlinger, 1982). Food is of great importance to children, and in groups it is a time-honored initiator of talk. As Rachman (1995) mentions, providing refreshments is seen as an integral part of a group therapy program, regardless of members' age, sex, education, or socioeconomic status,

or of the therapeutic setting. Schleidlinger (1982) states, "In work with la-
tency age children the group climate needs to be planfully structured toward constancy, nurturing, and feeding" (p. 138), and he includes actual
feeding in the form of a snack or even a full-fledged meal. He adds, "The
actual experiencing of gratification in this approach is most valuable" (p.
138). In this group, as the children came in for each session, they were
greeted with a spread of refreshments consisting of juice, fruit, and pretzels
at the low children's library table. The therapists soon also came to realize
how valuable it was for some children to be associated with the preparation of the food, no matter how simple their tasks were. On succeeding
weeks, young faces shone as the children were asked to wash grapes or
count pretzels. And as the weeks progressed, the insides of the children began to shine as well.

Development of the Group

In early October, a flyer from the principal went home with each child
at the local inner-city elementary school (which included kindergarten
through fifth grade), inviting parents and guardians to consider their children's participation in a children's grief support group, to meet once a
week for an hour for 6 weeks. The group would meet immediately after
school, and was meant to be helpful to those children who had experienced
a recent loss of a loved one due to death or separation and were in distress
(of whatever kind) because of that loss. When the tear-off responses came
in, there were 12 potential group members who fit the specific criteria of
recent experience of loss of a loved one due to death or separation. Of
these 12, 7 children attended regularly throughout the sessions, with no
dropouts. Five others who had been selected and signed up didn't attend
because of either reluctance on a child's part or transportation difficulties.

At the beginning, the children came in one by one; some of them were
quiet, others were nonchalant, but all of them were somewhat tentative. As
they gathered into a circle on the rug for beginning conversation, the children found a variety of comfortable positions. All of the children were in a
mood of anticipation, even the nonchalant ones. When invited to do so,
they introduced themselves in turn, and then the children were asked to
share the reason that brought them to the group. It was mentioned that
anyone could feel free to "pass," and one group member, Joey, 7, did. As
noted above, each of the group therapists had suffered the loss of a child,
and they spoke about this briefly. The children were very much interested
in their stories. It was important for them to see the therapists as models
who had experienced losses and had learned to deal constructively with
their feelings about these. The children were able to see that it was appropriate to put their feelings about the experience of loss into words, and that
this was a safe place for them to try to do the same.

The Children

Thomas, 8, had a father who was in prison for the third time. Thomas lived with his mother and grandmother. His father had been absent for most of his life, but on a few occasions he had taken Thomas to car races. At other times, the father's promises had usually gone unfulfilled. Thomas would become known to the therapists for his erratic moods and occasional aggressive behaviors.

Tameeka, 7, had witnessed the murder of her beloved older brother by her mother's boyfriend. She was badly traumatized, and she and her mother were now living temporarily with relatives. Her teacher reported that Tameeka clung to her and appeared withdrawn in the classroom, although she had had two angry outbursts with classmates, one of which involved a physical attack.

Marny, 9, had lived in three different foster homes since she was 4. Her grandmother had recently died in a fire in her home. The story was on television, but Marny did not acknowledge it to her classmates, although she had been very close to her grandmother and often spent weekends with her. Her demeanor was cool and in control. The therapists learned later that she would periodically explode in angry bouts of crying.

John, 8, had lived in a multifamily household with many changes in occupants, until his mother died of a drug overdose when he was 6. He now lived with his aunt, who had a disabling disease and had little patience with him. John told group members that his aunt worried about who would take care of him when she was no longer able to do so. He had a strong need for control and often picked fights.

Joey, 7, did not know that he was HIV-positive. He had been in foster care with the Patrick family since the age of 2. His mother, whom he never knew, died of AIDS when Joey was 3, and his father died when he was 7. He spoke of his father's many unkept promises, one of which was to bring him home. The Patricks took Joey to his father's funeral, where he met several cousins for the first time. He seemed pleased to be connected with an extended family. The Patricks' adoption of Joey would be complete 3 months after the start of the group.

Jamelle, 9, a winsome, talkative child who was overly eager to please, had spent her early years with extended family members; her teenage mother had left her at birth to live with a boyfriend (not Jamelle's father) out of state. At age 6, Jamelle was placed in foster care with the Demmy family, where there were three other foster children and one natural child. Mrs. Demmy was quiet and steady, with strong religious beliefs. Jamelle liked her religious training and spoke eloquently of the love of God, as well as God's judgment. She remarked often and bitterly about her mother's abandoning her. In spite of her religious inclinations, and her need to please, she had been seen to act in mean ways to the other children.

Rosie, 9, had often seen her father beat her mother. Once, in a drunken rage, he turned on the children, and they all had to run to their aunt's house. A month prior to Rosie's starting in the group, he died from complications of alcohol and drug use. The family had peace in the house now, but Rosie said that her mother cried a lot and didn't seem to know how to do anything.

Session 1: Getting Started

Not all of these stories were told in much detail during the first introductory circle. For the most part, the children were succinct in their description of their losses: "My mother died from drugs," or "My father is in jail," or "I'm in a foster home—I don't know where my mother is." It was yet too early for emotions; the children were probably defended against their own pain, or had been taught in a number of ways to "shut up," "be strong," or "move on." How many grieving children grow to adulthood with such unprocessed grief and trauma, only to suffer more severely and in multiple ways? There is a point at which children stop reaching out for support and comfort if it is not there. This amounts to a second loss for them and a most serious one.

Ground Rules

The therapists spoke of rules next, and the children were able to come up with some themselves: "Don't interrupt," "Don't call names," "Don't tease or make trouble," "Clean up after group." The therapists discussed what it might be like as the group members shared more and more. They stated, "Sometimes stories are not easy to tell, and everyone needs to remember that whatever happened, their feelings about it are theirs—not right or wrong but theirs, and okay, because they're real. And those who listen need to be serious about each person's feelings, no matter what they are." It was also important for the children to know that they were allowed to "pass" whenever they did not feel like talking. The therapists then talked about confidentiality and what it meant—that whatever the group talked about, it must remain "in the room." The therapists spoke of how adults and children alike can be very careless about this rule.

The therapists were concerned about how well the children observed this rule of confidentiality. The therapists did not learn much about confidentiality within the family setting, but they learned that within the school, because group members were not actually asked a lot of questions by their peers about the group, private material was probably not divulged. Based on feedback from the children's teachers, the therapists were fairly certain that those in the group did not initiate any talk about group content. This was a sign that group boundaries were being respected and that group cohesion was developing.

The Value of Talking

The children were curious about a colorfully decorated tree branch in a bag. John wanted to hold it, and the facilitators let him take it out to show the group. "This is a talking stick," they told the children. "It is just like those which were used by Native Americans when they got in a circle to talk. Whoever is holding it has the attention and respect of everyone else, because what is being said is very important to that person. For us, it means that no one else talks at the same time. It's a pretty serious idea, and we thought it would be good for our group. What do you think?" The group's interested response and quick "Yes" probably had as much to do with wanting to hold the "talking stick" as anything else about it. The therapists described how they would use it next week as they sat in the circle and had "check-in time"; for now, however, the children wanted to pass it around for inspection, and the therapists did.

The therapists then initiated a discussion about loss of all kinds and how it affects people, both young and old. They asked the children, "What are some of the things that can happen after the loss of someone we love?" There was a long silence, and then John asked, "What do you mean? Like the funeral?" "Well, yes, the funeral; but what about after the funeral?" John replied, "My aunt just said, 'Well, that's that' [making a rubbing motion with his hands], 'now let's get back to normal.' " "Is that how you felt too?" one therapist asked. "No, but when I began talking about the funeral and my mom, my aunt told me, 'Cut it out; nobody needs that talk.' " The therapists felt fortunate: John had helped them to get into just what they had planned. The therapists then guided the discussion into looking at how easy it seems to "put pain away" and *not* look at it. This discussion brought some stark observations from the children: "Yeah, who needs to be stabbed in the heart again?"; "Why talk about it? It doesn't help"; "When I cry, I upset my mother." There were some children who disagreed. Thomas said, "But I'm *so* mad! It stinks when you're told to 'stop talking like that'!" Jamelle said, "My foster mom says when I'm angry, it's the devil in me. Is that true?" Rather than responding to each comment, the leaders showed how impressed they were by the thinking of all the children—by the honest and sensible thoughts they expressed. The therapists went on to describe how the group would be a place to do some really good talking about those things. It was a safe place; the children would not be "put down" for anything they said; they could ask some really weird questions; they could share what hurt them and what helped them, even if it sounded strange.

The therapists had to remain aware that real help would lie not in their being "answer persons," but in listening. Especially with children, it is so easy to give a facile answer, which may even be correct but which becomes dangerously close to being didactic—a sure way to lose a group.

This does not mean that a therapist cannot bring up ideas that are helpful, but a group should do the exploring together, wondering and speculating about things as a group. A rather moving development is likely to result from this: The children find that it becomes possible to help one another. When this happens in a group, it is more than bonding—it is the beginning of caring and development of the capacity for concern about one another. The group becomes more cohesive as empathy for one another grows.

The Use of Activities

After this serious talk, the therapists planned a break for the group, which was an exercise involving movement and imagination: "How do we get our stuck feet out of this cement?" It was great fun. The children were free and un-self-conscious as they moved about and followed the silly scenario.

They then sat/fell into their chairs around the table. They were asked this question: "Would you like to make something next week that will be a way of remembering this group—and your lost loved one—and *yourselves?*" "Why us?" one child wondered. The therapists answered, "Well, you're the ones who are going to be doing all this thinking, and remembering, and wondering—and you ought to be able to include yourselves."

The therapists knew how important it was to help the children see that they were bigger than their pain, bigger than their loss. Every bereaved child has a self—a many-sided self—that went on in the world daily before the loss. That self still goes on after the loss, and the different "pieces" of it can be tapped into as the child moves toward healing: "Who am I as I make this box?"; "What do I think is beautiful?"; "What is my style?" These questions are not asked consciously by the child as he or she works, but they form an unconscious matrix for self-knowledge and growth—growth out of desolation and loss.

The therapists put it to the children: Would they like to make a piece of art, or a "Memory Box," or a special book—a journal or a scrapbook? The children were impassive (were they getting tired?—it had been 45 minutes). Then Marny said, "I would like to make a scrapbook if I could decorate it a certain way." This started a flurry of responses: "Can we use real photos?" "What would a Memory Box look like?" In the end, the group decided that each child would make a Memory Book, which would include photos, drawings, writing of all kinds, and any other creative ideas that the children might think of. Working on the books would be part of each meeting, but the group would be doing other things also.

The Closing

As they all entered the circle again for closing, the therapists invited the children to bring photographs of their lost family members (if they wanted to) or of their families, so everyone could get to know one another better. They reminded them to take good care of themselves, because they were so important! The therapists then suggested singing a song for ending and asked for suggestions. The children were quiet, or giggled, looking restless. Then Jamelle said, "Can we sing 'Amazing Grace'?" They all knew it; as they sang, holding hands, their restlessness subsided, and there was a perceptible feeling of calm and quiet. They passed around a handshake and parted until next week. The therapists had a sense of a good start.

Session 2: Continuing to Build Connections

Check-In

The second group session the following week had a pleasant feel of familiarity about it, as the children came in with questions such as "What are we going to do today?"; "Can I help with the snacks?"; "Where is the talking stick?" The therapists knew they would be doing something new—having "check-in" time—and the thought occurred to them that it seemed natural to do it at the table with snacks, because talk had begun to flow. They decided against it, however, because they suspected that one real risk would be that of abandoning structure when things "felt good." This did not mean that the role of intuition should be abandoned in any way; intuition is so important in working with children, especially in tuning in to "where they're at" emotionally at any given time. The therapists decided that "check-in" would be part of regular group routine, and that it would occur at circle time.

As the therapists explained this step to the children, now assembled on the rug in a circle, they told them that it mattered to them just how the week had gone for everyone, and that's why they wanted to "check in" with them. They asked each child in turn, "How was your week?" This was nonproblematic for all; in fact, the challenge was to keep updates short enough. The children enjoyed holding the "talking stick" as they recounted their news, and all members listening observed the silence rule quite well (so far!). The therapists made a modification: If one child had a question about another's "news," he or she could raise a hand to ask it. This occurred when Thomas described how he watched *Star Wars* two times at home while his mother went to visit his father in jail, and John wanted to know whether Thomas ever went with his mother on those visits. In a low voice, Thomas answered, "No, he said he doesn't want to see me." "Do you want to see him?" asked John. "Yes." There was pain in the answer as Thomas lowered his head. "That's tough!" someone was heard to say. The therapists wondered about some sort of helpful/comforting phrase, but sometimes (as in this case), silence itself speaks and honors the hurt.

Talking about Death

As the circle ended, the group went back to the library table once again. "What are we going to talk about?" asked Marny. "Death," was the one-word answer from one of the leaders. The therapists felt lucky that these children (like most children) could deal with straightforward answers. They would not "tiptoe" around difficult concepts with the children. They knew that they wanted to be sources of correct information if nothing else (of course, they wanted so much more!). As therapists, they knew they wanted to give consistent respect to the children, both in their attention to the children and in their presumption that they could deal with hard things. The children should never feel that the therapists were protecting them from harsh reality. This would actually be collusion in denial. Rather, as therapists, they would "walk with them" through whatever was likely to be hard.

The therapists embarked on a discussion of death by looking at the concept of "change" and its many forms in their experience. What changes were the children familiar with? Their answers included the seasons, their own growing up, and the difference between life and death in plants, insects, animals. "What does 'slow death' mean?" asked John. "My aunt says that's what she has." The therapists talked about the changes that disease brings—the many losses of physical ability—and how sad that is for sick people. They then talked of the permanence of actual death, and how many children growing up have a hard time realizing that there is absolutely no coming back from death. Jamelle said, "Mrs. Demmy says, 'Dead people fall asleep in the Lord.' " "Yeah, but they don't wake up," added John. "Well, then, why do they say 'fell asleep'?" asked Rosie. "It's kinda dumb." The group was able to talk then about some of the words people use for death, and about why they don't like to use the word "death" itself. "I always thought when people 'passed,' they were getting ahead of other people," said Tameeka. "Yeah, right," cut in John, "right ahead to the graveyard!" "My father," said Rosie, "he was a lot of times 'dead drunk,' said my mom. And guess what? He is really dead because he was drunk so much."

"So death is actually a pretty big change," the therapists observed, "from living to not living." "Forever and ever," said Joey quietly. He had not said anything so far, and both weeks he had looked very solemn and absorbed in his own thoughts. "That's saying it like it is, Joey," said one of the therapists, "and it's hard to say it that way, but we need to." "No big deal," he said, surprisingly. "My mother was 'forever and ever' away from me. I *never* saw her. So it was no big deal when she died." The children were quiet in the wake of this statement from the youngest member of the group. Their thoughts could almost be felt. "What must it be like to *never* have seen your mother?" Tameeka asked that question. Joey almost said again, "No big deal," but stopped and said, "Not great." "Man," commented John, "that's like *worse* than death." "Cut it out," snapped Thomas, *"you're* makin' it worse." "Thomas," the therapist intervened, "can you guess why John said that?" John jumped in: "I was trying to show *respect,* man!"

The therapists went on, in that heightened mood, to speak of what matters most when someone is in great pain from a loss. They wanted to bring out the importance of acknowledging that person in his or her sadness and pain. "We know we can't bring a dead person back, or make an absent person present, so what can we do when we're with someone who's had that happen?" "Shut up and not say something stupid," muttered Thomas. "Pretty smart, Thomas, but how do we show we care?" asked the facilitator. Thomas was at a loss. Other answers came: "Invite them somewhere" (Marny); "Say 'tough break, man'" (John); "Pray for them" (Jamelle). The therapists invited the children to do just that—literally say something to Joey—but he broke in and said quickly, "That's okay, I get it."

An Exercise Break and Work on the Memory Book Activity

This circle was longer and "heavier" than the therapists had anticipated. It was time for a break. It seemed a good idea to do the "cement shoes" routine again; it was so silly that it would do everyone good. When the children sat down to do the Memory Book activity, the therapists felt it would be helpful for them to have a rough structure to follow. Each child would do a title page naming him- or herself and giving some personal facts, especially about the loss and the loved one(s) the child wanted to keep in memory. (Titles chosen by the children included "The Book about Me and My Story," "Me and Mom," "My Memory Book about Tyrone" [Tameeka's brother]). Besides a title page, there would be a cover, and the facilitators knew that each child would decorate it carefully and elaborately. As the children defined what they wanted, they were focused on their own creativity—a strength, and a counterpoint to loss. They would remember that they were good and interesting persons in addition to bereaved persons— and that they could go on in life with sadness, with memories, *and* with self-awareness and strength.

The Closing

As the group drew to a close that day and the therapists asked for a song to sing, Marny said, "What about 'He's Got the Whole World in His Hands'?" It seemed very fitting; it also seemed as if everyone was helped by singing it. Enough verses were used to name each child, and then they named the therapists! A pretty good two-way support street!

Session 3: Sharing Painful Memories

The third meeting continued with a mix of circle talk (checking in); physical activity (this time, "Follow the Leader"); table talk (serious again; it seemed as if a climate of safety and acceptance had been reached early—the therapists felt so lucky); work on the Memory Books; and a farewell song and handshake (once again, "He's Got the Whole World in His Hands"—everyone liked it).

Circle talk on this day focused on memories, all kinds of memories: those of special times with the lost loved ones; those of the death and/or the funeral, in cases where loved ones had died; those about the rest of the family; or memories of anything else. They talked of good memories: "My father wasn't drinking and he was all dressed up nice when he came to my First Communion" (Rosie); "I used to go to the store for my grandmother, and she would say, 'Take 50 cents for yourself and get a candy bar'; she was *so* kind!" (Marny). They also talked of memories that weren't so good. Jamelle said, "I saw my foster mother on her knees praying once, and I asked her who she was praying for, and she said, 'Your mother.' " "That's an all-right memory," said John. "No, it isn't," responded Jamelle, "she said it wouldn't count probably, because she'll burn in hell. I kind of hate her [the mother] for leaving me, but I don't want her to burn in hell!" Tameeka then said, "I remember screaming at Richard to stop shooting my brother. It's an awful picture in my mind—I *hate* it!" "Wow," said Joey in disbelief, "I remember something bad, but it's not like a shooting. I remember the funeral of my father—I *hate* funerals." This raised a flurry of questions and observations: "Was the casket open?" "Were you told to kiss him?" "People say silly things to kids at funerals, like 'Have big shoulders for your mom.' Why do they talk about shoulders?" "My grandmother's casket had to be closed. She was so burned up." This from Joey: "Something *was* okay for me; I met some cousins who are neat, kinda cool. I didn't even know I had them for cousins!" He had a look of wonderment on his face.

All of this provided such a good opportunity for talking about ways of mourning—not only funeral practices, but the role of memory in people's lives. What was more heartening, though, was the openness with which these remarkable children expressed themselves, and the interest and caring they showed toward one another's stories.

By this session, the therapists observed the assuming of certain roles by group members. Marny, Thomas, and John emerged with a certain sense of authority—a responsibility, as it were, for the quality of the group and the well-being of its members. They filled roles as nurturers and expediters. Was this a function of personality or age? They were among the older members. Or had the path of their healing experience been one that had "toughened" them? The therapists felt thankful that these qualities had not been accompanied by denial; all three appeared to be looking at their feelings honestly.

Session 4: Feeling and Expressing Painful Feelings

At the fourth meeting, the therapists and children worked with feelings—it seemed a good time for it, and the children had already encountered some of their deeper levels of feeling. The activity chosen was a game of charades about feelings. The therapists had prepared a basket with several paper strips in it, each one identifying a feeling. On a flip chart, they had placed a large red cardboard heart—nothing else. Each child would take one strip and try to act out the feeling represented without using words. When the word was guessed, the strip would be pinned to the heart. The therapists hoped for some spontaneous talk about feelings as the guessing took place. Some of the words for guessing, and the exchanges that occurred, were as follows:

"Sad": Tameeka wiped her eyes and heaved her shoulders to show deep sadness. The other children guessed "crying," then "sad." Someone asked why she was sad. Tameeka paused as if not knowing how to say what she felt. Her face tightened and she said in a low voice, "I miss Tyrone; I want him back." She cried. Marny went to her, and together they sat down. John needed to say, "I'd be sad, but I'd be rippin' angry too—at Richard. I would be wantin' to get him." "Well, you're probably angry a lot," said Thomas, "because of what happened to you." "Yeah," replied John, "but you can't say to people, 'I'm so mad at my mother'—but I am." "Well, guess what? I'm mad at my father and I'll tell anybody, even him, especially him!" exploded Thomas. "He doesn't care about me; he doesn't even want to see me."

"Angry": It was so fitting that Thomas went next. He stomped around and punched the air. He made grimaces full of rage. He banged his fists on empty desks. "C'mon," he called to John, "you're angry too!" John followed and kicked some desks. He then got down on his knees and pounded the floor. He just stayed there, pounding the floor. It felt right to get down on the floor with him, so the therapists did. The children followed, and the group continued that way. Before leaving "anger," the therapists asked for some other words for it. Words came fast: "explode," "powerful," "hate," "want to scream," "scary," "head hurts." When the therapists brought up the question of how to express anger in ways that wouldn't hurt, the children gave all the right answers: "Use a punching bag," "Take a walk," "Count to 10," "Get in a private place." So often children can articulate correct responses, but how often can they do the pounding and kicking and be understood for the validity of that feeling, let alone do it together and *share* each other's feeling? In this case, as they all (therapists and children) knelt and pounded the floor, they were one.

"Grateful": Jamelle tried hard, but the group had a hard time figuring out the word. "Sorry," "praying," and "happy" were all guessed. She finally showed the word: "I was trying to show a fixed-up heart." "Do you have something to be grateful for, Jamelle?" the therapists asked. "Well," she paused, "I heard something awful the other day, and I'm glad—uh, grateful— she [my mother] didn't do it. I'm glad she didn't flush me down the toilet. But I still hate her for leaving me." "Why did she do that?" asked Joey, his eyes wide. "Mrs. Demmy says she didn't have good sense. She said she was scared to be a mother." "Well, I guess I'm grateful she didn't do it, too," exclaimed Rosie, who hadn't said much. The others each said something similar. Jamelle smiled.

"Empty": Tameeka wanted to add this word. She placed her hands in a circle over her heart. When the children didn't guess, she said, "It's a hole. I feel like I have a hole in me." Everyone understood and agreed with this.

The children added other words, and the acting out took most of the hour. They ended with *their* song: "He's Got the Whole World in His Hands." "Who wants a hug?" the therapists asked. No surprise: Everybody did!

This exercise was remarkable in many ways. Not only did it draw on the children's creativity and self-possession, but it was an opportunity for that important double task of *feeling* their feelings and of *expressing* their feelings. Because it was done in the community of their group, there was understanding and respect for each other's reality. The therapists knew that their plan to deal with feelings this week would include a certain degree of risk. The story of loss for each one of these children was so severe that touching those feelings could be too powerful, too harsh. Should they let this happen? What about their belief in the importance of "walking through the pain, not around it"? Did the therapists truly believe they could be with these children in the dark places, the broken places? Yes. If a reenactment of the original wounding was to happen, the therapists felt that the group was a strong enough holding vessel for that experience. They also knew that if revisiting the pain was too hard for some of the children, as revealed in their behaviors, the therapists would interpret this to the group. If the message from deep within was "Hey, I can't go there! Look at my silly behavior instead!," they could work on it together. Naming what was happening could be part of the healing process.

Session 5: Getting Back a Life

The next group session occurred right before Thanksgiving, and there was the benefit of three volunteers—a real luxury. The idea of giving thanks is more fitting than is often supposed for a traumatic loss group (as seen in Session 4, when the group worked on "grateful" with Jamelle). The children had absolutely no problem switching to the excitement associated with a holiday, especially one that is so connected with home and a very special meal. The children made some minibooklets of all the things they were grateful for. As they worked, each volunteer sat by the side of two of the children, while one therapist sat with Joey (who had gotten a slow start) and the other therapist "floated." The adults asked questions about the pictures that emerged. What happened in this process was felt by the therapists to be remarkable: As the children realized that there was genuine curiosity and interest in the particular practices of their *own* households, they became, as it were, spokespersons for the traditions of their families. The talk was quiet but nonstop, as just the right questions were asked: "You ate *how many* pieces of pie?"; "How does your mother ever get a turkey in the oven by 9 in the morning!?"; "How did you fit all those people around the table?" The children wanted to do intricate drawings of Thanksgiving scenes, including most rooms of their houses, along with family "portraits" of all (including extended family members). There were some lovely ways of portraying the lost loved ones (in a cloud over the house, in a heart-shaped picture frame on the wall of the dining room). The feeling was one of contentment, pride, and ownership—all as a counterpoint to loss. This was a rich and powerful step toward the goal of "getting back a life" (i.e., a child's knowing ways to be in the world that still surrounds him or her, and putting a value on whatever helps that to happen).

Session 6: Ending the Group

The sixth and last meeting meant that the children would finish their Memory Books and have some talk about ending. The therapists also planned to have a special guest—a musician, who came with her instruments, which were many and intriguing. At check-in time, the children gave their updates without much change to record. However, there was, if not behavior change, in fact some very clear change in viewpoints. Thomas said, "I have a feeling I'll have something to be grateful for soon—I think my father might want to see me on his birthday." He was smiling. Joey said, "On Thanksgiving, I said out loud at grace that I was glad to have my new cousins."

The children's Memory Books were remarkable collections of writings, drawings, photos, collages, and in one case an actual pop-up picture (Marny portrayed her grandmother in heavy colored paper in a rocking chair, which not only popped up but rocked!). Thomas cast himself as a Power Ranger who tore open his father's prison bars and brought him home. In the next picture, he gave a stark warning (complete with skull and crossbones): "NO MORE JAIL!" In the next picture, Thomas and his father were fishing.

The special guest, Melanie, came into the circle with her guitar, and the group sang a few songs together—some with motions, such as: "Did You See My Cow?" and "All God's Critters Got a Place in the Choir." She then brought in other instruments (tambourines, blocks, bell, triangles, drums, etc.) and did some wonderful African and Australian songs. The group members marched to "When the Saints Go Marching In." It was glorious to watch the children forget themselves and their burdens. As they sat down again, the leaders talked about ending. They urged all the children to feel okay about taking care of themselves. John began a "wise old man" act: "Now listen up, you all, remember you are bigger than 'it,' and you are gonna be okay, and if you forget how to take care of *you*, just come to me, and I'll give you my special help!!" Everybody laughed, and Rosie asked, "Do we have to make an appointment?" When they sang their farewell, it consisted of both "Amazing Grace" and "He's Got the Whole World in His Hands," this time with many, many verses: All of the people in the group, *and* all of their lost loved ones, were included. Needless to say, hugs were exchanged all around.

As the therapists watched the children leave together, they asked each other: "What, exactly, did the children learn? How did they change?" John's last words contained one of the biggest lessons: "You are bigger than 'it.' " How could he say that? How could the others laugh so knowingly, as if acknowledging common wisdom? It became clear to the therapists that one of the most important outcomes of group work with traumatized children is helping them find those other pieces of themselves—the pieces that are strong. In this case, the other children laughed affectionately at John's "wise old man" act only because they had all internalized the same wisdom. They could be "wise young people" to each other.

DISCUSSION

Summary of Group Sessions

What began as a collection of individual children suffering from grief and trauma, tentatively coming together, became a therapeutic work group in which the children helped one another heal their hurts. Some very important elements were put into place by the therapists to influence this outcome. Circle time was a crucial ritual that symbolically created the safe space needed to begin the group work each week. It set this time and place aside as different from the children's everyday environment. The ground rules laid the foundation for ways of communicating that were also qualitatively different from those in their daily world. The process of norm setting helped to define the group, giving it a structure in which trust could be built, especially around the respect that is essential for really hearing one another and holding that sacred sharing in confidence. This began tentatively the first week, but by the second week there was great eagerness in sharing. If the children did not feel ready to express themselves verbally, they were allowed to "pass."

In addition, the openness of the group therapists—their readiness to be real people, to show their vulnerability, to acknowledge that they did not have all the answers but that that they were truly present to walk with the children, and to be with them even in the hard places—helped to build trust not only in the therapists but in other group members as well. The children grew into the awareness that they were in this together. This was established from the first week, when the therapists opened the decision-making process to the children—"What project shall we work on next week?" It reinforced the concepts that the children had wisdom about what they needed for their own healing, and that they were bigger than their pain. The children learned that the group was a place they could have fun, too, as witnessed by their enthusiasm in playing games and singing. The realization that one can have fun while working on really hard things can be a pivotal insight into building resilience.

It was clear that things had "clicked" when the children gave themselves wholeheartedly to the group the second week. They happily helped with preparation of the snacks, and the circle discussion reached a deep level quickly. The group-building process had firmly taken hold. Already they felt a sense of safety and connection. They began their Memory Books with a flourish and enjoyed the predictability of ending the session with singing.

By the third week the children showed much interest in helping and caring for one another. They explored memories, both good and not so good, and in the process gained valuable skills in expression and in listening for meaning. Each week new territory was being blazed in regard to what it was safe to talk about and how they responded to another's heartfelt sharing.

The fourth week consolidated the children's learnings about feeling feelings and expressing these feelings in the community of the group. The fifth week honored what the children had to celebrate, especially as it pertained to the Thanksgiving holiday that week. This was a step toward normality, acknowledging what there was to work with and to build upon. In the sixth and last session, the work of the previous weeks had effected change in the ways that at least some of the children articulated their viewpoint of their reality. They were able to incorporate hopefulness as part of the bigger picture. The children's Memory Books held good solutions to each specific loss, whether it was in a particular way of memorializing their loved ones or in an answer to a family dynamic. In that process, they drew on the deepest springs of creativity available to each of them. This effected a transformation: They moved from pain to growth to a measure of peace.

In the end, the children saw themselves as more whole than fractured, and they mirrored that to one another. The group, collectively, was able to move beyond original wounding to health and a kind of wisdom. Some members "philosophized" about how important it was to care for themselves as they continued to heal.

Although there was no formal follow-up with this group of children, the therapists had fleeting contact with some of the children. When the therapists were present in the school for one reason or another in the ensuing months, group members who saw them flew to them for a hug and a "hello." In response to the question "How are you?," the children's answers would be "Fine" or "Okay." Unfortunately, there was no opportunity to ask further questions.

Throughout the group process, the therapists needed to be aware of what was going on in them and how these children were affecting them. They had come to care about (yes, "love") them, and they were buoyed at each sign of growing and healing that the children displayed. There were also some indications of countertransference at work. Both of the therapists recognized that Jamelle's frequent religious interpretations brought up feelings in them that were their own "stuff" about religion, and they needed to own those feelings. Similarly, Marny "reached" both of them in ways hard to interpret, both positive and negative. Was it because her grandmother had died and both the therapists were grandmothers? It was at once helpful, thought-provoking, and unsettling to realize how transactional the entire experience was.

Concluding Comments

As we look back on the clinical case study, it is possible to see the simple but powerful methods that provided the framework for the group's success. The specific methods are informed by an overall philosophy—that of meeting the children in a hard place and walking the way through it with them. Crucial to a journey of this sort are the following "ways of being":

1. Giving respectful and consistent attention to the reality of each child.
2. As much as possible, getting to know each child in his or her individuality.
3. Listening and engaging in empathic introspection.
4. Being a role model of openness and acceptance.
5. Trying not to be didactic (truths emerge in so many ways).
6. Developing group experiences/mutualities—a group identity.
7. Fostering the wholeness of each child (children *are* bigger than their losses!).

8. Looking for strengths ("catching them being strong").
9. Having a value that "Nothing is too awful to look at, because we are together and we will help one another."

There are many resource materials describing activities for use in groups of grieving and traumatized children. Some are listed at the end of the chapter. Comfortableness with a range of resources is important. The key is not to go into group sessions with a rigid plan, but to have a structure with a well-thought-out tentative plan that can be adjusted according to the creativity of the children and the therapist's ongoing assessment of their needs. The group is an ideal setting to effect change and heal some of the wounds of grief and trauma, especially for children—who tend to be naturally inclined to interact in groups. The important distinction to keep in mind in working with children is that they are still growing, and it is healthy for them to look at the therapist as an ideal parent and the group as an idealized family. They do not need protection from the harsh things of life that they have already encountered; rather, they need assurance that they will not be alone on their path to healing and that they have internal resources, which caring companionship on the journey can help to mobilize. It takes training and supervision to do this privileged work of entering into children's worlds, but equally as important are personal attributes that allow therapists to be comfortable with their own child spirits.

This work is not done in a vacuum. It is imperative to look at the larger landscape in which each child lives. It is recommended that concurrent groups for parents and guardians be offered whenever possible, to help them better understand their children's worlds and to help them with their own trauma and grief issues, which may prevent them from being emotionally available to support their children. Information, literature, training, education, and consultation for school staff, pediatricians, clergy, and other community members not only can aid them in understanding children's grief and trauma, but can help them make appropriate referrals for treatment. The need for addressing children's grief and trauma issues is vital. The potential for healing in the context of the group environment is extraordinary.

ACKNOWLEDGMENT

We dedicate this chapter to the memory of Mae L. Page. She was one of its authors early into this work, when her untimely death occurred. Her spirit permeates these pages. Her remarkable set of talents, along with her great heart, made beauty and healing happen. She was a friend, colleague, and bereavement therapist—who walked with those in pain, whose heart held them, whose gifts strengthened them, and whose vision changed both them and her, because the journey toward wholeness was also her own.

REFERENCES

Apfel, R. J., & Simon, B. (1996). Introduction. In R. J. Apfel & B. Simon (Eds.), *Minefields in their hearts: The mental health of children in war and communal violence* (pp. 1–17). New Haven, CT: Yale University Press.

Bowlby, J. (1960). Grief and mourning in infancy and early childhood. *Psychoanalytic Study of the Child, 15,* 9–52.

DeBellis, M. D. (1999, Spring). Biological stress systems and brain development in maltreated children with PTSD. *Traumatic Stress Points: News for The International Society for Traumatic Stress Studies, 13*(2), pp. 1, 5.

Freud, A., & Dann, S. (1951). An experiment in group upbringing. *Psychoanalytic Study of the Child, 6,* 127–168.

Garbarino, J., & Kostelny, K. (1996). What do we need to know to understand children in war and community violence? In R. J. Apfel & B. Simon (Eds.), *Minefields in their hearts: The mental health of children in war and communal violence* (pp. 33–51). New Haven, CT: Yale University Press.

Janoff-Bulman, R. (1985). The aftermath of victimization: Rebuilding shattered assumptions. In C. Figley (Ed.), *Trauma and its wake: The study and treatment of post-traumatic stress disorder* (pp. 15–35). New York: Brunner/Mazel.

Janoff-Bulman, R. (1992). *Shattered assumptions: Towards a new psychology of trauma.* New York: Free Press.

Johnson, D. W., & Johnson, F. P. (1987). *Joining together: Group theory and group skills* (3rd ed.). Englewood Cliffs, NJ: Prentice-Hall.

Pynoos, R. S., & Nader, K. (1988). Psychological first aid and treatment approach to children exposed to community violence: Research implications. *Journal of Traumatic Stress, 1*(4), 445–473.

Rachman, A. (1995) *Identity Group Psychotherapy with Adolescents.* Northvale, NJ: Aronson.

Rando, T. (1993). *Treatment of complicated mourning.* Champaign, IL: Research Press.

Rogers, F. (1979). *Talking with young children about death* [Brochure]. Pittsburgh, PA: Family Communications.

Schamess, G. (1993). Group psychotherapy with children. In H. I. Kaplan & B. J. Sadock (Eds.), *Comprehensive group psychotherapy* (3rd ed., pp. 560–577). Baltimore: Williams & Wilkins.

Schamess, G., Streider, F., & Connors, K. (1997). Supervision and staff training for children's group psychotherapy: General principles and applications with cumulatively traumatized, inner-city children. *International Journal of Group Psychotherapy, 47*(4), 399–425.

Schleidlinger, S. (1982). *Focus on group psychotherapy: Clinical essays.* New York: International Universities Press.

Siepker, B., Lewis, L., & Kandaras, C. (1985). Relationship-oriented psychotherapy with children and adolescents. In B. Siepker & C. Kandaras (Eds.), *Group therapy with children and adolescents: A treatment manual* (pp. 11–34). New York: Human Sciences Press.

Tuckman, B. W. (1965). Developmental sequence in small groups. *Psychological Bulletin, 63,* 384–399.

Webb, N. B. (1991). Assessment of the child in crisis. In N. B. Webb (Ed.), *Play therapy with children in crisis: A casebook for practitioners* (pp. 3–25). New York: Guilford Press.

Webb, N. B. (1993). The child and death. In N. B. Webb (Ed.), *Helping bereaved children: A handbook for practitioners* (pp. 3–18). New York: Guilford Press.

Wolfelt, A. (1983). *Helping children cope with grief.* Muncie, IN: Accelerated Development.

Wolfelt, A. (1996). *Healing the bereaved child: Grief gardening, growth through grief and other touchstones for caregivers.* Fort Collins, CO: Companion Press.

Young, M. A. (1996). *Working with grieving children after violent death: A guidebook for crime victim assistance professionals.* Washington, DC: National Organization for Victim Assistance.

Young-Eisendrath, P. (1996). *The gifts of suffering.* Reading, MA: Addison-Wesley.

RESOURCES FOR GROUP ACTIVITIES

Beckmann, R. (1990). *Children who grieve: A manual for conducting support groups.* Holmes Beach, FL: Learning Publications.

Cunningham, L. (1990). *Teen age grief training manual.* Panorama City, CA: Teen Age Grief.

O'Toole, D. (1989). *Growing through grief: A K–12 curriculum to help young people through all kinds of loss.* Burnsville, NC: Mountain Rainbow.

Perschy, M. K. (1997) *Helping teens work through grief.* Philadelphia: Accelerated Development.

Roseby, V., & Johnston, J. (1997). *High-conflict, violent, and separating families: A group treatment manual for school-age children.* New York: Free Press.

Salloum, A. (1998). *Reactions: A workbook to help young people who are experiencing trauma and grief.* Omaha, NE: Centering Corporation.

Ward, B. (1993) *Good grief: Exploring feelings, loss and death with under elevens.* London: Cromwell Press.

Webb, N. B. (Ed.). (1991). *Play therapy with children in crisis: A casebook for practitioners.* New York: Guilford Press.

Whitney, S. (1991). *Waving goodbye: An activities manual for children in grief.* Portland, OR: Dougy Center for Grieving Children.

Wolfelt, A. (1996). *Healing the bereaved child: Grief gardening, growth through grief and other touchstones for caregivers.* Fort Collins, CO: Companion Press.

Young, M. A. (1996). *Working with grieving children after violent death: A guidebook for crime victim assistance professionals.* Washington, DC: National Organization for Victim Assistance.

10

◄〇►

When Trauma Affects a Community: Group Interventions and Support after a Disaster

MARK L. DEMBERT
EDWARD D. SIMMER

A helicopter carrying many senior partners in a law firm crashes during a business trip, and all are killed.

A van with members of a high school band slides off a rain-slick highway and crashes into a tree, killing everyone.

A recently fired executive from a large company returns to the offices with a gun, killing several and wounding others before shooting himself.

A tornado touches down at night in a small town without warning, destroying most of the buildings and homes and killing or injuring most of the town's population.

During a championship middle school soccer game played in front of a large crowd of families from both schools, one of the boys trips and falls directly against the metal goal frame. He collapses, suffers a cardiac arrest, and dies, despite the resuscitative efforts of two doctors attending the game.

Traumatic events like the examples above—by no means an inclusive list—cast a wide net involving families, communities, businesses, and government. Although the medical community's recognition and treatment of individuals suffering the devastating emotional and psychological aftereffects of such events have markedly improved over the last half century, the recognition and treatment of small or large groups of such individuals have only developed over the past two decades (Farberow & Frederick, 1996; Mitchell & Everly, 1996; Peuler, 1988; Young, 1998). These groups fall into two basic categories: acute interventional debriefing groups used immediately after a disaster, and various support groups that provide valuable services for months or even years after a disaster. Neither of these is a psychotherapy group in the sense of fostering intrapsychic change, resolving neurotic conflict, addressing past histories of developmental or early trauma, or changing maladaptive character traits. Members of these groups are generally healthy people who are having normal responses to an abnormal situation. Those who conduct groups for this work thus regard themselves as "group counselors," "facilitators," or "leaders"; these are the terms members use.

How, then, can the traditional group therapist begin to understand the nature of this work and the nature of his or her role in this process? This may initially seem difficult. However, the underlying goal of disaster work is the same as that of traditional group therapy: alleviating suffering and improving function. And although the approaches used in postdisaster groups are somewhat different, many of the techniques used in this work are similar to those used in short-term therapy groups. These concepts become clear in the examples and discussions that follow.

ACUTE INTERVENTIONAL
DEBRIEFING GROUPS

In a factory room containing 20 employees, a steam pipe explosion seriously burned two workers and caused lesser burns to others. Those present who provided emergency first aid to their seriously injured colleagues were confronted with the horror of seeing their severe thermal burns and hearing their painful screams. After learning that one of the two severely burned men died after being taken to the hospital, several of the workers later refused to return to work and enter that room. All described themselves as being very emotionally shaken by the event.

A Critical-incident stress debriefing (CISD; see below) was held 2 days after the incident. The workers in the group were able to discuss what happened, each from his own perspective. By hearing each other's perspectives, they were able to get a better cognitive and emotional understanding of the entire event; even more importantly, they learned about the expectability of their reactions. Information about possible physical, emotional, and cognitive responses to a traumatic event was presented briefly. Ways to deal with the loss, including memorializing their dead colleague, were then reviewed.

After this intervention, all of the employees were able to return to work in this room. Only one required follow-up mental health counseling.

The group therapist who wishes to be involved in disaster mental health work should have training in acute interventional debriefings and should be well versed in issues of stress, posttraumatic stress disorder, psychotrauma, crisis intervention, the nature and functions of emergency services work, and biopsychosocial aspects of disasters in general (Mitchell & Everly, 1996). Acute interventional debriefing groups can be used both for responding emergency workers and for direct survivors, as well as for indirectly affected victims of disasters.

Critical-incident stress management (CISM) programs, which include prevention-oriented stress management strategies of psychoeducation and CISD, developed out of an awareness that disaster workers and emergency personnel can experience a wide array of social, psychological, and physical reactions to stressors inherent in disaster work. These consequences include formal stress disorders, job "burnout" and job loss, family and marital disruption, psychiatric disability and suicide, medical illnesses, and substance abuse.

CISD involves a defined and concise local program of contact with individuals assembled in groups within 24–72 hours after they have provided response and rescue services. These group debriefings may last up to 3 hours each and are led by a team of trained peer support and mental health personnel. Each debriefing follows a seven-step process described in more detail elsewhere (Mitchell & Everly, 1996). In brief, the first phase ("introduction") sets the stage for the rest of the debriefing, with guidelines fully explained for the entire process. The second phase ("fact") allows each group member to introduce him- or herself, to describe where he or she was when the disaster occurred, to indicate his or her job or role, and to describe what occurred to the best of that person's knowledge. The third phase ("thought") allows each member to describe the initial thoughts that occurred once the immediate reaction was over; this process provides a transition from the cognitive experience to the emotional experience. The fourth phase ("reaction") allows the members to describe what was emotionally the hardest to experience about the disaster; this usually leads to a wide variety of freely expressed emotions. The fifth phase ("symptoms") provides a transition from the emotional domain back to the cognitive domain, with a focus on members' experiences of stress-related symptoms. The sixth phase ("teaching") is very educative in approach and allows for much discussion and education about stress survival techniques, including self-care and reintegrating with families, friends, and coworkers. The seventh phase ("reentry") brings closure to the debriefing: Final questions are answered, summary statements are made, and the transition to future thinking and a return to daily life routines are facilitated.

Community disaster response teams, another part of CISM, hold postdisaster debriefings for nonemergency worker populations in the community, such as citizen groups, schools, and businesses (Mitchell & Everly, 1996).

Related postdisaster group interventions used as part of CISM include "defusings" and "demobilizations." Defusings are used for selected small groups, perhaps six to eight persons working as a team, who are exposed to severe trauma during the disaster. It is done within hours of their experience. It provides an opportunity for those exposed to a horrible event to talk about the experience before they have time to later rethink the experience and erect cognitive and emotional barriers to processing it appropriately. Demobilizations can be used for larger numbers of persons than can defusings or debriefings (10 to 30 or more). These are done after the end of the first two or three shifts for emergency workers responding to a large-scale disaster or very traumatic event. These are two-part processes: The first part is a brief talk that presents information on understanding and managing expectable reactions to the stress of the work just experienced, and the second is the provision of food and rest at a demarcated place. Demobilizations provide a transition from the traumatic event to the routine within a short period of time. Defusings and demobilizations can also be provided for others who are not emergency workers/disaster responders, including survivors.

The National Organization for Victim Assistance (NOVA), founded in 1975, conceptualized and put into practice in the 1980s the community crisis response team (CCRT) process (Young, 1998). These teams, composed of emergency management peer support members, clergy, other lay personnel, and CCRT-trained mental health care providers, are invited to community-wide crises and provide acute interventions similarly focused on individuals assembled in groups. Like CISD, these interventions are used in an attempt to reduce later morbidity. The process for these debriefings follows a multiphase framework similar to that of the CISD model. CCRT interventions have been used for emergency response and rescue personnel as well as for victims and survivors, involved medical personnel, local government leaders, construction and utilities repair personnel, and members of religious and community service organizations. Involvement with the news media, psychoeducation, and postdisaster planning are among other unique CCRT duties.

SUPPORT GROUPS

In 1996, two major hurricanes struck the coast of North Carolina within a 3-month span. Although few people were injured or killed, extensive damage occurred, and many people lost both their homes and their livelihoods.

Support groups were started 1 to 2 months after the second hurricane. These groups were timed to start after the initial cleanup was mostly complete. These groups were initially led by mental health professionals, but attendance was very poor.

Discussions with trusted leaders in the community indicated that the likely cause was stigma attached to attending a group thought to be for those with mental disorders, because the leaders were mental health care providers. As a solution, interested community leaders were trained to be cofacilitators of these existing groups. As a result, the perceived stigma was replaced with beneficial images, and group attendance greatly increased.

The groups successfully served to allow people to discuss their reactions to the disaster and also to share solutions to many practical problems. Eventually, the mental health professionals were able to phase themselves out of the groups, which then became more like combined support and self-help groups.

Whereas both CISD and CCRT are traditionally used right after a disaster for both emergency response workers and traumatized survivors, support groups are usually begun many days or weeks after a disaster and are primarily organized for traumatized survivors and other members of the affected community. Emergency response workers whose lives outside of the direct practice of their skills have also been affected can participate in such support groups as well.

Support groups constitute one of the mental health interventions of choice for traumatized individuals (Janoff-Bulman, 1985) and the community after a disaster. The beneficial objectives of these support groups are to a great extent concordant with many of the "therapeutic factors" described by Yalom (1995), including instillation of hope, universality, imparting information, altruism, group cohesiveness, and existential factors. Postdisaster support groups also foster a sense of normalization (the reactions members are experiencing are considered to be expectable reactions to an abnormal or unexpectable event); a sharing of resources, which promotes cohesiveness; an optimizing of recovery, so that members can approximate their predisaster daily functioning; and prevention or amelioration of possible disaster-related psychological morbidity (Bradford, 1994).

Wee (1994) provides an excellent comparison of basic types of support groups. The first type consists of the standard support groups, which provide psychological education with emotional support as the primary function over many weeks or months. The phases of the standard support group, compared to those of CISD, are as follows: "recovery goals," "remembrance," "cognitive mastery," "mourning," "stress management," "teaching/resources," and "follow-up." Groups of the second type are referred to as "topic groups." These are organized around recovery topics (e.g., completion of paperwork for damage and insurance claims; advice on how to pick a building contractor or architect) and may meet once or twice and allow for group interaction, support, and networking. Groups of the third type are called "event groups." These groups bring large groups of disaster survivors together for a single occasion or event to address an entire community's needs (e.g., an anniversary commemorative event).

In addition to the types of support groups that can be developed after a disaster, the mental health provider who plans to work with or begin one or more support groups must take many other issues into consideration (Peuler, 1988; Wee, 1994). The first is evaluating the need for support groups. A broad spectrum of specific populations with unique needs within the community should be considered for separate support groups. These include but are not limited to children, the elderly, ethnic groups, sexual minorities, renters, homeowners, members of various professions and interest groups (e.g., nurses, artists, domestic workers, therapists), those who lost pets, those with physical disabilities, disaster response and recovery workers, those who lost loved ones, and the chronically mentally ill (Speier, Thomas, Carter, DeWolfe, & Rubin, 1996). Also affecting the need for a support group and the type of group chosen are such issues as the overall short-term and long-term impact of the disaster on the specific community, and the extent and magnitude of damage, death, and injury experience among community members (Herman, 1992).

Once the need for support groups has been evaluated, and the types of groups and target populations have been selected, the groups' utility and effectiveness can be maximized through attention to a variety of factors. First, the population of the affected community must be looked upon as a composite of many predominant subgroups stratified by age, socioeconomic status, marital status, religion, ethnicity, race, occupation, health, and geography of residential areas, to name some common ones. An effort must be made to match planned group leaders with salient characteristics of the likely members of these groups. As a corollary, cultural aspects and practices of these subpopulations must be respected when such groups are planned. For instance, food and drink provided at meetings must not conflict with cultural or religious dietary sanctions followed by the members, and group meetings should not conflict with a religious sabbath or church worship schedules, if at all possible.

Second, depending upon the effects of the disaster and the populations it has affected, group leaders may be more concerned (especially at first) with practical matters: arranging temporary housing, providing basic food for families, immediately starting loan or mortgage applications or insurance assessments of home damage and loss, and/or providing contractor or self-help services for the immediate repairing of homes or of wells or septic systems.

Third, support groups must be held in locations that maximize the transportation assets and abilities of community members. Flooded or damaged highways or local roads, washed-out bridges, debris that block roads, and areas of high damage to homes all influence members' attendance. The emotional attachment to lost or damaged homes may keep many members from making long or arduous trips to a noncentralized group location. If a local building of any type is chosen for group meetings, it should be in a central area. Transportable meeting places, such as trailers or recreation vehicles, may need to be used. Individuals or car dealers who own four-wheel-drive vehicles may be pressed into providing taxi services.

Fourth, the group schedule must take into account the other urgent needs that community members have in recovering from the disaster. Immediately after the disaster and for several weeks afterward, damaged homes and injured family members take precedence in the psychological and physical priorities of individuals. A weekly group schedule may be too demanding, but an every-other-week schedule may be feasible. The time and day of the week chosen for group meetings are also important factors, which are influenced by the geography, the weather, the integrity of the roads, the availability of child care, the occupations of the local community members, and so forth. Nighttime meetings may inculcate a sense of fear and resistance to attendance when there are poorly lighted or damaged roads. If individuals in the community are able to go back to work, then a balance has to be struck between weekday work schedules and the need for weekend time to regroup and recover mentally, physically, and emotionally with family members.

Fifth, disasters easily conjure up in the minds of the suffering the idea of vulnerability and need for safety. This has to be factored into providing available group locations with nearby parking, as well as very visible protection from crime both outside and inside the meeting area. Such group meetings should be held in areas usually devoid of crime, if at all possible.

Sixth, consideration must be given to providing child care services at the site of group meetings, so that adult members can feel free to express their feelings and concerns in the shared privacy with other adults, without being interrupted by children's situational needs.

As far as the actual mechanics of setting up groups are concerned, many groups seem to work best as open groups, with community members being able to participate when possible. This works best with support groups dealing with topics such as home repairs and other self-help issues, local governmental issues, resumption of community and utility services, and so forth. Other support groups fare better as closed groups, whose leaders may choose to do a pregroup screening for each individual to ensure compliance with basic rules of privacy and confidentiality and participation, as well as to rule out evidence of severe or impairing mental disorders that indicate a need for immediate treatment. These latter groups have been used in the aftermath of disasters involving significant loss of life, especially when such disasters have been caused by an accident (e.g., an airliner crash), intent to harm others, or negligence. In these disasters, examples of which are described below in more detail, the emotional reactions (anger, numbness, shock, etc.) are persistent and at times overwhelming; the call for justice may be overarching; and the intense grieving may endure for months and years. All of these factors necessitate an enclosed, safe, trusting, and containing group environment. The duration of support groups remains flexible in most situations, driven by the unique characteristics and needs of each specific group of individuals; some last a few sessions, some last several months, and some can last years. Last, group rules are usually minimal; however, depending upon the type of disaster, the open or closed nature of initial membership requirements, and the needs of the participating members, additional rules described commonly (Yalom, 1995) may be instituted.

Promoting the group requires consideration of (1) developing flyers; (2) contacting key persons and organizations in social networks; (3) seeking publicity through newspapers, radio, and television; and (4) promoting referrals from other disaster survivors as well as health care providers.

Piper, McCallum, and Azim (1992) provide a good theoretical and clinical basis for incorporating loss and mourning into short-term groups. Session-by-session issues in support groups are well described by Paolercio (1993). Basic themes in facilitating support groups are addressed in the case examples below. When and how to refer a seriously disturbed group member for urgent or emergent care needs to be considered, as well as what to do if a group member later dies by suicide, illness, or injury. Anniversary dates are extremely important to acknowledge and plan for in the group (Myers, 1994). The group leader must have an understanding of when documentation and reporting are mandatory for issues brought up in group.

Termination strategies need to be thought out ahead of time. Issues to be considered include (1) preparing the participants; (2) deciding how to continue individual relationships after the group; (3) making referrals to other resources as needed; (4) inducting new support group facilitators; (5) continuing the support group as a self-help group; and (6) providing follow-up to individuals or the group as a whole when funding for the group ceases, such as a federal or local grant for a specific time period of group sessions.

SPECIFIC DISASTER TYPES
AND RELEVANT SUPPORT GROUPS

The type of disaster and its inherent themes often shape the nature, content, processes, and schedules of the support group(s) used (Lystad, 1988). In this section, five types of disasters are described: natural disasters; accidental disasters (transportation and technological accidents are common); disasters caused by intent to harm others; business or industry disasters; and disasters that directly or indirectly traumatize children and adolescents. Particular issues in the formation and facilitation of relevant support groups are illustrated in case examples reported by mental health care providers involved in postdisaster groups.

Natural Disasters

Issues to Consider

Even with the inevitable loss of property and possible loss of life, a natural disaster brings up issues of fate and luck. Individuals often turn inward and search their souls for why the disaster happened. Family members often endure the disaster together. There is usually an expectation that all victims' remains will be recovered for burial and emotional closure. Memorial sites may be erected, and these should be readily accessible to community members. Despite the tragic nature of such a disaster, the sense of future is based upon a perspective of relocating (if necessary), rebuilding, and starting a life over.

As noted earlier, logistical factors may complicate conducting support groups after a natural disaster. For instance, many persons may be isolated by floods when roads and bridges are destroyed. Contacting these persons directly, as well as finding ways to enable them to come to a group, can be extremely difficult. Support groups can be started in a shelter even while the natural disaster is ongoing; this allows for very early intervention and paves the way for people to come to more long-term support groups later. Finally, some natural disasters may recur not long after the initial event (e.g., earthquake aftershocks, mudslides, brush fires, floods). This expectably heightens community fears and also requires flexibility in relocating support groups.

Example: Santa Cruz County Floods and Mudslides

In January 1982, a disastrous winter rainstorm hit Santa Cruz County, California. Floods and mudslides took numerous lives and caused extensive property damage. A community support group was formed 3 weeks after the storm in the village of Soquel, and it continued weekly for over

1 year. There was a core group of 10 members; the maximum attendance was 13; and new members were taken in as the group progressed.
Jack Peuler, LCSW, formerly of the Santa Cruz County Department of
Mental Health Services and former director of Project COPE (Counseling
Ordinary People in Emergency), and a colleague have described this
group (Peuler & Ritter-Splain, 1983). The following is taken from that
report:

> The first four to eight weeks were marked by a sense of the group mem-
> bers being "in shock." Most were emotionally detached and thankful to
> be alive, while some were euphoric at being alive. These mood states
> seemed to protect the survivors from the devastating reality of their losses
> until they were more able to address them.
>
> Group members, without exception, reported poor sleep patterns and
> nightmares. Many seemed preoccupied and restless. Parent-members were
> often in denial that their children may have suffered.
>
> In the initial phase, group members most wanted to tell their stories
> and repeatedly vent their feelings. Many expressed survivor guilt in the
> form of a magical belief that in some way they had caused the disaster to
> happen. By the end of the first phase, the members' realization that their
> losses were even more devastating than they had initially perceived began
> to set in. There was a sense of a loss of identity, loss of a sense of home
> and refuge, and loss of a community of neighbors.
>
> The next six to twelve weeks were colored by group members' anger
> and frustration over the obstacles in receiving assistance from various
> governmental agencies. Often there was indignation that after paying
> taxes all their lives, they got so much less than they needed or expected.
>
> Group members reported feeling vulnerable and out of control. There
> was a great need to have others who were affected less or not at all by
> the disaster understand how traumatic their own experiences had been.
>
> Four to six months after the disaster, a remedy phase began. Group
> cohesiveness was very evident. Individuals became actively involved in
> their own recovery efforts. They exchanged practical information with
> others inside and outside the group. At the same time, anger over unan-
> swerable demands for accountability surfaced. Bad dreams persisted al-
> most without exception. Often, these nightmares involved being caught
> or trapped by something or having walls crash down.
>
> Six months after the disaster the group considered disbanding. Mem-
> bers experienced themselves as having survived the crisis and now having
> a sense of future to embrace. However, they realized they weren't truly
> ready to stop. They redefined their needs and goals and continued on. Is-
> sues of personality changes, spirituality, control and autonomy, and de-
> pendence versus independence were discussed. It was also at this point
> that parents in the group became truly aware that their children had been
> affected by the disaster and problem solving sessions focused on how to
> help their children.
>
> During the ninth through twelfth months, new members joined the

group as recurrent storms activated anxiety among original survivors who had not first sought support. The anniversary date brought relief and celebration, with sadness over memories of losses.

Personality traits which are culturally reinforced by sex roles created observable differences in the impact of the disaster on men and women and the types of interventions needed from the facilitators. Women tended to placate, to put others first, and to feel overly responsible for the welfare of others. These served as obstacles to giving themselves permission to grieve their own sorrows, to regain self-trust, and to tend to their own needs. Key interventions included encouragement to set limits on others' demands, to assert their own needs, and to validate their abilities to trust themselves.

Many men found it difficult to acknowledge and express feelings of helplessness and sadness. They described feeling as failures in their roles as family protectors and providers by "allowing" this devastation to strike their families. For some, the threat or actual occurrence of physical injury jeopardized their sense of "manhood." Facilitators encouraged men to accept and express feelings of vulnerability and/or helplessness as human inevitabilities and to make realistic assessments of their own strengths and limitations. (Peuler & Ritter-Splain, 1983, pp. 8–11)

Accidental Disasters

Issues to Consider

In an accidental disaster, such as a transportation disaster or technological disaster, there can be a sudden, devastating loss of life and property. Surviving family members or friends of the victims can experience haunting survivor guilt; in particular, they may blame themselves for making the victims take a certain airplane flight or go to work for a certain shift. An effort to affix blame as to the cause of the accident is also quite common. Any suspicion that the accident was due to terrorism or specific intent to harm others fuels the outrage until such causes are officially investigated and suspicions are laid to rest. When there may have been an error in judgment, negligence, or a design defect that led to the disaster, these possibilities will be heavily scrutinized by families of victims and investigatory agencies.

A family's hierarchy can be instantaneously transformed by such a disaster, especially when a spouse or child is the victim, and family cohesiveness, grieving, and problem-solving capacities can be seriously impaired. A large number of victims' remains may not be recoverable if the accident was totally obliterating or if it happened at sea. Especially in a transportation accident, there may not be a community sense of loss from which survivors can derive support, as victims may have been brought together by chance from many parts of the country. There may not be a memorial site to visit later, especially if the disaster occurred at sea or in another country.

Example: USAir Flight 427 Crash

On September 8, 1994, USAir Flight 427 crashed near Pittsburgh, Pennsylvania, killing all 132 passengers and crew members. The essential obliteration of the aircraft and bodies created a highly traumatic experience for victims' families, rescue and relief workers, and counselors. Pittsburgh was the termination of this flight from Chicago; thus many of the victims were from the Pittsburgh area and left spouses with children. After CISD was accomplished with emergency response workers and family groups, subsequent support groups focused on families, adults, children, and adolescents. Facilitators from funded public agencies and private practices alike conducted support groups.

Grace M. McGorrian, MD, a psychiatrist in private practice who herself had lost a brother to a commercial airplane disaster overseas many years before, led one such support group for 16 sessions over a 1-year time period (McGorrian, 1995). The following description of her experience is from G. M. McGorrian (personal communication, September 1998) and is modified from her 1995 unpublished document.

Shortly after the CISD interventions and many funerals were held, McGorrian sent out individual letters with personal notes to families in a demarcated area of interlocking neighborhoods, inviting them to attend a support group. She followed up with telephone calls to interested families. These calls served several purposes. First, they provided personal condolences. They also allowed her to describe her reasons for forming the group, its goals, its scheduling, and other information (this group was held at no cost to the members, as she volunteered her time). Furthermore, they allowed her to find out more about the impact of the crash on each family. Finally, they allowed her to do a rough screening for significant depression or anxiety that would indicate a need for additional treatment.

The group started less than 4 weeks after the disaster. The membership was closed at 10 members after the third week; members were informed of the closed nature, in case other survivors approached members later for admission. The group was to run for 8 to 10 sessions, with an option for the group to vote later to extend it.

Since members were from similar neighborhoods, cohesiveness and networking outside of the group began early. Sessions were conducted at a group therapy suite in a physicians' office building (which was centrally located for all members) and were held from 7:00 P.M. to 9:00 P.M. (a convenient time).

McGorrian found it exceedingly helpful to gather as much information on the crash from media sources, and as much information about victims and surviving family members as possible; these details assisted her in the facilitator role. A list of names, addresses, and phone numbers was made for all group members to share. Basic group ground rules were established.

Confidentiality was stressed; and McGorrian's responsibility to decide when a member should be referred for outside mental health evaluation and treatment was stated.

McGorrian found it important to uphold boundaries on time, consistent participation, and her personal information, with the exception of anecdotal details of her own prior bereavement process. She did inform group members of her brother's death. They appreciated her disclosure, seeing her as an "insider" who could comprehend what they were facing in their lives. When she encountered a group member in a public setting, the interaction was friendly and supportive.

She encouraged group members to participate in memorial services, to visit the memorial to all crash victims that was constructed at a nearby cemetery, and to visit the gravesites of loved ones interred there. She made herself available to accompany group members, if asked.

During the course of the group, media coverage of other disasters, especially those similar to the group's disaster, brought about expectable transient recurrences of initial symptoms and some forms of individual or group regression.

Members were encouraged as the group progressed to investigate relevant national support groups, such as Compassionate Friends or Parents without Partners, for additional specific networking.

The group was actually conducted for 1 year and was terminated formally after the 1-year anniversary. The first 10 sessions were conducted over 3 months; Sessions 11 and 12 were monthly; Sessions 13, 14, and 15 met every 2 months; and Session 16 met right after the anniversary date. The members and McGorrian maintained telephone contact long after the group's termination.

The following is a summary of relevant themes seen over time:

Sessions 1–3: Members were in a stage of emotional shock and grief over the sudden deaths. There were feelings of deprivation and injustice regarding the perceived preventability of the crash or loss of lives.

Sessions 4–5: These were more emotional, tearful, and outwardly grieving sessions.

Sessions 6–8: The group began to talk of the future and to express hopes of feeling better some day.

Sessions 9–10: These sessions were marked by evidence of members' strengthening important relationships at home and in the community.

Sessions 11–13: In these sessions, legal aspects of the disaster were discussed. Some members had decided to settle out of court, whereas others wanted to proceed with jury trials. Guilt and ambivalence regarding either type of decision were described.

Sessions 14–15: Group members were aware of the impending anniversary date of the crash, as well as the termination of the group. Attempts were made at emotional closure, as well as at realistic coping after the anniversary.

Session 16: This was the final session, held several days after the anniversary. The mood was upbeat and celebratory, born out of the realization of how strong in caring and support the members had been for each other. Individuals expressed optimism for the future and a desire to network among themselves.

Disasters Caused by Intent to Harm Others

Issues to Consider

Violence by one or more human beings against others casts a shadow of incomprehension, rage, insecurity, and distrust across a community—a shadow that can best be likened to a permanent stain in clothing. It really never leaves the collective fabric of the community unconscious or the minds of the individual survivors. Everyone's personal sense of trust and safety in day-to-day society is shaken. There is a fear that a similar incident could happen again in the community, and that it might even be caused by the same perpetrators if they have been released from confinement. A strident demand for justice is common. If the perpetrators are never caught, then for many survivors there is an even greater sense of distrust, loss, and anger that never goes away.

Consideration must be given to starting new support groups months or years after the disaster. It is not uncommon for other community members who were peripherally involved in but nevertheless exposed to the trauma (e.g., witnesses, those who discovered remains or personal effects away from the disaster site, funeral home staff who prepared or embalmed whole bodies or remains) to come forward for emotional support or mental health treatment long after the disaster. This reluctance to participate in support groups can be due to fears of "I will be thought of as crazy if I tell someone how I feel," cultural biases against revealing strong emotions outside of a close-knit community, a need to support loved ones or friends first over time, or fears of losing a job if one is identified as needing emotional support or counseling.

Example: Bombing of the Alfred P. Murrah Federal Building

On April 19, 1995, an intentional bombing of the Alfred P. Murrah Federal Building in Oklahoma City, Oklahoma resulted in the death of 168 individuals in the building, including 19 children. Two suspects were subsequently apprehended and found guilty after jury trials. One was initially sentenced to death and one was initially sentenced to life imprisonment, but both sentences were then appealed. At this writing, the appeals are still pending.

Both CISD and CCRT acute interventional practices were immediately utilized over the next several days after the bombing. After initial American Red Cross response and involvement with disaster workers, survivors, grieving families, and citizens involved as witnesses and rescuers, many types of support and loss groups were quickly formed. Project Heartland was established to coordinate this community-wide counseling response, and it continues to the present.

Edith King, PhD, a clinical and forensic psychologist in Oklahoma City, volunteered her professional time to initiate two support groups for U.S. Department of Housing and Urban Development workers and Social Security Administration workers who survived the blast despite being in the building. These two groups have run continuously since their inception in the late spring of 1995 and are expected to continue for many more years. Information relating to the disaster, and the descriptions of these groups, are presented below from E. King (personal communication, November 1998).

The members of these two groups were terribly affected by the disaster. They were coworkers and close friends of the deceased; a strong sense of family existed in the two organizations before the disaster. Many of the survivors were injured by the blast, and most were haunted by visions of being near coworkers who suddenly disappeared in the explosion. Intense survivor guilt was an immediate consequence that has lasted throughout the groups.

The two groups began within a few weeks of the disaster. Each group had a core number of 7 to 8 routinely attending and participating members. Because membership in the groups was open, the attendance for a single session could attain 15–17. Group sessions were weekly and lasted for 90 minutes. They were conducted at "safe" places far removed from the disaster site, which was an ever-present reminder of loss, anger, and intense grief.

Each group could be conceptualized as going through initial, middle, and later phases. During the initial phase, members described being in a state of shock or emotional numbing, along with disbelief or suspended reality. Time sense was lost. Importantly, members described cognitive difficulties: forgetfulness; getting lost while driving; losing items in the home; or even memory gaps for simple information such as addresses, phone numbers, and birth dates. These difficulties continued into subsequent phases.

During the middle phase, intense emotions were characteristic. Tremendous subjective fear generated by a single thought or sensory perception was common, as were marked periods of depression. Rage and demands for justice in the form of execution of the perpetrators surfaced. The loss of friends and coworkers became magnified as group members tried to reassemble their lives as family members and workers. Loss of confidence in abilities as spouses, parents, or family breadwinners was marked. The fears of being out of control, having no control over one's life, and losing one's mind were themes that required continued processing in the group. Crying, sometimes for days or weeks on end, was observed in many.

The later phase (which is still continuing) has been a refined progression of existential awareness to the realization that a survivor can begin to rebuild a life; that others in the group do have a vested interest in and care about the welfare of each individual; and, most importantly, that a survivor will never become the person he or she used to be before the disaster. There can be no return to life as it was before the disaster; instead, over time, each member has begun aspiring to "reach a new normal" day-to-day life.

As observed in the groups, significant changes in personality, thinking, and private world views developed after this disaster. Members came to accept that others had truly died and would not return. Denial was a particularly adaptive defense mechanism against grief and loss; it allowed members to experience a sense of hope and optimism over small but important events in their lives.

The group counselor has had to be supportive and realistic, to foster cohesiveness, and to convey honest optimism and altruism. She has had to support the quite obvious group needs for reassurance that members could regain a sense of control and mastery in their lives and that they were not "going crazy." Psychological, emotional, and physical strengths and capabilities were (and are) the focus of emphasis at all times. Past traumatic events as they surfaced and were reported in the group have been acknowledged as previously important in the group members' lives, but the focus has always been on the present ("here and now") and the immediate future.

The lengthy trial process and the publicity surrounding it were constant stimuli for group members' anger, as well as for fears that the perpetrators would be found not guilty and released. Despite the guilty verdicts and stringent sentences, the appeals process remains as an ever-present stimulus for these same emotions.

Finally, no real "closure" has been attained by these survivors. The horrific and incomprehensible nature of the perpetrated disaster has irreversibly altered the lives of survivors—probably more so than in any other disaster type.

Business or Industry Disasters

Mental health care involvement and access to businesses and industries whose personnel—corporate executives, employees, and their families—are affected by a disaster can be quite limited, for obvious medical, legal, union, and disability compensation concerns. Issues of causation and liability may remain indeterminate for long periods of time, and investigations into these issues are sensitive corporate matters. Recounting of specific events, catharsis of strong emotional reactions, survivor guilt, and private philosophical views about fate and responsibility are common themes during acute interventional debriefings, but participating individuals may fear that their job security and pensions, or possible future claims for disability, will be jeopardized by their openness. Provision of any postdisaster mental health services is solely a decision by the company or industry or its insurance company.

The group therapist who wishes to make his or her services available to an industry or corporation for postdisaster work needs to have a well-based connection with the corporate medical department, the human resources department, and the employee assistance program prior to the incident (Myers & Wolfe, 1996; Sperry, 1996). Time spent working with these departments in the areas of mental health prevention and consultation (e.g., psychoeducation, developing written programs, speaking to worker groups, dealing with psychological aspects of downsizing, etc.), as well as developing a private mental health care practice for the referral and treatment of employees, greatly enhances credibility and the likelihood of being contacted for postdisaster services. Concurrently, group therapists may contact and work with the insurance companies underwriting the specific industry, in the areas of mental health prevention, consultation, and treatment; again, this is with the aim of developing credibility and thus availability in time of disaster. Issues of confidentiality and documentation of care, with explicit understanding of to whom the therapist reports, must be agreed upon.

The more flexible the group therapist can be in terms of advertising to a company his or her ability to design the appropriate interventional debriefing or support group in accord with the company's wishes, the better. The processes observed and the themes discussed in any interventional debriefing or follow-up support group will be influenced by the basic type of disaster (natural, accidental, etc.) that has befallen the company.

Disasters That Traumatize
Children and Adolescents

When a population of children and adolescents is especially traumatized in a disaster, they are the primary focus for all of the community, including grieving and surviving adults.

Disasters That Directly Traumatize: Issues to Consider

After an incident that directly kills or injures children or adolescents, consideration in forming debriefing groups and support groups within a school should be given to preexisting bonds between: (1) classmates/close friends of the deceased; (2) children injured in the incident and their classmates/close friends; (3) uninjured children who were involved in the incident; (4) siblings of deceased/injured children and the siblings' classmates/close friends; and (5) school workers, faculty, and school administrators. Acute interventional debriefings and possible support groups should also be considered for (as examples) a bus driver or bus company, a train crew or airline company, personnel of the construction company that built a school, medical personnel who cared for injured and dying children at the site or at the hospital, and responders who recovered bodies.

Example: Cary–Grove High School Bus–Train Crash

On the morning of October 25, 1995, a commuter train hit a stopped school bus carrying 38 students to Cary–Grove High School in Cary, Illinois. Seven students were killed and 31 students were injured, several critically. After acute interventional debriefings were completed, two types of support groups were initiated. Philip Kirschbaum, MSW, a therapist in private practice, worked closely with students and staff at the high school and cofacilitated both types of groups. Information on the disaster and the groups described below are from P. Kirschbaum (personal communication, August 1998).

The first group type was a set of concurrent 8-week closed-membership support groups that began within 3 weeks of the crash. There were 8 to 10 students in each group, all of whom were closely affected by the crash. Groups included survivors of the crash and friends and siblings of the deceased students. Members were selected for specific groups on the basis of existing bonds to a specific victim or victims, and the groups mixed all four of the grade levels (9–12). Basic assumptions were conveyed to group members that they would be given support and empathy, that they were to continue learning and progress through the school year, and that they would reintegrate with the rest of their classmates psychologically and emotionally over time. Coleaders for groups included one member from the school (psychologist, guidance counselor, nurse, or teacher) and an outside consultant/therapist.

In these support groups, there was an emphasis on two important areas: (1) telling and retelling what was seen or experienced as a survivor, witness, close friend, or sibling; and (2) sharing coping strategies. These strategies were for such common problems as completing school homework and taking tests, resolving conflicts at home with family members, and reducing symptoms of stress (poor sleep, emotional lability, inappropriate anger, and social isolation). Group members kept journals and shared their entries.

Difficulties within families were commonly described. For instance, many of the older students were at an age range where independence from families was being negotiated and navigated. Although they needed their families for emotional support and reassurance of a general world view of safety, at the same time they chafed at parents and family members who hovered overprotectively for their own needs of reassurance and safety. Many parents who knew the deceased or injured were traumatized themselves by the nature of the disaster. Many group members were also outraged at the intense media (especially TV) involvement, and the perceived intrusion into the privacy and grief of so many students and families.

Symptoms of acute stress disorder were reported. Many students experienced poor concentration, inattentiveness, disorganization in their schedules, forgetfulness, impulsiveness, hyperactivity and inability to sit still, difficulty in completing tests and homework, low frustration tolerance, and poor performance on tests. These symptoms were transient, but the school provided tutoring for students who were especially impaired.

These groups were held in school and during regular class time. The members were fed bagels and juice during the groups, and the refreshments were well appreciated. Midway through the 8 weeks, group facilitators held a meeting with parents of the group members. They briefed the parents on the basic issues discussed in the groups; at the same time, parents could describe to what degree their children appeared to be coping and significant problems that remained.

Issues of loss and mourning over the victims, as well as the impending termination of the group, were brought back into focus at the seventh and eighth sessions.

After the Christmas holiday period passed and the time-limited support groups were completed, some of the members elected to continue in newly formed long-term support groups. These groups had closed membership, with seven to eight students each. These students included (1) ones who needed continued support over unresolved grief and other school or social issues; and (2) ones who had been seriously injured in the crash and thus could not attend the initial 8-week groups because of required medical stabilization and recovery. Special attention was given to selecting seniors, who would be graduating at the end of the school year. The groups have continued, as students who were freshmen at the time of the crash could continue to participate for the duration of their high school years. The groups did not meet over holiday periods and summer vacations.

Family grief support groups were formed not long after the accident. These were cofacilitated by workers from a local hospice as well as school staff members.

Over the many weeks following the crash, expected and unexpected themes emerged in the various groups. Parents of the deceased, as well as survivors of the crash, wondered whether they had caused the crash by some indirect or direct action on their part; conversely, some parents asked over and over what they could have done to prevent the crash or to prevent their children from taking the bus that morning. Survivor guilt was reported by many crash survivors and classmates. Several survivors later re-counted seeing such phenomena as a white haze, angels, or floating figures dressed in white hovering inside the bus in the minutes following the crash and while trapped in the bus. Finally, many cited a sense of spiritual dis-covery, belief in a personal god, or religion as a component of recovery.

As the first anniversary of the crash approached, members of ongoing groups, as well as students from the previous short-term groups, reported a resurgence of stress disorder symptoms (e.g., high subjective anxiety, startle reactions, hypervigilance, poor concentration, and easily provoked states of apprehension). These symptoms resolved with processing in groups, one-on-one counseling, and the passage of time.

Disasters That Indirectly Traumatize: Issues to Consider

When there is an incident that causes death or injury to family members of a large number of children or adolescents, among the primary consider-ations are the needs of the grieving children separate from the surviving adults. There may not be preexisting bonds between the children and ado-lescents, as often the nature of such an incident involves families from many neighborhoods in a large city or from many disparate communities. Acute interventional debriefing groups may be conducted centrally, such as at a transportation hub where families gather, or peripherally at commu-nity centers or schools. Subsequent support groups may be conducted pe-ripherally but at locations convenient for a number of communities to use. Group cohesiveness is a special challenge for the facilitator working with children and adolescents in these situations.

Example: USAir Flight 427 Crash (Children's and Adolescents' Support Groups)

A child or adolescent is a traumatized survivor when an accidental disaster takes the lives of one or both parents, one or more siblings, or extended family members. Sue Wesner, MSN, from University of Pittsburgh Medical Center's Services for Teens at Risk (STAR) Program, led support groups for children whose family members were killed in the crash of USAir Flight 427. These groups were based upon the program's work in schools affected by sudden deaths (Kerr, Brent, & McKain, 1997) and are described below (S. Wesner, personal communication, October 1998).

Children aged 4 to 8 years, and those aged 9 to 16 years (predomi-nantly 13 to 16 years), constituted two separate populations from which to draw support groups. Each group was run weekly for a time-limited block of eight sessions, but they were then repeated in subsequent 8-week blocks. The groups for the younger children generally lasted for two to three of these blocks. The group blocks for the older children/adolescents were repeated over and over for approximately 18 months, as, developmentally, their experiences of loss and mourning required a much longer, more adult-like period of processing.

In all groups, fostering a sense of safety and security was a basis for then encouraging the members to talk about their families, what they themselves were doing at the time of the crash, what happened in their households and their schools after the crash, and how others reacted around them. This allowed for a shift from the facts of loss to feelings of grief and sadness. As the groups progressed, discussion of feelings was supplemented by discussion of worries and concerns. These included fears that a surviving spouse and children would become poor, especially if the deceased parent had provided the main source of income; worries about whether a surviving parent would ever remarry (and, if so, that the surviving parent would forget, in the eyes of a child, the deceased parent); and frustration and anger that everyone expected a child or adolescent to do well in school and in activities as if nothing had happened. As noted earlier, some victims' remains were never identified; thus some children could not visit a specific family gravesite.

The longevity of the groups (repetitive 8-week blocks for 18 months), the ability to recall and rework issues of loss and abandonment, the space and time to process initial feelings, and the need to come over time to accept the actual death(s) of the parent(s) were all allowed to be experienced again and again through the repetition of the groups. This led to a progressive mastery of developmental obstacles and emotional hurdles resulting from the disaster.

Anger at USAir for causing the loss of the children's parents was a very palpable emotion in the groups. One innovative way this was dealt with was in a specific ritual 6 months after the disaster: The members jointly created a large poster of USAir and then threw balled wet paper towels at it in anger. This seemed to aid in creating a sense of power over their grief and anger at the question most angrily asked in these groups: "Why did this happen to my [parent]?"

Suicidal ideation was not common, but did appear at times in a member's wanting to die, so that the deceased parent would not have to be alone any more. Realistic support along with gentle probing of the feelings behind the wish were helpful in ensuring that such ideation did not develop into worrisome proportions.

A sense of sadness was described by many members when they described how a deceased parent's extended family stopped visiting over time. This led to discussions in the groups of a sense of confusion and further loss, especially when there were close attachments to extended family members.

Reappearance of grief and sadness, as well as difficulties in school and learning, were transient but expected at the time of important family holidays and birthdays, and especially as the 1-year anniversary of the crash approached. At that anniversary, the groups visited the memorial constructed at a large nearby cemetery where many victims were buried. Some children read letters to their deceased parents; some planted small trees in remembrance; and some left important belongings that were felt to provide a special connection and accompaniment for the deceased parents.

Other positive aspects of the support groups were the social connections that they allowed the members to make. Friendships developed over time, and some of the group members kept in touch long after the formal groups had stopped.

THE GROUP THERAPIST IN DISASTER MENTAL HEALTH WORK: LIFE, PRACTICE, AND TRAINING CONSIDERATIONS

A group therapist should be in good physical health, because physical endurance is challenged when many single-session acute interventions are required for potentially long hours at sites of disasters, far from the comforts of an office and in possibly harsh environments. Adaptive aspects of mental and emotional health include a stable personality; the capacity for controlled reactions to stressful life situations in general; a minimum of current life stressors, such as family or professional strife or change; and a past history of personal exposure to traumatic events that has been sufficiently resolved over the passage of time, as well as with personal therapy if needed.

Considerations for professional practice include the type(s) of practice the therapist currently conducts; the flexibility for making sudden changes to practice schedules (salaried vs. private practice); the types of patients seen in the practice, and their general ability to adapt to sudden therapist absences; and the financial needs and goals of the therapist balanced against sudden changes to schedules. A therapist who is more comfortable with a narrow focus of practice and relative control over clinical situations—for instance, analytic groups or long-term psychodynamic groups—may not be well suited for much disaster mental health work. In contrast, a group therapist who remains eclectic and adaptable to conducting different types of groups (both short- and long-term), and can weather unpredictable patients and clinical situations, is likely to be better suited for this work.

Other professional considerations include specific skills in disaster mental health work—in particular, past training in conducting acute interventional debriefings and accumulated experiences in previous civilian, government, or military disaster or trauma work with individual patients or groups. Skills in providing organizational leadership, public speaking, and working with the media are important as well.

Also helpful are consultant positions or therapy practice arrangements with emergency response organizations (police, firefighters, emergency medical technicians); community disaster response organizations such as the American Red Cross; social services or community mental health organizations; school districts; local transportation industries with disaster potential (airports, railroad centers, shipping ports); industrial corporations or factories with disaster potential (e.g., chemical or munitions manufacturing, foundries); nuclear power utilities; and military bases with an emphasis on weapons installations, ships, air transport, and hazardous duty training commands.

Geographical or environmental considerations, especially if the therapist lives and/or works in areas and communities vulnerable to extremes in weather or other natural phenomena, can be very important.

Finally, a group therapist who is a survivor of a disaster (e.g., family members are injured or killed, a large number of patients are injured or killed, a home or office is destroyed) should in general shed the therapist role, and instead should participate in acute and subsequent groups as a survivor and allow other therapists to facilitate the groups. In contrast, a group therapist who has not been personally affected by the disaster should be able to function as a group facilitator.

Myers (1994) provides a valuable and comprehensive discussion of the preparation, roles, work, and self-care of mental health workers in a disaster setting. She also addresses the extremely important issue of group leaders'/facilitators' being debriefed themselves periodically throughout the practice of acute interventional debriefings and support groups. This process of "debriefing the debriefers/facilitators" was utilized in all of the postdisaster group settings described in detail in this chapter.

The field of disaster group mental health work continues to develop. The type of disaster and demographics of those involved will help determine the types of interventions that will be most helpful. In a general sense, however, in virtually every situation, a combination of acute interventional groups followed by support groups will benefit those who are affected by the incident. For the mental health professional with the motivation and temperament for it, disaster group work can be very rewarding and is an excellent way to serve the community.

ACKNOWLEDGMENTS

The efforts of the following persons are greatly appreciated for their direct assistance in regard to various topics discussed in this chapter:

Acute interventional debriefing groups: Cheryl Tyiska, National Organization for Victim Assistance, Washington, DC.

Acute and posttraumatic stress disorders and postdisaster support groups: Bruce H. Young, LCSW, disaster services coordinator, National Center for PTSD, Department of Veterans Affairs, Palo Alto, CA; (650) 493–5000, ext. 22494.

Loma Prieta earthquake, Oakland–San Francisco, CA; East Bay firestorm, Berkeley–Oakland, CA; California winter storms, 1997, and El Niño storms, 1998; Hurricane Andrew, Dade County, FL: David Wee, MSSW, disaster mental health coordinator, City of Berkeley Mental Health, Berkeley, CA; (510) 644–8562, ext. 223; Michael Paolercio, MPA, CEAP, San Francisco, CA.

Santa Cruz County, CA, flood/mudslide disaster: Jack Peuler, LCSW, former director, Project COPE (Counseling Ordinary People in Emergency), Sacramento, CA.

USAir Flight 427 crash, Beaver County, PA: Kenneth Thompson, MD, Western Psychiatric Institute and Clinic, Pittsburgh, PA. Grace M. McGorrian, MD, Cranberry Township, PA. Sue Wesner, MSN, Services for Teens at Risk (STAR) Program, University of Pittsburgh Medical Center, Pittsburgh, PA.

Alfred P. Murrah Federal Building bombing, Oklahoma City, OK: Gwen Allen, MSW, MPH, director, and Jim Norman, MEd, counselor, Project Heartland, Oklahoma City, OK. Edith King, PhD, director, Forensic Psychology Services, Oklahoma City County Crisis Intervention Center, Oklahoma City, OK. Bruce H. Young, LCSW (see above).

Business or industry disasters: Michael Paolercio (see above). Diane Myers (see below).

Cary–Grove High School bus–train crash, Cary, IL: Philip Kirschbaum, MSW, Gurnee, IL.

Finally, the unique assistance of Diane Myers, RN, MSN (a national consultant on trauma intervention, disaster management, and CISM, Royal Oaks, CA; telephone (831) 768–1101) in providing general information and points of contact, as well as in reviewing the draft of this chapter, is gratefully acknowledged.

The views expressed in this chapter are our own and do not reflect the official policy or position of the U.S. Department of the Navy, the U.S. Department of Defense, or the U.S. Government.

RESOURCES

Group therapists interested in acquiring training in acute interventional debriefings should contact either the International Critical Incident Stress Foundation (Unit 201, 10176 Baltimore National Pike, Ellicott City, MD 21402; (410) 750–9600) for CISD qualification (local city, regional, or state disaster management or emergency response services may also sponsor CISD training), or the National Organization for Victim Assistance (1757 Park Road N.W., Washington, DC 20010; (202) 232–6682) for CCRT qualification.

The National Mental Health Services Knowledge Exchange Network (P.O. Box 42490, Washington, DC 20015; (800) 789–2647; ken@mentalhealth.org)—sponsored by the U.S. Department of Health and Human Services (DHHS), Substance Abuse and Mental Health Services Administration—provides numerous free-of-cost, excellent DHHS publications and videotapes on many aspects of disaster mental health services and programs. The Knowledge Exchange Network will send a catalog from which orders can be placed.

All persons listed in the "Acknowledgments" section are willing to be contacted directly in writing or by telephone for specific information; some have provided telephone numbers above for ease of contact. Some citations in the "References" section are especially noteworthy for their comprehensive discussion of theory and practice in disaster mental health (Lystad, 1988; Myers, 1994), support groups of all types (Wee, 1994), and session-by-session description of the entire life of a support group after a natural disaster (Paolercio, 1993).

REFERENCES

Bradford, E. (1994). Support groups. In D. Wee, *Support groups in crisis counseling programs: Training handout* (Vol. 1). Berkeley, CA: Project REBOUND, Northridge Earthquake Crisis Counseling Assistance and Training, Regular Services Program (FEMA 1008-DR-CA).

Farberow, N., & Frederick, C. (1996). *Training manual for human service workers in major disasters* (DHHS Publication No. SMA 90-538). Washington, DC: U.S. Government Printing Office.

Herman, J. L. (1992). *Trauma and recovery.* New York: Basic Books.

Janoff-Bulman, R. (1985). The aftermath of victimization: Rebuilding shattered assumptions. In C. Figley (Ed.), *Trauma and its wake: The study and treatment of post-traumatic stress disorder* (pp. 15–35). New York: Brunner/Mazel.

Kerr, M. M., Brent, D. A., & McKain, B. (1997). *Postvention standards guidelines: A guide for a school's response in the aftermath of a sudden death* (3rd ed.). Pittsburgh, PA: University of Pittsburgh, Services for Teens at Risk (STAR) Center.

Lystad, M. (Ed.). (1988). *Mental health response to mass emergencies: Theory and practice.* New York: Brunner/Mazel.

McGorrian, G. M. (1995). *After disaster strikes: A workbook on supportive group therapy.* Unpublished manuscript.

Mitchell, J. T., & Everly, G. S. (1996). *Critical incident stress debriefing: An operations manual for the prevention of traumatic stress among emergency services and disaster personnel* (2nd ed.). Ellicott City, MD: Chevron.

Myers, D. (1994). *Disaster response and recovery: A handbook for mental health professionals* (DHHS Publication No. SMA 94-3010). Washington, DC: U.S. Government Printing Office.

Myers, D., & Wolfe, D. (1996). Critical incident stress management. In J. Mattman & S. Kaufer (Eds.), *The complete workplace violence prevention manual* (Vol. 2; pp. 75–107). Costa Mesa, CA: James.

Paolercio, M. (1993). *We're still quakin'. . .* Hayward, CA: Theodon Books. (Available only through the author at 568 Prentiss Street, San Francisco, CA 94110)

Peuler, J. N. (1988). Community outreach after emergencies. In M. Lystad (Ed.), *Mental health response to mass emergencies: Theory and practice* (pp. 239–261). New York: Brunner/Mazel.

Peuler, J. N., & Ritter-Splain, S. (1983). *Project COPE (Counseling Ordinary People in Emergency): Final report.* Santa Cruz, CA: County of Santa Cruz, Community Mental Health Services.

Piper, W. E., McCallum, M., & Azim, H. F. A. (1992). *Adaptation to loss through short-term group psychotherapy.* New York: Guilford Press.

Speier, T., Thomas, M., Carter, N., DeWolfe, D., & Rubin, M. (1996). *Responding to the needs of people with serious and persistent mental illness in times of major disaster* (DHHS Publication No. SMA 96-3077). Washington, DC: U.S. Government Printing Office.

Sperry, L. (1996). *Corporate therapy and consulting.* New York: Brunner/Mazel.

Wee, D. (1994). *Support groups in crisis counseling programs: Training handout* (3 vols.). Los Angeles: Project REBOUND, Northridge Earthquake Crisis Counseling Assistance and Training, Regular Services Program (FEMA 1008-DR-CA).

Yalom, I. D. (1995). *The theory and practice of group psychotherapy* (4th ed.). New York: Basic Books.

Young, M. A. (1998). *Responding to communities in crisis: The training manual of the NOVA crisis response team* (2nd ed.). Washington, DC: National Organization for Victim Assistance.

11

<o>

Group Psychotherapy
for Victims of Political Torture
and Other Forms
of Severe Ethnic Persecution

ANDREAS VON WALLENBERG PACHALY

What cannot be talked about can also not be put to rest, and
if it is not, the wounds continue to fester from generation to
generation.
                    —BRUNO BETTELHEIM (1982, p. 11; my translation)

When we work with victims of torture, we must always consider two factors: (1) The utmost destruction of personality, including the destruction of
the good internal holding group, is one of the goals of torture; and (2) in
order for a person who has been tortured to achieve distance from and to
demarcate him- or herself from the internalized torturer, it is necessary to
repeat, relive, and work through the pain of torture and the feelings of revenge within a protective therapeutic setting. The aim of therapy is to rebuild a good, containing, holding, and protecting internalized group to
achieve an end to the devastating effects of torture on the victim (and ultimately, on his or her offspring).

From a therapeutic standpoint, small and large groups (including social systems) constitute the most effective settings for containing and reversing the effects of trauma. In what follows, I explore the individual and
group dynamics of political torture and of the victims of torture, and examine how they are revived and repeated within the group psychotherapy

setting. I also discuss the therapeutic possibilities that the group offers to alleviate the pain and heal the tremendous damage that torture has done to a human being. I believe that many of the points made here about group therapy for torture victims can be applied to the group therapy of severely traumatized patients in general.

THE RELEVANCE OF TORTURE
TO AN UNDERSTANDING OF OTHER
SEVERE TRAUMATIZATION

Therapists treating narcissistically injured patients (including those with borderline and narcissistic personality disorders, major depression, and many psychotic disorders), as well as victims of rape and of sexual and physical child abuse, regularly find in such patients' histories cumulative violations of their bodily as well as their psychic borders. Such therapists find multiple episodes of scapegoating; denigration by their most important figures of reference; and sexual, physical, and psychological exploitation. At a very early age, many of these individuals have been exposed to life-attacking, life-forbidding stimuli in a totalitarian manner. By this I mean that such children are completely dependent for affection and love on the same figures that attack them. In the worst cases, there is no other human contact available, and the child victim experiences the traumatizing human and family environment as the universe in its totality.

Importantly, these traumatizing atmospheres are easily reestablished in the transference relationship with the therapy group, where (ideally) they can be gradually countered by a more life-sustaining, growth-enhancing group experience.

> For example, in one such group, it was noticeable that Geraldine spoke very quickly and that the longer she talked about herself, the more restless, nervous, self-conscious, and obviously uncomfortable she felt. She increasingly expressed the feeling that because she seemed to monopolize the group time, she made others, especially the women in the group, jealous and envious of her. Frequently she would tell the group about her sister, who she felt was much more intelligent, prettier, and more skillful than she was. Soon she felt inferior to all but one woman in the group. Interestingly, her negative feelings were not accessible for correction by the shared perception of the other group members. That she felt inferior was beyond debate, and when the other women insisted that they were not jealous, she refused to believe it. Gradually, the group learned that she had been raised in a family where her mother, supported by her much more aloof father and her older sister, had established a dramatic, black-and-white polarization between the two girls. Geraldine's sister had always been the intelli-

gent star of the family, while she had been the one who was thought to be "stupid" and backward in her development. In fact, she had been taught that she had an obviously inferior genetic disposition. Bit by bit, with the help of the group, she could look at her family history and began to recall many instances when she had been denigrated, denied recognition, and ridiculed. Eventually, a clear picture evolved of a parenting system in which the older daughter had become the container of the idealized unfulfilled wishes of the parents, especially of the mother, whereas Geraldine had become the container of the unwanted, despised, rejected sides of the mother. This split had provided a comfortable balance of mind for the parents, who felt a permanent need to compare themselves with the rest of the world, because they as individuals were lacking stable, true selves.

In such cases of family dysfunction and devaluation as Geraldine's, the traumatizing effects usually result from the inner psychic needs of the reference figures and are not intentionally planned. Torture as an expression of organized state violence, however, is a planned attack on the identity and psychological life of its victims. It represents the most extreme and clear-cut form of traumatizing behavior. Since it is frequently exerted on individuals who were psychologically healthy before torture, it provides an opportunity to elucidate the effect of traumatizing influences on previously relatively mature personality structures (Bettelheim, 1982). At the same time, it furnishes insights that are relevant in the treatment of other severely disturbed patients who carry with them the effects of traumata, because both the psychodynamics and group dynamics resemble each other and function along similar lines. The difference between a traumatized patient who has not been tortured and a torture victim is that in the former instance a fragile self is exposed to perhaps not such extreme trauma (with the exception of the most severe child abuse), whereas in torture a stable, mature self is exposed to trauma of the utmost severity.

One of my chief aims in this chapter is to illustrate how work with victims of torture enriches our understanding of group psychotherapy with other traumatized individuals. Specifically, it provides an opportunity to learn in depth how projective mechanisms are addressed, real trauma is explored, superego pathology is confronted, and the external and internalized dynamics of life-attacking group formations are countered by life-supporting and life-affirming group dynamics.

DEFINITION OF TORTURE

According to U.N. Resolution No. A/30/3452, adopted on December 9, 1975, "torture" is defined as follows:

1. "[Torture includes] every act by which a person, by a carrier of state power or induced by [state power], is submitted to intentionally strong bodily or psychic pain or suffering in order to force him to give a testimony or a confession concerning a deed he committed or is suspected to have committed, or to punish him, or to frighten him or other persons" (United Nations, 1976, p. 91).

2. "Torture is an extreme form of intentional, cruel, inhumane, or denigrating treatment or punishment" (United Nations, 1976, p. 91).

In addition, it is important to emphasize that the act of torture is deliberately intended to destroy the victim's personality.

Torture is usually motivated by a desperate pathological striving to preserve the identity of a political, national, and/or ethnic group. Torture tries to preserve the perpetrator's group identity at severe cost to the identity of a member of another group, or an entire ethnic group. Volkan (1991) has discussed the social and political dimension of this dynamic and has explored the function of a national or ethnic identity "tent," which strengthens and protects individual and subgroup identities in times of identity diffusion or global threat to the sense of self. The metaphor of the "tent" suggests an enclosure-like ego-protective function of identity, as well as its tendency to be profoundly affected by environmental and cultural changes (just as a tent can be affected by stormy weather, etc.). This metaphor for identity preservation and identity disturbance is yet another insight from work with torture victims that is valuable and instructive for work with other extremely disturbed patients, who underneath a facade of severe symptomatology carry within themselves the psychic and bodily traces of traumatic and cumulative traumatic experiences.

TORTURE'S AIMS AND MEANS

An essential part of torture is the total assault not only on an individual's entire personality, but even on the somatic integrity of the body as a living system. Not only the mind, but all the systems that coordinate and organize the biological functioning of the human organism, are attacked. At a time when the capacity for feelings and thoughts is already wiped out and a psychic state of numbing has been reached, the torturer's attacks on the limbic system and on the autonomic nervous system in general continue.

A political prisoner is a human being with strong beliefs and political convictions. In order to force such a prisoner to give up his or her convictions, to change the relationship between ego and superego, the ego has to be brought out of balance. The prisoner has to be confronted with a dilemma: either to submit to the torturer or to lose his or her mind. The director of the prison "Libertad" in Uruguay summarized it thus: "If possible, we do not kill them; eventually we have to let them go. Therefore we have to use the time to rob them of their minds" (quoted in Espinola, Gil, Klinger, & Gil, 1985, p. 34; my translation).

A major objective of torture is, through ongoing physical and psychological attacks, to deprive the victim of any sense of security, reliability, or dependability. The victim's internalized containing, holding group is destroyed. Améry (1977, p. 73) has vividly described the consequence of this loss of the good internalized group object as "not feeling at home any longer in this world" (my translation). Whether the torturer succeeds in this goal depends on whether the torturer can isolate the victim from his or her reference group, which provides holding in the here and now. Only then will the victim experience the world as offering no more alternatives to the world of the torturer.

An example of this objective at work can be seen in the mass rape of Bosnian women (and their subsequently being forced to carry the resulting pregnancies to term). This was intended to destroy their belonging to their own group or any other, as well as their children's capacity to belong to any group. Their children will not be Serbs, nor can they be accepted as Muslims by the Bosnian Muslim community. These women and children are condemned to a life outside any identity-protective cultural tent. Moreover, the Bosnians' entire cultural network of relationships has been attacked for generations to come.

Two other major aims of torture are as follows: (1) to destroy the victim's basic beliefs about life (Janoff-Bulman, 1992); and (2) to generate an extreme yearning for dependency and its corollary, pathological loyalty.

POSTTORTURE DISTRESS SYNDROME

I conceive of the "posttorture distress syndrome" as a diagnostic entity in which victims of torture manifest at least several of the following symptoms: anxiety, depression, feelings of resignation, sudden weeping bursts, apathy, fear, suspiciousness, feelings of guilt, aggressiveness, intensive rage, irritability, suicidal attempts, introversion, drowsiness, exhaustion, memory difficulties, lack of concentration, disorientation, sleeping difficulties, paresthesias, sexual disturbances, and psychosomatic disturbances (e.g., gastrointestinal disorders, skin irritation, heart problems, and specific pains after specific forms of torture). (See also Roth, Lunde, Boysen, & Kemp Genefke, 1987.) These symptoms may occur immediately after torture, but can occur even decades after the actual act of torture, along with paranoid ideas, hallucinations, and alcohol and drug abuse.

In my opinion, posttorture distress syndrome should be distinguished from other forms of posttraumatic stress disorder (PTSD) as defined by DSM-IV (American Psychiatric Association, 1994), because both the traumatic events and their effects are often more severe.[1] Victims of torture have usually been exposed to extreme stressors over very long periods of time, often continuing into the present (years of persecution, multiple imprisonments, torture proper, a perilous period of escape, the cultural shock of exile, and retraumatization in exile), whereas some other forms of PTSD may be caused by a single, circumscribed traumatic event. In addition, PTSD may be caused by a natural disaster (an earthquake, a hurricane, etc.), a technological disaster (an airplane crash, a car accident, an industrial accident, etc.), or a human-made disaster (a hijacking, physical or sexual abuse, etc.). Of these three types of disasters, the human-made disaster is often the most challenging to survivors' sense of safety and of a just world—and torture is the most extreme form of human-made disaster. Its effects are accordingly even more severe than those seen in other forms of PTSD, as various authors have pointed out.

In an attempt to differentiate forms of PTSD according to their severity, Herman (1992) has developed the profile of "disorder of extreme stress not otherwise specified" or "complex PTSD." Herman's formulation takes into consideration lasting, repetitive traumata that occur within interpersonal relationships and lead to significant disturbances in the following areas:

1. Regulation of emotions (continuous depressive moods; extreme repression of rage and aggression, alternating with eruptions of these emotions; loss of sexuality or inadequate seductive sexual behavior).
2. Awareness (amnesia, dissociation, depersonalization).
3. Perception of the self (shame, guilt, self-accusations, isolation).
4. Perception of the perpetrator (permanent thoughts of revenge; the apparent paradox of thankfulness toward the perpetrator, taking over his or her value system and beliefs).
5. Relations with others (isolation, withdrawal, destruction of relationships with spouse and family, suspiciousness, loss of the capacity to protect oneself).
6. Systems of belief and faith (loss of faith and trust, feelings of hopelessness and despair).

Van der Kolk, Roth, and Pelcovitz (1992) have further developed this profile of "complex PTSD" or "disorder of extreme stress." They describe symptoms specific to victims of torture and other forms of extreme stress, including difficulties coping with anger and rage; self-harming or suicidal behavior; impulsive, risky behavior; chronic pain (psychosomatic pain); idealization of the perpetrator/torturer; taking over of the perpetrator's/torturer's values and beliefs; incapacity to trust others or oneself; the tendency to become a victim again; and the tendency to victimize others. Victims of torture, like patients with milder forms of PTSD, frequently develop comorbidity (i.e., other severe symptoms, such as depression, obsessive–compulsive behavior, suicidality, substance abuse, eating difficulties, and somatization).

The final definition of posttorture distress syndrome is still not generally agreed upon. It is further complicated by the facts that it defines the pathological suffering of a formerly reasonable, sane individual, and that it has to be considered as a result of extremely destructive social and political forces.

TRAUMA AND AVOIDANT BEHAVIOR

It is not a traumatic act as such that is traumatic; rather, the feelings related to the traumatic act are what have to be fended off, because they are so painful. They also engrave their traces deep in the patient's biochemical matrix. This results in various avoidant behavioral strategies, which can be extreme at times. Since the basic brain structure, the limbic system, has been fiercely attacked in torture (and, to a lesser extent, in other traumatic events), we can observe deeply engraved psychosomatic reactions as evasive reactions to an aversive stimulus. These reactions, however, are maladaptive in the sense that they perpetuate the basic disturbance, the trauma. Here the role of group psychotherapy becomes decisive, because it provides a safe container for the avoiding behavior as well as for the previously warded-off traumatic feelings.

> Mary, a victim of torture, had recently joined the group. Another patient was having his last session after 3 years of successful group analysis. The group engaged in an intense exchange of feelings of affection, sadness, and separation. The patient had been an important group member, and all would miss him, though there was a common feeling that it was the right time for him to go his own way. After 30 minutes, Mary stood up and said that she would "wait outside and read a book." She insisted that these feelings of loss had nothing to do with her. The group asked her back in only when they shared a glass of champagne to celebrate the other patient's departure. Some months later, Mary could verbalize how important it had been to avoid all the feelings of separation, abandonment, and rejection evoked inside herself by the other patient's departure. It had been equally important to be able to "wait outside" and to feel that she was not rejected, but could regulate and manage the situation to escape from her unbearable feelings of powerlessness in the face of feelings she could not have shared yet at that time.

DEFENSE MECHANISMS
IN TORTURE VICTIMS

While under torture, a victim will have to develop special defense mechanisms to protect his or her ego from disintegrating, in order to make a desperate effort to preserve the good objects and to save the good, containing, and holding "internal group," both of which are attacked by the torture process.

Torture itself causes regression to the paranoid–schizoid position. This process is induced by the victim's position of extreme dependence within the totally controlled environment. The first defensive step is to regress to splitting. The victim thinks, "We [the group of victims—e.g., the members of my political movement] are all good, and they [the torturers] are all bad." Torturers who succeed in breaking down this splitting defense will succeed in their aim, because the torturers will be able to take the place of the holding group. I discuss this point in more detail later in regard to sexual torture (see the third of the "Three Cases," below).

A prominent defense mechanism, even years after torture, is self-harm. It manifests itself not only in physical violations, but in the symptom in which the ego floods itself with horrible pictures to protect itself from even more pain. Self-generated pain and self-mutilation can actually rescue the victim from other, seemingly unbearable feelings.

The obsessive focus on bodily symptoms serves the purpose of avoidance of the feelings connected with the trauma. Avoidance may be further reinforced by the insecure situation in which a patient lives; for example, it may underlie excessive concern about a residency permit. This concern supports a strategy of warding off the unbearable feelings connected with the trauma, and at the same time of permitting the patient to flee from the here and now.

In the group, the patient often plays a withdrawn, ego-restricted role. He or she may feel persecuted or, conversely, may take over an attacking role—identifying with the former aggressor, the torturer.

TASKS OF GROUP THERAPY
WITH TORTURE VICTIMS

The first major task in the psychotherapy of survivors of torture is to "give the victim a hand" and to lead him or her into the here and now. Otherwise, the symptomatology will become chronic and the avoidant personality structure will become petrified. A degree of "collusion" with and acceptance of the victim's view of the world (however distorted it may be) is necessary, to let the feeling grow that therapy is a safe space. By "collusion" in this context, I do not mean experiencing oneself as a victim, but taking the victim's side and attuning oneself empathically to his or her state of mind.

Before the therapist and the group can relate adequately to the victim, he or she has to overcome a gigantic wall of shame. These feelings represent not only shaming by the ego ideal or blaming a "fallen" ego; they are also an expression of the incapacity to link and to relate. Eternal isolation of the victim is what the torturer has striven for. This has been done through gruesome attacks on linking. Destroying the links between and among ideas, objects, and persons has been described by Bion (1959) as a primitive mechanism for coping with painful emotions. In torture, the torturer robs the victim of familiar holding and containing links with beloved and valued others by denigrating the victim's attachment to them, and by trying to foster attachment to the world of the torturer during a state of absolute dependency. (The victim of torture in turn can fend off feelings of absolute annihilation by attempting to hold on to these links, as I discuss in regard to the first of the "Three Cases," below.) Shame about and disgust with one's body and one's whole being are devastating effects of torture: "What kind of a person am I that this happened to me?" "My body is ugly and spoiled; I hate my body," "My whole life is destroyed; I can't tell anybody what I experienced." "My psyche is sick, and my head is crazy."

And yet, despite therapists' best efforts, they cannot help becoming persecutors at some moments in their work with victims, because in certain regressed ego states a question, a gesture, or a therapist's mere presence may represent torture to a victim. In such a case, a group matrix in which a positive feeling for a fellow patient may survive gains tremendous importance. The compassionate empathy of a fellow patient may at times bring back the soothing of the fellow inmate. (At times, a therapist must also follow this compassionate line and help the victim cope directly with painful symptoms by recognizing their crippling extent and assisting him or her in finding alleviation via catharsis or at times via cognitive and behavioral techniques.)

Group therapy has to open up a space for the patient to share his or her violations, denigration, and abandonment. When the victim comes in touch with these unbearable feelings, there may be times when words cannot express his or her pain and grief adequately and sufficiently, and the group's collective mourning and shedding of tears may be the most appropriate and sometimes the only possible way to express not only the victim's but the group's overwhelming feelings. At the same time, this process may create a bond that can become an early step toward mutual consolation and recovery.

Finally, group therapy must work through the deficient self-esteem, the self-accusations, the dependent character, and the basic insecurity of the victim and other group members. Group therapy gives us opportunities beyond those that are possible with an individualistic model such as Melanie Klein's, which is founded on the dynamics of libidinal and aggressive drives. Internalized life-preserving and life-forbidding group dynamics become externalized in the group setting. We can conceptualize the group as a web of object relations—as a web that contains a certain amount of energy in its knots, cells, and links. The web can contain, hold, and generate positive social energy (von Wallenberg Pachaly & Griepenstroh, 1979), or it can strangulate, imprison, and suffocate. The web can also lack cells and links, resulting in insecurity. The group can now, in a manner analogous to a heart transplant, become such a network of links and cells with which the victim can link and bond. Gradually a holding web may be "transplanted" (i.e., internalized) as healthy new psychic elements within the selves of the members.

> Consider, for example, the case of a patient who again and again was flooded by anxieties, felt bodily paralyzed, panicked, and let himself be rushed to the hospital for an injection of a sedative. This habitual pattern in turn reinforced his conviction that he was unable to bear his feelings, and he felt increasingly dependent on his medication. After the group had explored and put into words the context of his "sudden" attacks of anxiety (whenever he felt deserted), and as he realized through the group's interaction that he was able to take a stance against others, he felt less fearful and increasingly empowered. He became able to take a stance against his own anxiety. He could now tolerate such feelings and share them with the group.

The therapeutic group may provide the safe space within which it becomes possible for the victim to look once more at the feelings that are chronically numbed because they were initially experienced as so overwhelming. The fended-off traumatic feelings include especially extreme feelings of loneliness, isolation, abandonment, loss of trust in one's own perception, total powerlessness, and dissolution of self. Therapy can succeed when these traumatic feelings are accepted and contained. It offers a chance for the victim to regain some familiarity with the everyday, reasonably secure world, because group psychotherapy carries the power to support, sustain, and reinforce the good internal objects.

Finally, group therapy can help the victim to discern between his or her premorbid personality and the life-destroying group dynamics he or she has internalized under torture. This will free the victim of crippling feelings of guilt. A note of caution is in order, however: Efforts can be made in therapy to help the victim to try to reconstruct what was destroyed, but what remains is a certain emptiness in face of the experienced loss of humanity.

TECHNICAL CONSIDERATIONS
IN SETTING UP GROUPS

When a victim of torture begins group therapy, several points have to be considered. In the beginning a series of individual sessions is usually helpful, to open a space for the patient's feelings of shame. Homogeneous groups may be of greater help for victims of ethnic cleansing than for victims of individual torture. These groups, in my experience, have the quality of solidarity groups concerning the difficulties of living in a foreign country and/or of continuing a political fight against the torturing system from abroad. To the degree that they foster solidarity and holding, they improve the chances for success in the endeavor of group psychotherapy. However, I personally prefer to work with heterogeneous groups (see point 4 below).

The use of drugs should of course be very time-limited and has to be carefully judged in relationship to the abuse of psychotropic drugs a victim may have been subjected to under torture. Hospitalization is usually only appropriate in an emergency situation—not only because the hospital frequently reminds a victim of prison, but also because the treatment period will be too short. In my experience, therapy with a victim of torture takes from 6 months to 4 years. It cannot be completed in a few weeks.

Other technical considerations in setting up groups for torture victims, or groups that include torture victims, are as follows:

1. It is my experience that a certain degree of a healthy capacity for ego demarcation is necessary for a victim/patient to be able to integrate into a heterogeneous therapy group.

2. Therapists should bear in mind the concept of "critical acculturation." That is, a patient's cultural background needs to be respected, and the patient should be supported to keep it alive and to build bridges gradually with the culture of the "guest country" (Barudy, 1989). The patient should certainly not be expected to discard or deny his or her cultural background; otherwise, there is the danger that the patient will perceive living in the host country as a repetition of the torture scene.

3. In regard to group composition, it is my experience that there should always be at least one other severely traumatized patient in the same group. Facilitating identification with a fellow patient prevents an early dropout, because it reduces the danger of scapegoating as well as of idealization by the other group members, and reduces the victim/patient's fear of abandonment.

4. I prefer to work with heterogeneous groups because they correspond to the reality of life, are much richer in their mutual therapeutic possibilities, and also offer less disturbed patients a chance to come into contact with deeper layers of their personality structure. The overwhelming

traumatic material, in my experience, can very well be contained and worked through in a heterogeneous group—provided that space is opened up for the nontraumatized members to communicate frankly about their emotional reactions, and that these are accorded respect and importance. The therapist may utilize the fact that even nontraumatized patients can understand trauma in some respects, since, thanks to television and other media, nearly everyone is vicariously familiar with such experiences! If trauma is understood as a result of a flooding of the self with excessive feelings, it can be explored gradually. This helps to build bridges with nontraumatized fellow patients, as well as with those who have been traumatized but not tortured. After an initial phase in which the whole group has to learn to tolerate and to address trauma and related feelings, it is my experience that the integration of severely traumatized patients furthers group cohesion.

5. Communication with the victim's "large-group system" should start as soon as possible, because frequently this is a prerequisite for a successful realization of psychotherapy. (See "Social Systems Therapy," below.)

6. Special attention has to be paid to ensuring that tortured and other traumatized patients, with their special emotional sensitivity, are not exploited by other patients to contain feelings that the latter are not yet able to experience.

KEY ISSUES, CONCERNS, AND DIFFICULTIES IN GROUP THERAPY

The following is an overview of some of the key issues, concerns, and difficulties that will be experienced in running a psychotherapy group for torture victims (a homogeneous group) or a group that includes victims of torture in the membership (a heterogeneous group). Either type of group evolves from an aggregate of strangers with an unknown history, to establishment of personal histories and expressions of anxiety, to a recurrence of the fusion that took place between torture victims and victimizers (with mutual projections), to empathy and the reconstruction of trust and the capacity for closeness. The victim's damaged personalities must be restructured, and society must cooperate in the task of acknowledging the atrocities and helping these individuals.

1. The psychotherapeutic work starts out in a foggy twilight, where the original personality structure, the experience of torture, and the resulting personality deformation (or even destruction) of a victim/patient are very much interwoven. It becomes the group's task to get an understanding of (a) who this person was before torture; (b) why he or she experienced torture in this particular way and not in another way; (c) how he or she

was in fact abused, tortured, and maltreated; and (d) what effect the torture had on his or her personality.

2. Since a torture victim has experienced a real preexisting traumatic or cumulative traumatic event, and not merely a fantasy as such, therapists should never forget when working with such individuals that encountering them should prevail over analyzing them. Therapists can accompany them in confronting the often unspeakable nightmares of torture once more—in their efforts to free themselves from the ghosts of the past. But these ghosts were real humans and did real injustice, force, and violence to these patients. And, worst of all, torture is the absolute, inescapable proof that there exist humans and human institutions that leave humanness completely behind them—the real barbarians.

3. Tortured humans don't trust their own perceptions anymore. They have incorporated their torturers' view of the world, and at the same time have lost their confidence in their own views of other people. Here, of course, the psychotherapeutic group can be of great help, as it represents an arena for training victims to check and trust their perceptions. Moreover, the group can provide the experience that a humanity beyond torture continues to exist. The group may open a transitional space where the life-destroying group dynamics can be recognized and confronted with life-giving and life-protecting dynamics.

4. The group is a place where the effects of torture can be explored. It can provide an empathic mirror for reconstructing the truth. A victim/patient (and other group members) can begin to see how the victim's ego boundaries have been blurred, even the border between torturer and tortured; how, during the regressive ego states that go along with torture (anxieties of annihilation, of total abandonment, and of absolute rejection of a psychotic quality), a fusion of ego boundaries has occurred; and how, sometimes quite suddenly, the victim can become the perpetrator.

5. In group psychotherapy, the notion of "fusion of ego boundaries" becomes especially important, because the fusion recurs with the entire group. It is as if suddenly—triggered by perhaps a casual remark, facial expression, or gesture—the victim/patient feels victimized, persecuted, and tortured by the entire group. At times then, in turn, the victim/patient starts persecuting the entire group, becoming a "persecuting victim." My understanding of such dynamics is that they occur in moments when the victim is overwhelmed by the terror of fusion—of becoming swallowed up, overwhelmed, and extinguished.

Peter kept complaining that the group members, and particularly the therapist, did not like him. The group noticed that at the same time he felt intense needs for closeness. He began to attack the group and the therapist vehemently, thus destroying any feelings of closeness. Several times he "seduced" the group into violently counterattacking him, accusing him of destroying any feelings of closeness and affection. Eventually, some group members worked out the understanding that the very closeness he wanted so much must seem so threatening to him; only after this could he recall and discuss several instances when his torturer had established a seemingly close emotional relationship with him. This closeness had then been brutally abused and destroyed, to make him even more dependent and "broken."

6. Thus, on the spur of the moment, projective mechanisms may prevail. The psychotherapy group is then challenged to demarcate itself against the life-attacking forces exerted on it, and to understand and empathize with the extreme anxieties, agony, and feelings of abandonment that underlie the projections. The potential destruction of the life-preserving, life-giving, sustaining, and holding internalized group must be recognized and if possible "confronted" with the life-protecting group dynamics of a well-functioning psychotherapy group.

7. The group becomes a container for unbearable feelings. At times the group will have to tolerate feelings of abandonment, isolation, and agony. The members will need just to sit and attend, and not to run away.

8. The members' genuinely and authentically relating within the group is the key to dealing successfully with projections and to containing painful feelings. The matrix of mutual relations—the members' tolerance of one another—forms the soil in which empathy, instead of pity, can grow. If the group members succeed in relating their genuine feelings and even "countertransference feelings" about each other, then this process will counteract the destruction of linking and will alleviate the damaged feeling of belonging. I think of several tortured patients (as well as other severely traumatized patients), who, upon feeling rejected in the course of a group session, vehemently attacked the group. Their own feelings were inaccessible to emotional correction through the shared perception of fellow patients. Only as each of these patients succeeded in creating a feeling of complete helplessness in all other patients and myself, and after we shared this feeling with each patient, did the patient him- or herself feel relieved and no longer rejected, but understood and accepted. The group in such a process can be conceptualized as a "digesting container" for originally unbearable feelings, which can then be survived without a traumatizing effect.

9. The psychotherapeutic group as an empathic mirror can help a victim to find his or her posttorture personality, which must strive to integrate the experience of torture for the rest of the person's life. In this process, the limits of therapy are felt most painfully. Therapy in many cases can only alleviate the effects of torture; it cannot heal them, much less undo them. The container, a deep-rooted feeling of basic trust, is broken and can be repaired only partially. It is in this area of extreme traumatization that we can diagnose the "broken personality" of the torture victim.

10. As I have discussed above, in the process of reestablishing the borders, reality has to be reconstructed as far as possible, has to be acknowledged, and has to be made public. The group thus becomes the first public space where the capacity to demarcate oneself from the world of torture can be developed. Pathological loyalty to a traumatizing system, which I have found in many of these patients, can be resolved.

11. In this context, victims' bonding with institutions like Amnesty International means that they preserve a reference group separate from torture. In this way, good and bad are kept in their respective places and a complete blurring of borders can be prevented, or at least borders can be restored. This is a phenomenon I have seen in many severely disturbed patients. Their chances for integration into social life and for emotional growth increase as they succeed in joining and creating groups that are important to them. (Elsewhere, I have discussed this as the group-dynamic understanding of the ego function of social participation; see von Wallenberg Pachaly, 1983.)

12. It is my understanding, however, that group psychotherapy alone cannot accomplish this task. The process of group psychotherapy for victims of persecution, torture, and ethnic cleansing can be greatly facilitated (or greatly hampered) by processes in society at large. For example, at present, all the old files of the former East German secret state police are open. Now all victims of persecution by the secret police have the right to learn what information once was stored about them, how their lives were destroyed, and which destructive influences were exerted on them in what ways. A whole administration has been created (called the Gauck Administration, after its chairman, a highly respected clergyman of the former East Germany) that scrutinizes, administrates, and deciphers all available records of the former East German secret police. And every German citizen has the right to ask for a full record of everything that is available on any oppressive, destructive activities that were carried out against him or her. The South African Truth Commission serves the same purpose. Such society-wide developments can be of immense therapeutic benefit for victims of torture.

13. Healthy superego development is dependent upon a sincere, loving parent–child relationship. The group dynamics of torture, however, "prove" to a victim that ideals may be lethal. Differing somewhat from ethnic cleansing, torture proper also attacks ideology, beliefs, and ideals. During torture, the victim's ideals prove disastrous. Ego ideals crumble, and treachery leads to a loss of morale. A corrupt superego may result. The adult ego blames a corrupt superego, neglecting the fact that at times of torture there is no adult ego. From this, a terrorist superego and a feeling of total powerlessness may develop. The frequent "seemingly irrational" feelings of guilt are reactions to feelings of absolute dependency and total impotence. If the victim feels guilty, this allows him or her to feel active, rather than com-

pletely powerless and overwhelmed by external powers. At least the victim can view him- or herself as the cause of everything bad that has happened. Leon Wurmser (1999) discusses similar ideas. The group can help to put such things in a realistic perspective.

14. In a certain way, tortured individuals are like victims of rape. They too were raped; they frequently blame themselves; and yet the part of the self that survives torture is like the helpless "infant self" stemming from the act of rape. Can victims of torture still love themselves, or must they hate themselves, since they are products of the violence of torture? The primary task of the group is to take each victim back into the human family. This is a task that, in my experience, is valid for many severely disturbed patients.

15. Victims of ethnic cleansing have been robbed of their homeland, and a fierce attack has been made on their ethnic "tent." In my experience, the rebuilding of this tent has to be supported; simultaneously, the integration of the victims of torture, rape, and mutilation back into the ethnic community has to be accomplished.

THE BURDEN OF THE BARBARIAN WITHIN US: EXPLORING PROJECTIVE MECHANISMS AND COUNTERTRANSFERENCE FEELINGS

Victims of torture in therapy groups nearly always come from another country, and frequently come from a completely different culture. They often represent the aliens/scapegoats upon which even professional clinicians project all that is "evil" within them. Chattopadhyay and Biran (1997) have reported on a meeting of group psychotherapists (International Group Relations and Scientific Conference: Exploring Global Social Dynamics) where this process was studied. But therapists need only look at their own professional group processes—for example, the ways in which rival psychotherapeutic schools frequently attack and shame each other.

Projective mechanisms are relevant to the question of pity versus empathy. Pity allows therapists to keep their distance and serves to reaffirm their prejudice toward others as inferior barbarians. As empathy grows, they are disturbingly confronted with the barbarians within themselves.

The initial countertransference feelings in response to a victim of torture are shame and sadness in the presence of a broken man or woman. This frequently leads to countertransference feelings of wanting to repair and to revenge the atrocities. Consequently, the danger of enmeshment for the therapist becomes a paramount challenge. Nontraumatized or nontortured group members, too, will be torn at first between doing repair work to the tortured group member and fantasizing about the striving for revenge.

The group's countertransference responses to the somatic destruction of the patient (the awareness of the physical harm and somatic problems due to torture) often include rejection, avoidance, and denial.

George kept repeating his complaints and descriptions of his somatic pains again and again. His stereotyped behavior usually resulted in a politely listening group that soon ended up bored and without interest. Sometimes however, George not only reported his somatic pains, but unwillingly (it broke out of him, though he wanted to suppress it) conveyed the horror, agony, and fears of annihilation underneath the somatic pain—that is, the psychic pain he had taken in under torture. In those moments the group became frightened, sad, and silenced. For George, it was not possible to view this as a friendly reaction; he experienced it as rejection. He stiffened up and withdrew into silence. The frozen pain of torture—frozen within the somatic symptoms—could be melted by giving the group members a space to share their feelings in reaction to George's somatic symptoms. This in turn helped George to become able to tolerate, live through once more, and demarcate himself from the psychic pain that had been intolerable for him under torture.

As a reaction to the victim's loss of trust in humans, and to the destruction of basic trust, the group itself may feel petrified and absolutely powerless.

David, who had been kidnapped from home, had been extensively tortured for some months, and had been at the verge of death several times, had also been submitted to extensive brainwashing and indoctrination techniques. When he reported how he had been shown indoctrinating films for hours and hours, with his eyes fixed on the screen in a completely powerless physical and mental position of absolute dependency, the group realized that at times he obviously also sometimes experienced the group like a film. His hypnotic states, but also his lack of capacity to trust and to believe in the perceptions of the group, made the members feel absolutely powerless and petrified in the beginning. Later they tried to "persuade" David of their view of the world—that they were trustworthy, and that he was valuable. They did this in vain, of course. Only as they could start to share their feelings of absolute powerlessness, paralysis, and rejection could David, in turn, start sharing his feelings under this specific mind-exterminating torture.

Envy of and identification with the aggressor can be observed within the group, as a defense against the extreme feelings of powerlessness and helplessness.

Last but not least, I have observed in my own practice and in supervision work that if a therapist who becomes overwhelmed by traumatic feelings may sometimes regress him- or herself and identify with the victim/patient's projections. That is, the therapist may become the aggressor and verbally attack the patient.

THREE CASES

In this section I discuss three cases at greater length, to illustrate my understanding of the group dynamics of torture and how these can be challenged.[2]

The Life-Attacking Group Dynamics of Torture— Inside and Outside Confinement

The first case demonstrates the group dynamics effective under torture; the influence of a torturing political system; and the way in which such a system becomes internalized in the life-attacking, identity-destroying group dynamics that prevent an individual from coming to terms with his or her own past, or from being able to link up and bond with other fellow beings and with him- or herself in the here and now. It demonstrates the core issues that must be addressed in group psychotherapy, as well as what we can expect will be relived in that context.

Victor, a very sophisticated, academically trained patient, came to my office because one of his children had become drug-addicted and because of an increase in his own symptoms of sleeplessness, nervousness, depression, recurring nightmares, and constant restlessness. He had been acknowledged as a political refugee, and his status in Germany was secure. His internalized isolation and life-forbidding, relationship-cutting, link-attacking forces were so strong, however, that therapy proper was not possible for him.

Victor had been imprisoned for 2 years and had regularly been physically and psychologically tortured; among other forms of torture, he had been subjected to several mock executions. He had been confined to a cell of 15 fellow inmates, all of whom had been similarly tortured. He described his relationship with his fellow prisoners as a source of intimacy that helped him to endure the drag of torture and to contain the pain; it allowed for a closeness that was a clear counterweight to the loneliness experienced under torture. The other prisoners were humans who understood his suffering. Solidarity in the cell was a source for sharing—if not by words, then by looks or touches. This closeness protected them from isolation, which most humans are not able to endure. It helped them to maintain the conviction of being on the right side, and it confirmed the importance of remaining truthful to oneself. Thus a minimal degree of containing could be preserved. Victor's recollections of his prison life give us a first hint of how group psychotherapy might work as a holding, secure, reassuring container that allows life to be.

Unfortunately, when a victim forms a relationship with other human beings, torturers know this and try to destroy the life-preserving group system by enlisting spies within the group. In Victor's case, this actually happened not while he was in prison, but later. After his release from prison, Victor was still obliged to report to the state police once a week, telling them with whom he had met and what he had talked about. This meant that every person whom he contacted now automatically became a suspect too. In a psychological sense, he was infected with a deadly disease, "torture," that could be transmitted by the slightest social interaction. There remained no one he could talk to without running the danger of becoming a torturer himself. This led to a cruel isolation, which he experienced as greater mental pain than the physical and psychological torture to which he had been submitted in prison.

We can assume that this period of continuing traumatization resulted finally in the destruction of Victor's holding and containing internal group dynamics. Each time he felt close to a person, when he felt the need for warmth and closeness and the need to communicate, such nurturing was prohibited by the "social control" of his torturers.

We can draw parallels to a child who is exposed within the caretaking environment to "torturing" abuse and attacks on his or her physical and psychological integrity, and yet feels the need to approach the "torturer" for recognition, affection, and holding. Again and again, such a child is suddenly attacked. This dynamic stands for the torturing system's ultimate attack on linking. Fragmentation[3] of the self and the objects remains the last resort for preserving a rudimentary feeling of existence in the face of this totalitarian annihilation. In efforts to reverse the process of fragmentation by reintegrating the self and the objects, the arising anxiety must be contained. The therapeutic group can offer such a strong and reliable container.

Finally, 2 years later, after having arranged the flight of his wife and his children, Victor succeeded in escaping to Germany. However, he found out that he was not totally safe even here. He learned of some mysterious assassinations of fellow fugitives, who had become victims of the secret service of his home country operating abroad. This caused a deep conflict. On the one hand, he felt the urge to inform the world about the atrocities that were being committed in his country; on the other hand, he felt that he would be in danger if he exposed himself too much. We can here observe how the prohibition against disclosure is brought to its extreme.

Within a few diagnostic sessions with Victor, several central points that exemplify the group dynamics and psychological position of victims of torture became very obvious:

1. Victor still lived in the past; his trauma still kept him a prisoner.

2. His family's present life was a mess—a condition for which he held himself responsible. His life-attacking group dynamics, introjected during the experiences of torture, became projected into the dynamics of his family.

3. Feelings of guilt and shame were central in our contact. Victor felt responsible for the emotional state of his family. He felt shame and guilt that he had not been able to tolerate the situation in his home country any longer, and he believed he had betrayed and abandoned his compatriots.

4. The question of who he had been before torture (his "premorbid personality") became increasingly highlighted.

5. Lurking beneath his doubts as to whether he should be allowed to benefit from psychotherapy was the question of whether he could become capable of confronting his horrible feelings: the unbearable solitude of isolation, the grief over the lost solidarity of his fellow inmates, the pain of torture.

Unfortunately, Victor refused to become a member of a therapeutic group. I was not strong enough to encourage him to join a group, which would have provided a life-supporting, containing, holding, and growth-enhancing environment. One of the reasons was probably that I had been too fascinated and intrigued by the content of what he had recalled, and had not addressed sufficiently, in the initial phase of our encounter, his feelings of shame in the relationship with me. There was some corner deep in his psyche where he felt guilty for everything he had suffered, which led him to reenact the torturing scenes again and again. I should also have addressed his feelings toward his wife and children, and the fact that to enter therapy for him in this moment paradoxically meant to abandon them. These topics should also have been addressed in the initial phase of group psychotherapy.

Isolation, Withdrawal, and Inner Immigration[4] of a Former East German Dissident

The second case illustrates how life-supporting, life-affirming group dynamics can challenge the internalized life-attacking, identity-destroying group dynamics by opening a space to share the extreme isolation, loneliness, and feelings of abandonment the victim has suffered. The group can thus lead the victim of torture away from the pathological development of avoidant personality disorder.

Sonja had been imprisoned for 18 months in the former East Germany. She was "bought into freedom" by the former West German government (for about $50,000) and finally released to the former West Germany. (During the division of Germany into East and West, many thousands of political prisoners were "bought into freedom" by the West German government. As noted earlier, all the files of the former East German secret police are now open, and everybody has the right to find out, through the research of the Gauck Administration, who spied on him or her and what subtle or overt pressure was applied.)

In the former East Germany, Sonja had been subjected to continuous observation and harassment, because she had engaged in nonviolent activities opposing the system. When she could not bear the pressure anymore, and it became clear that there was no professional future for her, she tried to escape, but was captured at the then heavily guarded border. (For a detailed discussion of the effect of the former East German system, see von Wallenberg Pachaly, 1995b.) During her stay in prison, she was physically and psychologically tortured. She entered therapy after her release because of recurring depression, free-floating anxiety, inability to focus her attention, prolonged difficulties at work, obsessive–compulsive thinking, and eating difficulties.

In the course of participating in a standard group analytic setting twice a week, Sonja decided to participate in a 3-week-long, time-limited psychoanalytic therapeutic community (von Wallenberg Pachaly, 1992). She perceived how it offered the fellow patients in her group a chance to feel more secure. During her stay in the community, she would have the opportunity to be seen, perceived, and perhaps understood in her entire existence. This expectation became true to the degree to which in the community she reenacted the internalized dynamics of persecution and isolation.

She first put her dynamics on stage within her work group of six members, whose task was to build a greenhouse. She managed to participate in the group's work, but only at a distance (although she was in view of the others); she fixed windows, yet worked completely for herself. Her fellow patients tolerated her "satellite" participation, but felt hesitant to cross the imaginary border she drew around herself.

In turn, of course, Sonja's suspiciousness and lack of trust caused a countertransference feeling in her fellow patients of wanting to keep their distance from her. They sensed how easily hurt she was, but her social withdrawal caused suspicion and hurt in others. Similarly, at a later phase of her therapy within the community, Sonja was prone to becoming a scapegoated outsider by avoiding involvement. Because she was identified with the resisters against a terrorist regime, she also represented a very strong ego ideal, which was at times experienced as a terroristic superego.

It was only when the community members went on an excursion to an art exhibition that Sonja could make visible how she really felt. That day she again appeared isolated and withdrawn. At the entrance to the exhibition, she was asked by a guard to leave her bag in a locker for security reasons. Suddenly she looked utterly bewildered and paralyzed, as if her whole self had collapsed. A fellow patient, who shared a bedroom with her, discreetly told me that inside the bag was her teddy bear. Out of what could be called "informed therapeutic intuition," I firmly intervened and told the guard that inside the bag was a life-saving medical apparatus, which this person needed to have with her all the time. The other community members, too, spontaneously insisted on not entering the exhibition unless Sonja was allowed to take the bag with her. The guard was so baffled that he allowed her to take the bag with her, without further questioning its content. The "life-saving apparatus" was a transitional object—a little teddy bear that was most important to giving her a feeling of security and belonging!

It was through this action that the community group could understand the full extent of the lack of trust and the isolation from which Sonja was suffering. At the moment she was asked to hand over the bag, she felt as overwhelmed and as impotent as when she had been imprisoned and tortured by a powerful state that had tried to rob her of her innermost convictions, beliefs, perceptions, and identity, and had destroyed her basic feelings of security toward the world in general.

In the group session that evening, Sonja could finally begin to share her feelings of total abandonment and absolute powerlessness under torture. That the group had spontaneously backed her up, and that I had stood up for her, counteracted this devastating experience. Originally the relationship with her teddy bear represented a comforting relationship that gave her power. Now the relationship with the group instilled power and confidence in her.

When the bag was about to be taken away from her, Sonja had been flooded with feelings of unreliability, an absolute lack of power, and overwhelming anxieties. In subsequent sessions, it became possible for her to convey her feelings of absolute helplessness and to share them with the group and myself. These emotions were utterly painful and hard for the group to tolerate. But only through this group process, where pain really had been shared, could she step out of her isolation and her "satellite" position in the group.

The destruction of basic trust, of dependability, and of reliability in interpersonal relations is one of the basic elements of torture; indeed, the torturer's destruction of the internalized life-sustaining, holding group can be understood as the essence of torture. It explains why the reaction of the group to this patient touched her so positively and implanted the seed of healing within her.

Seduction, Abduction, and Sexual Torture

The third case involves the effects of sexual torture, which is indeed the most extreme form of torture, because here positive and negative stimuli are so intertwined that total dependency is provoked. Such torture resembles the situation of a child who is abused, maltreated, and "tortured," and yet is totally dependent on the "torturer" for any positive affection. In the worst-case scenario, the torturing situation represents the total and only available universe for the person.

Sexual torture, according to Agger (1988), can be defined as "a relationship between torturer and victim characterized by ambiguity, containing aggressive as well as libidinal elements" (p. 233; my translation). Not only pain is inflicted; in addition, positive sexual stimulation is used to foster shame, dependency, and the destruction of the personal and sexual identity.

Central in sexual torture are the breakdown of splitting as an identity-saving mechanism, and the evoked fusion of good and bad self and object. By this, I mean the fact that the victim internalizes not only through identifying with the aggressor, but through introjecting the torturer via this more primitive psychic process, wherein the boundaries between self and other are blurred and disappear. The tortured thus becomes the torturer.

This process is induced by the victim's extremely dependent position within this totally controlled environment. The victim is totally dependent on the torturer for his or her (usually her) most basic needs. Food and water are supplied at the torturer's whim, as are light, sound, and heat or cooling. Whether the victim may see at all or is blindfolded, whether she may go to the toilet, or whether she may wash depends entirely on what the torturer wants. Frequently the victim has to defecate or urinate in her clothes. Every mutual, reliable relationship is annihilated, and the victim is thus driven into an extremely regressive psychic and physical state. In this state she becomes incapable of relating to her body, to the outside world, and to other human beings, because the torturer attacks her private self (like a sadistic superego) and instills feelings of guilt, mocking and denigrating her (Amati, 1990).

The regression to splitting is a desperate, adaptive attempt to save the good self, the ego ideal, and the good internalized objects. My clinical experience has shown that the devastating extent of the traumatic consequences correlates with the torturer's capacity to stimulate the victim sexually (in a psychophysiological sense). The reason is that if in the paranoid–schizoid position the victim reacts to sexual torture with physical and psychological sexual arousal (consciously or unconsciously), then this results in her experiencing the relationship with the torturer as ambivalent. When the victim is sexually stimulated at an ego state of extreme regression, early libidinal bonds with the mother can be revived and projected onto the torturer. The ambivalent reaction to the torturer makes it psychologically impossible for the victim to fend off the "bad," the torturer, as it generally still is psychologically (though not physically) possible in rape. This process is accomplished by using the "bad" and the "good" torturer—the latter of whom provides warmth, holding, and friendly skin contact, as well as positive sexual stimulation. The processes of splitting and projection break down; the victim's ego boundaries dissolve; and she re-gresses to a state of complete dependency. The victim incorporates the bad and feels "finished." She starts looking at the world through the eyes of the torturer and feels guilty, because she has been subversive and fought against the political system and its representatives. Both the personal iden-tity and political identity of the victim are destroyed.

After torture, shame and guilt are generated as the predominant, over-whelming feelings and threaten to stay with the victim forever, because she has submitted to the torturer. In treatment, talking about sexual torture is associated with extreme feelings of shame and social taboo. For example, it took Clara (see below) a full year of therapy in the group until she could express the first hints that something like sexual torture could have hap-pened to her. The other group members in turn "missed" her first two hints; they initially heard only plain physical torture and denied the sexual quality because it obviously seemed too painful and dangerous.

In rape, the victim is usually more psychologically able to maintain a demarcation between herself and the perpetrator. Although the assault is also traumatizing, the fusion between good and bad, perpetrator and vic-tim is not accomplished by the perpetrator of rape, as it is by the torturer. Male victims of torture usually are not confronted with this extreme disso-lution of ego boundaries, but their sexual organs are destroyed more fre-quently. In sexual child abuse, quite obviously, the fusion we find in sexual torture can occur too. The results of course are as devastating.

Clara, age 22, came to treatment via the recommendation of her law-yer after she had made her fourth suicide attempt. Though she was not a political fugitive, she had a history of sexual torture. After a few individual sessions, she joined one of my analytic groups.

In her experience, rape and sexual torture were combined with com-plete economic dependency on her torturers and the impossibility of leav-ing them behind. The torturers at the same time seemed to promise security from existential anxieties, starvation, and abandonment. In her transfer-ence relation with the group, Clara felt completely ashamed and guilty, but also absolutely dependent upon the group. Her fifth suicide attempt, made at an early period in therapy, was a total effort to reestablish her ego boundaries, a rudimentary self-esteem, and dignity. She was striving to re-gain her capacity to split the world again into good and bad, and to throw the bad inside her out—to rid herself of the bad introjects, and simulta-neously to establish borders between the self and the outside world.

In the following group sessions, there was another foreign group mem-ber who also had a history of sexual abuse, so Clara did not feel so "strange" and isolated from the rest of the group. This addresses the ques-tion of group composition—in my experience, there should always be at least one other severely traumatized patient in the same psychotherapy group as another traumatized patient.

During the sessions, it became gradually evident that Clara's seductive behavior had evolved more and more as desperate and the only available way for her to make and keep contact with other humans and to satisfy her dependency needs.

Within her analytic group, this behavior soon became obvious as well in her relationship with group members, and the group confronted her with this. It was difficult to balance between not pushing her into a deep depression by not gratifying her needs for recognition and helping her enter into a genuine communication with her true self, and share the psychic pain she had undergone.

Later she could verbalize that the erotic approach she instinctively chose in order to be intimate was her way of controlling the situation. It seemed that what tortured her most, at the same time had been a rudimentary source for gratification. She was finally able to discover that it was possible to be close without sexualizing her relationship.

Supporting the victim-patient to regain sexuality as a satisfying way to relate remains a challenge since frequently the time necessary for such a process is not available, in part for financial reasons, but also because of the impending exile of the patient by the government.

SOCIAL SYSTEMS THERAPY

Victims of torture; other fugitives from totalitarian, persecuting, or fascist political systems; and, incidentally, many other severely disturbed patients are frequently caught in a network of "helpers" (social workers, lawyers, volunteers), legal authorities (police, court officials, prison administrators), and administrative bureaucracies. This societal network of significant others may be conceptualized as a "large-group system" (A. von Wallenberg Pachaly, 1997; S. von Wallenberg Pachaly, 1997), which represents the individual patient's life space. This may include the patient's residential group (family, partner, friends); a psychiatrist with medical responsibility for prescribing and monitoring medication; one or more psychotherapists; coworkers or coparticipants at a sheltered workplace; during times of acute crisis and subsequent hospitalization, the hospital staff; the representatives of the social welfare agency that provides the financial support for the social work input; and representatives of other bureaucratic institutions. Such a "large-group system" is not convened purposely and will never meet as a group. However, if for the sake of argument this network of significant others is conceptualized as a sort of large group, whose members consciously and unconsciously relate to the patient and each other, it becomes clear how a therapist can work with these interactive dynamics and understand disturbances in communication within this system as a mirror of the patient's psychic processes.

Victims of torture (especially within the large-group system setting of their unknown host country) may regress to the psychic states they first experienced under torture and may reexperience the same traumatizing feelings. This is not only because small stimuli may trigger the memory of torture, but also because the "large-group" effect of the social system itself may cause identity diffusion and regression, due to the anonymity involved and due to the fact that barriers and misconceptions are harder to break down than in small groups.

Since the large-group system is characterized by the fact that face-to-face communication is usually not possible, it easily arouses persecutory anxieties and reinforces the defense mechanisms of projection, projective identification, splitting, and fragmentation. This has been frequently discussed in the recent literature—for example, by Kernberg (1995). Striving to integrate a knowledge of large-group system processes with a knowledge of the psychic mechanisms working in an extremely regressed self (e.g., in a victim of trauma) may open up new possibilities for therapists to make use of the former processes in a healing way.

It is my experience that understanding the large-group system is a means of getting in touch with the psychotic nucleus of groups as well as of individuals. From a developmental, psychodynamic, and group-dynamic point of view, feelings experienced in the large-group system by a self in a regressed ego state appear to date back to an early developmental period in the life of the infant, where the differentiation between me and you, self and other, the inner self and the external world is at best blurred but certainly not yet fully established. The establishment of a mature sense of identity is *in statu nascendi*, and feelings of omnipotence alternate with feelings of helplessness and impotence. Projective identification is a major means of the infant's communication with the mother, and, for the infant, persecutory anxieties alternate with feelings of oceanic well-being, complete containment, and ecstatic fusion. Similar processes can occur in the large-group system, as well as in a large group proper and in social institutions (a hospital, etc.).

Hypotheses about Large-Group System Dynamics and the Constructive Use of Them

The following hypotheses are attempts to challenge our conventional knowledge relating to large-group system processes and to facilitate a dialogue that will explore the conditions under which they become constructive and healing. It is also a response to Kernberg's (1985, 1993) discussion on the disruptive power of large-group processes. The hypotheses I wish to propose are as follows:

1. Large-group system dynamics are prone to be experienced as threatening and persecutory, thus evoking projection, projective identification, splitting (in the case of patients with borderline personality disorder),

and fragmentation and fusion (in the case of patients with psychotic disorders).

2. Parallel processes can be observed occurring within the large-group system's dynamics and within the psychotic, pre-Oedipal nucleus of the individual personality (Bleger, 1972). Agazarian (1994) has discussed similar ideas on containment from a systems-centered perspective.

3. If, as an influential member of the large-group system, a therapist succeeds in fostering a change in the prevailing group dynamics toward the dynamics of a mutually holding relational matrix that fosters tolerance, respect, appreciation, communication, and containment, then, as a result, split-off, fragmented feelings and aspects of personality become perceivable and discernible. They can thus become contained, verbalized, worked through, and integrated. A sense of security and a feeling of becoming master of one's own fate—of being able to survive and transcend the catastrophe experienced by the self—grow within the patient.

4. These feelings will grow in the other members of the large-group system, too. They will become more able to tolerate feelings of impotence and helplessness in the face of the "landscapes of death" (Benedetti, 1992) of the patient's self. They will be less compelled to manage and control the patient; instead, they will become facilitators of emotional growth and accompany the patient on his or her therapeutic journey.

A skilled group therapist working with the large-group system may obtain the leadership of the group and cope with the destructive communicative disruptions from within it. These disruptions frequently mirror the patient's predominant defensive organization, and can be understood as an expression of his or her deep-seated conflicts arising from the traumatic feelings experienced under torture. Such an approach provides impressively forceful insights that enable a deeper understanding of the traumatic scenery the patient carries within him- or herself and has not yet succeeded in leaving behind, to become fully able to live his or her own life.

Case Example of the Therapeutic Use
of the Large-Group System

Said, pending trial, had sewed up his mouth because he faced deportation to his home country. He had been tortured brutally there, and he believed that if he returned, he would face instant execution. He had been imprisoned in Germany on drug-related charges, and German policy is to expel such persons. Large-group system psychotherapy in this case meant, first, building a network among the various individuals who were involved with Said and fostering a common understanding of his personality and predicament. It also meant containing the anxieties of those persons involved who feared that Said was a liar, that he would fool them, that he was psychotic, or that he was simply seductive. Finally, it meant containing their own alternating, overwhelming feelings of anxiety, powerlessness, and almightiness in the face of the traumatic feelings associated with the fact that Said really had been cruelly tortured.

Working with a victim of torture confronts the therapist as well as group members and members of the large-group system with questions such as "What would I have done in such a situation" and "What has really happened?" Answering these questions was the decisive point in Said's therapy. As his therapist, I had to fight this out not only with him, but also with the significant societal figures in his life, such as his prison social worker, his lawyer, the judge, and the minister of internal affairs. Eventually we all reached the same point: It became clear that there was only his testimony to rely on, and nothing else. To believe or not to believe meant for him to be or not to be.

Importantly, and in contradistinction to the traditionally more passive role of the psychoanalytic psychotherapist, clinicians can be therapeutically effective with victims of torture and severe trauma only if they are willing and able to take a firmly supportive stance. Otherwise, therapy will merely result in another in the series of traumatic destructions of the victims' personalities. Only a recognition of the injustice suffered and a position of clear-cut support for the victims will make reconstruction, mourning, and "healing" of their wounds possible. At a certain point, therapists become the fellow human beings who must accompany the victims of torture and persecution through their mourning for their lost faith in humanity, their lost dignity, their psychic and physical pain, the destruction of their psychic structure, and their existential fears.

Psychotherapy with Said addressed his superego pathology by working through his hatred of authority and the institutions he identified with his torturers, and simultaneously by empowering him to demarcate—not only to say "no" by sewing up his lips, as in anorectic behavior, but to become able to say "yes" without fearing the destruction and annihilation of his self. The final goal was to revive a containing internalized group. For Said this became possible because the large-group system evolved in such a way as to contain both *his* and *its* own anxieties. He could return to the society of the here and now, and he did not have to rely any longer on "psychotic" behavior or to continue living in his world of torturers of the "there and then." Eventually he received the relatively mild punishment of probation, and was to obtain a permanent residency permit.

In my experience of daily clinical work with severely disturbed, regressed patients. who frequently too are caught up in a large social system, this knowledge about large-group system processes and how to cope with them facilitates group therapy proper; indeed, it may sometimes be necessary to make the latter possible. The managed care approach to psychotherapy, too, can be analyzed from this perspective: Are processes of fragmentation, for example, to be understood as coming from within the patient's internal mechanisms, or does a relatively nonempathic large-group system limit or harm the patient's emotional growth?

CONCLUSION

As Malcolm Pines (1994) has noted, group analysts today not only treat more severely disturbed patients then ever before (patients with borderline personality disorder, severe narcissistic personality disorder, and even schizophrenia and other psychotic disorders); they are also more aware of the fact that their patients have suffered real trauma and that beyond confrontation, interpretation, containing, and setting limits, an empathic approach that provides holding and soothing is necessary. Informed empathic mirroring, holding, and emotional sharing go beyond pity and mere supportive psychotherapy in the following ways.

1. Such empathetically attuned therapy challenges the therapist's capacity to share—to let him- or herself get involved and "used" as a container and as a "part-object" by the patient—and yet to demarcate him- or herself again and to survive as a therapist. The group as well is challenged to survive, and not to fall prey to pity or to become a revolutionary revenge committee.

2. The working through of retraumatizing situations—living them through in the group, containing them, and learning to distinguish the there and then from the here and now—becomes the first opportunity for the patient to live life in the present. The development of avoidant personality disorder may be reversed. This applies to a wide range of traumatized patients.

3. Psychosomatic reactions can be integrated into the group psychotherapeutic process. A therapist can translate them into dialogue. They are prominent, not only because the pain is unspeakable, but also because torture attacks the personality at such a profoundly regressed level that the entire being is attacked. The memory of torture is preserved at the physical level, too. The clinician may receive a certain hypochondriacal impression, or hysterical, dissociated ego states may be perceived. This means that the victim/patient is as yet incapable of integrating the feelings connected with the traumatic experience into his or her psyche.

4. The dissociation between the use of civilized speech and the destruction of civilization and humanness is what strikes us in cases of torture. Within the group context, dissociated feelings can be recovered. The traumatic emotional impact of torture associated with expressions such as *telefono* (i.e., strokes on the ears), *submarino* (i.e., submersion in a stinking

liquid to the point of near-drowning), and *papagai* (i.e., tying a person's legs and hands together and suspending him or her) is recovered. The overwhelming feelings that went along with the traumatic interactions can be integrated and eventually put to rest.

5. Primitive psychic defensive processes such as splitting, projection, fragmentation, numbing, and dissociation can be recognized, recovered, and even worked through. The ego regains the strength to survive and to live on.

6. Therapists who work with torture victims develop a heightened recognition and consciousness of the *children* of these victims—children who, as we know, carry the unspoken within themselves. Victims of torture undergo group psychotherapy not only for themselves, but for their offspring and for subsequent generations.

7. Victims of torture teach therapists, group members, and other "observers" that what gets in the way between them and the victims is the observers' own pain.

The treatment of torture victims represents significant progress in the evolution of a therapeutic group culture. It acknowledges the reality of traumatogenic social conditions and takes full psychotherapeutic, social, and political responsibility for the patients. It is yet another application of the "group-dynamic understanding of structural violence" (A. von Wallenberg Pachaly, 1995a).[5]

The psychotherapy group explores truth. What really happened with this person? Where did his or her own responsibility end? Where did he or she become a victim? How did the patient react? How was he or she able to survive? What did the torturer and the life-attacking small- and large-group dynamics do to the patient? The therapy group is also a quest to understand what torture did to the patient's inner world of internal objects, group dynamics, and the capacity to relate to and bond with him- or herself and others.

To be confronted with a victim of torture—the severest form of human-made trauma—confronts a therapist with questions such as, "Would I too have behaved like this?" and "What are my ideals?" The group psychotherapy of victims of torture opposes any ideology that there is no "absolute truth." To put it simply, human-made physical and psychological death *is* absolute truth. The treatment of torture victims calls for a global perspective; it demonstrates the great need for common symbols that unite humankind, and for common laws that set standards for humane behavior.

Finally, the treatment of victims of torture makes it clear that any human being can be destroyed physically, mentally, and emotionally very easily, and that only a holding, containing group can assure such a person's survival. This form of therapy creates hope for the future: When the traumatic wounds of torture are challenged, they will not have to be transmitted to the next generation with their destructive, revenge-seeking, life-attacking impact.

NOTES

1. There is no diagnosis or subdiagnosis of posttorture distress syndrome in the DSM-IV. Rather, it is diagnosis formulated by those who work with torture victims.
2. For reasons of confidentiality, but also to protect the physical security of patients still under threat, the case examples are heavily disguised and also several group and psychodynamically similar cases are condensed in one. However, I feel they are still powerful enough to convey the underlying group dynamics at work.
3. I consider fragmentation as a primitive psychotic defense mechanism that saves the patient from total annihilation and dissolution in face of an object that otherwise would be experienced as totally overpowering and overwhelming.
4. "Inner immigration" is the process of maintaining one's true convictions, one's true self, and one's identity, but concealing them from the outside world. The alternative is to run the risk of being destroyed, even physically. In Germany, "inner immigration" is a commonly used expression for people who did not emigrate from Nazi Germany (e.g., Thomas Mann), but instead kept their regime-opposing convictions to themselves.
5. At the end of the 1960s, Oslo social scientist and peace researcher Johan Galtung (1975) defined "structural violence" as the cause of the difference between (or of the failure to reduce the difference between) the actual and potential achievement of an individual, as well as of a whole group. Taking his ideas further, I (A. von Wallenberg Pachaly, 1995a) consider all group dynamics that encourage the isolation of an individual or of whole groups, and that hinder their ability to enter into lively contact with others and to undergo further development, as manifestations of structural violence. Conversely, I consider all group dynamics that encourage differentiation of individuals and the differentiation of group structures (internal differentiation, as well as differentiated relationships to a variety of other groups) as factors opposing structural violence. Structural violence wants to keep the balance of power as it is. It wants to control the needs and wishes of individuals and of whole population groups. A group's capacity to sense its own needs and to live within its own identity is a permanent threat to the wielders of structural violence.

REFERENCES

Agazarian, Y. M. (1994). The phases of group-development and the systems-centered group. In V. L. Schermer & M. Pines (Eds.), *Ring of fire* (pp. 36–85). London: Routledge.

Agger, I. (1988). Die politische Gefangene als Opfer sexueller Folter. *Zeitschrift für Sexualforschung, 1,* 231–241.

Amati, S. (1990). Die Rückgewinnung des Schamgefühls. *Psyche, 8,* 724–740.

American Psychiatric Association. (1994). *Diagnostic and statistical manual of mental disorders* (4th ed.). Washington, DC: Author.

Améry, J. (1977). Die Tortur. In J. Améry (Ed.), *Jenseits von Schuld und Sühne* (pp. 46–73). Stuttgart: Klett Cotta.

Barudy, J. (1989). A programme of mental health for political refugees: Dealing with the invisible pain of political exile. *Social Science and Medicine, 28*(7), 715–727.

Benedetti, G. (1992). *Psychotherapie als Existentielle Herausforderung.* Zürich: Vandenhoek & Rupprecht.

Bettelheim, B. (1982). *Erziehung zum Überleben.* München: Kindler.

Bion, W. R. (1959). Attacks on linking. *International Journal of Psycho-Analysis, 40,* 308–315.

Bleger, J. (1972). *Symbiosi y ambigüedad.* Buenos Aires: Paidos.

Chattopadhyay, G. P., & Biran, H. (1997). The burden of the barbarian within. *Free Association, 7*(2), 151–170.

Espinola, M., Gil, D., Klingler, M., & Gil, E. L. (1985). *La vida diaria en un carcel politica como sistema tortura.* Paper presented at the Seminario Internacional: La Tortura en America Latina, Buenos Aires.

Galtung, J. (1975). *Strukturelle Gewalt.* Rowohlt, Germany: Rheinbeck.

Herman, J. (1992). Complex PTSD: A syndrome in survivors of prolonged and repeated trauma. *Journal of Trauma Stress, 5,* 377–391.

Janoff-Bulman, R. (1992). *Shattered assumptions: Towards a new psychology of trauma.* New York: Free Press.

Kernberg, O. (1985). The couch at sea: Psychoanalytic studies of group and organizational leadership. In A. D. Colman & M. H. Geller (Eds.), *Group relations reader 2* (pp. 399–411). Jupiter, FL: A. K. Rice Institute.

Kernberg, O. (1993). Projective identification, countertransference, and hospital treatment. In A. Alexandris & G. Vaslamatzis (Eds.), *Countertransference: Theory, technique, teaching* (pp. 165–187). London: Karnac Books.

Kernberg, O. (1995, February). *Bureaucracy and ideology as social defences against paranoid aggression.* Paper presented at the Arbours 25th Anniversary Conference, London.

Pines, M. (1994). Borderline phenomena in analytic groups. In V. L. Schermer & M. Pines (Eds.), *Ring of fire* (pp. 128–148). London: Routledge.

Roth, E., Lunde, I., Boysen, G., & Kemp Genefke, I. (1987). Torture and its treatment. *American Journal of Public Health, 77*(11), 1404–1406.

United Nations. (1976). *General Assembly official records: Declaration on the protection from being subjected to torture and cruel, inhuman or degrading treatment or punishment* (Resolution No. A/30/3452, 30th Session, Supplement No. 34 [A/10034]. New York: Author.

van der Kolk, B. A., Roth S., & Pelcovitz, D. (1992). *Field trials for DSM-IV posttraumatic stress disorder: II. Disorder of extreme stress.* Washington, DC: American Psychiatric Association.

Volkan, V. D. (1991). On chosen traumas. *Mind and Human Interaction, 3,* 13.

von Wallenberg Pachaly, A. (1983). The capacity for social participation and the capacity for peace: Thoughts on the dynamics of large social groups. *15th Symposium of the German Academy of Psychoanalysis.*

von Wallenberg Pachaly, A. (1992). The time-limited therapeutic community. *Therapeutic Communities, 13*(4), 193–207.

von Wallenberg Pachaly, A. (1995a). A group-dynamic understanding of structural violence and group psychotherapy. *Free Associations*, 5(2), 221–238.

von Wallenberg Pachaly, A. (1995b). "The German marriage": Intrapsychic, interpersonal, and international dimensions. In M. Ettin, J. Fidler, & B. Cohen (Eds.), *Group process and political dynamics* (pp. 189–215). Madison, CT: International Universities Press.

von Wallenberg Pachaly, A. (1997). The large group and the large group system. *Therapeutic Communities*, 18(3), 223–229.

von Wallenberg Pachaly, A., & Griepenstroh, D. (1979). Das energetische Prinzip bei Freud und Ammon. In G. Ammon (Ed.), *Handbuch der Dynamischen Psychiatrie* (Vol. 1, pp. 213–232). München: Ernst Reinhardt Verlag.

von Wallenberg Pachaly, S. (1997). The odyssey of sheltered living in the therapeutic community within the community. *Therapeutic Communities*, 18(2), 27–37.

Wurmser, L. (1999). *Magic change tragic change.* Paper presented at the 5th Steprather Symposium on Visions of the Psychotherapy of Psychosis, Geldern-Walbeck, Germany.

12

◄◌►

Group Psychotherapy in the Treatment of Dissociative Identity Disorder and Allied Dissociative Disorders

CATHERINE G. FINE
NANCY E. MADDEN

The advent of the new nomenclature of "dissociative disorders" (DDs) goes back to the DSM-III (American Psychiatric Association, 1980); it was at this time that conditions that had existed for centuries in the German, French, and even English encyclopedic medical literatures were crystallized by the U.S. psychiatric community. The following 20 years in the field of DDs have involved the development of strategies and methodologies, both individual and group, for better understanding and more effective therapy of these complex conditions. This chapter reviews some of the essential findings on the nature and treatment of these psychiatric conditions; particular attention is paid to dissociative identity disorder (DID), because it is the paradigmatic DD. This means that if therapists can understand and treat DID, they can treat any of the less complex dissociative and posttraumatic states. The primary focus of this chapter is on the use of groups in the treatment of DDs. Our aim is to delineate with clarity, precision, and deliberateness the purpose, structure, and processes of groups for individuals with DDs. Though some of our considerations may seem overly obsessive to therapists unfamiliar with this diagnostic category, over a decade of successful group work with patients in this category suggests that the keys to therapeutic effectiveness in these groups may be their extreme structure and their minimization of regressions.

Although DID continues to be a controversial diagnosis within the field of psychology, a recent survey by Rossel (1998) notes the increased incidence of this trauma-based diagnosis over the last two decades. This diagnostic dispute is neither new nor readily settled. The historically phasic nature of the emergence of the diagnosis of DID is evident in the medicopsychological literature of the last two centuries, ranging from Petetin (1775), Despine (1840), Janet (1886), and Prince (1919) to more recent work by Thigpen and Cleckley (1957), Wilbur (1984), Kluft (1984), and others. The ebb and flow of this diagnosis and the other DDs are as much a function of the rise and fall of theories and conceptualizations in psychology (e.g., magnetic somnambulism, hypnosis and mental desegregation, the ego state model[1]) as of the sociopolitical climate of different eras (in the current era, the feminist movement, the Vietnam war, and the theory of false-memory syndrome have played differing roles). Each reemergence brings with it a more complete understanding and perhaps a novel perspective on the continuum of DDs and their treatment.

Even though it remains understood that individual psychotherapy is the unquestionable treatment of choice for DID and other DDs, nonetheless the use of diagnostically homogeneous groups is a valid and helpful adjunctive modality. (We should emphasize here that though physical or sexual abuse in childhood, or both, are the self-reported traumata in the childhood of 97% [Kluft, 1985] to 98% [Putnam, 1989] of patients with DID, and though many therapists and treatment programs support the sole use of groups to heal survivors of physical/sexual abuse, our direct experience with decompensated patients in outpatient and inpatient settings has led us to refuse to treat such severely abused individuals without the essential and primary involvement of individual psychotherapy.) Inpatient programs for patients with DDs commonly make use of homogeneous group psychotherapy (Buchele, 1994) along with other group formats, such as art therapy groups (Jacobson, 1993) and movement therapy groups (Baum, 1993).

Curiously, psychotherapy groups geared toward support, clarification, and learning for these patients are still rarely available on an outpatient basis. This rarity is intriguing, in light of the reported effectiveness of group psychotherapy in general (Yalom, 1983) and its positive usages in the treatment of traumatization resulting from causes such as rape, incest, and war (van der Kolk, 1987). Also, regrets are frequently expressed by former inpatients with DDs who cannot find a group to support their individual work once they leave the hospital. Putnam (1989) reports a congruency between patients with DDs and therapists in endorsing outpatient homogeneous groups for such patients. It appears that this agreement may have much to do with the additional holding environment offered a patient by the group, as it may (perhaps in a parallel process) better sustain a therapist, who may thus more successfully ward off the sequelae of chronic "compassion fatigue" (Figley, 1995). However, there are fairly clear supraordinate requirements or cautions that need to be in place before a group format is offered to patients who have such fluid identities, affects, and behaviors.

Failing to recognize or honor the fundamental dynamics of patients with DID or other DDs (Kluft, 1985; Putnam, 1989) may have thwarted the efforts of well-intentioned but poorly informed therapists. For example, one common misconception about these patients that interferes with stabilization of the group climate (Roback & Smith, 1987) is group therapists' confusion about what the patient's primary defense is. Group therapists naive to the dynamics of DDs (elaborated in Kluft, 1985, and Lowenstein, 1991) believe that splitting is the primary defense used by these patients, whereas therapists who commonly work with this population must deal with their actual primary defense, which is dissociation. Another scenario for the breakdown of groups for patients with DDs is that the group experience becomes sufficiently noxious to the therapists and/or the group participants (because of intragroup acting out, such as self-injury, attacks on others, etc.) as to have the therapists reconsider and review their hopes/designs for the group.

It is essential for any therapist who does group psychotherapy with DDs to be fluent in the treatment of these disorders on an individual basis (Madden & Fine, 1990; Putnam, 1989). A therapist unfamiliar with trauma-based disorders may be understandably challenged by tracking one patient with DID in individual psychotherapy; tracking a group of such potentially labile patients pooled together, with the resulting exponential increase in mutually reflected affective experiences, can be overwhelming. When therapists new to the field of DDs encounter disinhibited patients in a group setting, the common consequence is a group where spontaneous and uncontrolled abreactions prevail. These are retraumatizing to the individuals having the actual flashbacks as well as to the other group members; they interfere with group cohesiveness (Lego, 1984) and do little to reinforce "reality-centered behaviors" (Klein, Hunter, & Brown, 1986). The anticipated and repetitive outcome of such a group is a "domino effect" of uncontrolled affective bridges and collapse of the group—over and over again. Though this scenario no doubt tells the story of the family-of-origin dynamics, it is nonetheless retraumatizing to the individual group members and impedes learning. Groups conducted in this manner do not promote the important notion for the patients that today's reality (where they may "feel" abused) is different from yesterday's reality (in which they were actually being hurt). When these patients are regularly retraumatized in group psychotherapy, past and present collide. Fundamentally, under these conditions, past and present feel the same.

The problem of retraumatization within the group is one of a number of predictable snafus in homogeneous groups for patients with DID or other DDs—problems that will go against the overall treatment goal for these patients. The goal of therapy for a patient with DID or other DDs has been discussed at length elsewhere (Kluft, 1985; Fine, 1988, 1990), but it can be summarized as the congruence of purpose and motivation among the various personalities/parts of the mind, according to Kluft (1985). Fine (1991) describes the treatment goal as a unification of all behaviors, affects, sensations, and knowledge across traumatic and nontraumatic experiences for all parts of the mind, in order to restore continuity of past and present experience. So the prime directive for this chapter is to explore some key factors of relevance to homogeneous groups for patients with DDs that will support the stated treatment goal.

THE RATIONALE FOR GROUP PSYCHOTHERAPY FOR DDs

Given the complexity and fear-based personality development of patients with DDs, combined with the difficulties inherent in negotiating the trauma response (which guarantees a protracted course of individual psychotherapy for these patients), group psychotherapy can be a controversial treatment for DDs. Our rationale for group psychotherapy for these disorders is based on our view of (1) the characteristics of patients with DDs, and (2) the purposes of a group for these patients.

Patient Characteristics

Patients with DID or other DDs share a complexity rarely found in neurotic, psychotic, or even personality-disordered individuals. They seem not to fit into any prescribed or commonly anticipated categorization, since such categorizations ignore the impact of trance states, hypnotic phenomena, and hypnotizability. Thinking of these patients as primarily having Axis II disorders—for example, misinterpreting them simply as demanding, complex, chronic patients with borderline personality disorder—reflects the countertransference of therapists and their frustration with these patients to a greater extent than it reflects the patients' actual characteristics. Though a comorbid Axis II diagnosis can coexist with an Axis I diagnosis of a DD, it is helpful for the individual therapy dyad to have achieved some diagnostic clarity before individual treatment goals are delineated. Subsequently, the individual therapist can make a referral to a psychotherapy group and appropriately inform the group therapists (see the discussion of confidentiality later in this chapter). Again, group therapists must be informed practitioners of individual therapy with these patients to maximize the benefit of group contact.

As a reminder, clinicians think of patients with DID as having "personalities," whereas patients with other DDs are said to have "polarized ego states." (The term "DDs" encompasses all of these disorders, regardless of the specific diagnostic nomenclature.) Personalities can be understood as personified adaptational strategies; they are representations of conflicts, fears, and wishes. Ego states (Watkins & Watkins, 1997), like personalities, can have strong and differentially impermeable boundaries. These boundaries, like the membrane of a cell, can be selectively and differentially permeable to affects, sensations, and knowledge of the host personality (primary ego state) or other alternate personalities (alters) or ego states. These amnestic boundaries will define the communication streams that exist between the personalities/ego states. Their permeability needs to be modified if changes in the system of mind are expected. This permeability can be affected both by individual therapy and by group inclusion.

Hence, a therapist must get to know a patient's personalities/ego states, or else the patient will be minimally understood and the defensive structure will remain puzzling. The therapist must (1) understand the conflicts of the parts; (2) learn with whom these personalities/ego states, in the sphere of their inner world, relate to, speak with, and share; and (3) grasp whom the personalities/ego states avoid and whom they fear. Individual and group therapists alike must take healthy advantage of the fact that patients' systems of personalities/ego states are not stagnant, inert, and unmoving. Patients' inner lives, as defined by their personalities/ego states, are forever evolving and relational (Kluft, 1999). Therefore, a patient's developing a trusting and predictable relationship with an individual therapist, and then being able to extend the relationship to group therapists and group members, expand the hypothesis testing necessary for modifying traumatic expectations. The personalities/ego states within the patient have, in the group, a holding environment that allows them to augment their often restricted interactional sphere and discover that there is a place for them in the world today. Such a patient can, through a group, learn that current reality is different from and better than past reality.

Homogeneous group therapy is particularly helpful and empowering in enabling patients with DID or other DDs to note, assess, and change the faulty beliefs from their past. The group provides a way for these patients to devise a structure and a predictable system of verification (Klein et al., 1986). This methodology borrows from the Socratic process, which is valued in the experimental model championed by most cognitive therapies. The group, through the mere self-generated questioning or exploratory exchanges of its members, fundamentally promotes dissonances within and between traumatically entrenched beliefs. The microdisequilibrations that occur when such dissonances are instilled are followed by temporary restabilizations as the group members support one another. Eventually the evolving beliefs and goals of the personalities/ego states will crystallize in a parallel direction and will coalesce as the dissonances between them decrease.

Therefore, dealing with the dissonances within and between the personalities/ego states serves several functions (Fine, 1990, 1991): (1) it helps the personalities/ego states begin to notice their internal and external realities; (2) it subsequently helps them establish hypnotic duality, which is a prerequisite for abreactive work in individual therapy; (3) it brings to the forefront, and to patients' attention, the dissociatively established double binds and the complex double–double binds that have been promoted since their childhoods; and (4) it becomes a dynamic foundation that is mastered over time and that enables the personalities/ego states to reflect, deliberate, and progress. The message is that change is not necessarily bad (the traumatic expectation) and can actually be good. It is invaluable for a patient not only to hear this from the individual therapist, but to receive feedback from other patients who have "been there." In addition, group therapy can contribute to restoring hope in alters/ego states who lack a sense of self-efficacy and future orientation (Madden & Fine, 1990). The therapist-monitored reciprocal influences on group members decrease the incidence of decompensation related to significant impairment of self–object differentiation (Klein & Kugel, 1981).

Purposes of a Group

Though a group may be homogeneous from a diagnostic perspective, different group members are at differing stages of their individual therapy and self-development. Those group members who are further along in their overall therapy work can be role models for those patients who feel that no progress can ever be made, because no one ever gets better. They can help in the "enculturation and socialization" (Klein et al., 1986) of the patients who are newer to therapy. Their mere presence in the group instills hope; it means that the newer patients do not have to be constantly reassured that things can change for the better. On the other hand, those patients who have yet to learn how to negotiate the trials and tribulations of therapy remind the more advanced members of the group by their comments and behaviors how far they (the more advanced ones) have come themselves. Indeed, patients with DDs learn better when they can pool their own observations and experiences. Therefore, another purpose of a group is to support the group participants in owning the path already traveled and tracing the upcoming course. This grounding and these reality-centered observations enhance the continuity of experience.

Group psychotherapy for patients with DDs also helps banish the notions that "I am alone in the world" and that "No one has ever gone through or known what I have known." The traumatic ordeals that 97% of patients with DID (Kluft, 1985) have endured are related to physical and sexual abuse prior to the age of 4½ (Schultz, Braun, & Kluft, 1989). The attacks usually happen in secret and in isolation; the child who is abused in this manner is often sworn or threatened into secrecy, increasing the aloneness. The dissociative defense that comes into play under these overwhelming circumstances—in other words, the trauma response proper—is also designed to isolate the experience from the mainstream of awareness. Consequently, it necessarily chips away at the child's connection with the world. By the time the patient with a DD is an adult, the mind has recreated the sequestered world associated with this trauma response. Feeling alone in the world is one of the hallmarks of a trauma survivor; a diagnostically homogeneous group can begin to modify this complex module of experiences and help these patients overcome social isolation.

In addition, the group can provide an opportunity to engage in or learn about relationships where there is "give and take." Individuals diagnosed with DID or other DDs have a history of dysfunctional relationships, as well as the capacity for developing relationships that place them in positions of being revictimized (Kluft, 1990). The group process provides such patients with the potential to develop healthier relationships as they examine their relationships (both in the world and within the group) with one another and the therapists. As described by other authors (Klein & Kugel, 1981), the group can begin to modify maladaptive interpersonal intragroup responses. It compels patients who have difficulties in attending to actual goings-on in the moment to pay attention to the interpersonal exchanges in the group, so that these will not go far awry. Furthermore, many patients with DDs are both rageful and afraid of others' rage. Their phobic response to perceived criticism and anticipated rage is paralysis. Therefore, the group format will allow for corrective feedback and modification of maladaptive symptoms. This feedback will in the beginning be initiated by the therapists, who can serve as role models and positive selfobjects, but it will eventually be continued by the group participants. Listening skills are cultivated, empathic attunement is developed, and rebuttal skills are learned.

To clarify and expand this point further, patients with DDs often do not listen to what they are being told by either therapists or other people in their world. They are so convinced (all the while denying it) that they "really know" what people mean or are saying that they trust their affective responses to what outsiders begin to say, rather than hearing those persons out completely. This leads to much confusion and many misunderstandings for the patients. Whether this is stated out loud or not, these patients typically preempt in their understanding what other people are saying. Fairly commonly, their affective responses are based on the past and on other people, rather than the persons with whom they are currently interacting.

The group psychotherapy allows them to be presented with their rapid and false interpretations, as other group members gently confront the confused members or clarify for them what they (the other members) actually meant, rather than what the confused members "heard."

Empathic attunement implies that a patient with a DD will be able to "walk in someone else's moccasins" and respond to that person accordingly. Therefore, it implies that such patients must have some mastery over their narcissism and the impact of their dissociated personalities/ego states. Though many patients with DDs are typically capable of being empathic with others under certain circumstances, unfortunately the attunement typically reflects "complete identification," rather than "trial identification." Trial identification allows a patient to understand and temporarily "feel with" the other person, yet maintain some objectivity. Complete identification suggests that the observing ego is nowhere to be found and that the affective response dictates the rejoinder. The group therapy allows for the objectification of empathic comments based solely on self-identification, rather than on poised reflection informed by affective understanding. For example, it is not uncommon for a group member with a DD to recount an event in his or her current life that is unfair and may have been promoted by someone who reminds the group member of a past abuser. The recounting of the event is often embellished by interpretations that are about the original abuser and not about the other individual currently under scrutiny. Once "launched" in this direction, the group can easily fall into bashing of that other individual without any data. The group can readily crystallize surrounding an attack of an innocent (though perhaps foolish) individual, reinforcing yet again the notion that the world is an unsafe place. Patients are often indignant when their individual therapists attempt exploration of this tendency, whereas they often report feeling that the group therapists don't quite "get it" (already a less toxic response) and seem to be able to hear the actual concern when a group member gets confused about who he or she is actually talking about in the present—the protagonist in the current story or a past abuser. Therefore, again, the group can help detoxify knee-jerk trauma-based reactions.

The rebuttal skills and willingness to correct false statements are learned very gradually in the group. A group member always takes a risk when contradicting the interpretation of another group member, especially if it is perceived (and denied) that anger is near the surface. Group therapists are invaluable in role-modeling gentle but clarifying confrontations that will facilitate appropriate questioning and desirable elucidations. Taking this rebuttal skill into the nontherapy world is priceless for patients with DDs, who often tend to capitulate in the face of confrontation and then proceed to seethe or feel victimized.

Therefore, as in most groups, the fact that individuals in similar circumstances are sharing with and supporting one another is invaluable. Although individuals with trauma histories may often discount and dismiss recommendations offered by others (including their therapists), discounting and dismissing what others with similar histories offer is more difficult.

> For example, a group member noted that another group member often returned from visiting her parents (her alleged abusers) in a more destabilized condition than she had been in prior to the visit. The first member suggested that the destabilized group member might weigh the evidence related to whether there was a connection between these visits and the destabilization; she added that she had had similar experiences at one point in her life. The ensuing discussion helped both conversing members directly—one to learn new data, the other to further "own" her life. It also helped the group indirectly, because it is often the experience of one group member's responding to another that makes the unspeakable speakable for the group as a whole.

Weighing the evidence to support or refute a point (reality testing) is one of the common cognitive therapy techniques routinely employed in these groups. Patients with DID or other DDs typically hold to fixed internal trauma-derived beliefs that they do not question (Fine, 1988, 1990, 1996a). The group can further the task of the members' individual psychotherapists by helping create more cognitive dissonance (Fine, 1991) within the typically unyielding rules by which these patients live. Their unchallenged cognitive rigidity usually translates in the world into strong edicts to which they hold themselves and others. Much as patients with obsessive–compulsive disorder do, individuals with DDs use rituals and routines to try to organize the world outside of them to match their internal reality, in the hope of gaining some measure of control. Individuals with DDs who either are not in psychotherapy or have only just begun it make repeated attempts at decreasing the dissonance in their outside world and are typically very controlling. Increasing their internal cognitive dissonance will allow them to become more realistically connected to the world outside themselves; homogeneous group psychotherapy for DID or other DDs promotes this notion well.

Therefore, the groups that we champion for patients with DDs differ in very important ways from what many patients expect from a group (and perhaps many therapists as well). The groups that we conduct, though not bound to any one theoretical model, straddle several modalities; the overarching rule is that no abreactive work will be encouraged in the group setting. The primary purpose of the group is energetically to support abreactive work in the individual therapy. That is, the group will help patients anticipate and prepare for abreactive work, and will help them process this work after the fact. The group format is not affect-driven, but rather affect-informed in both theory and structure.

THEORETICAL CONCEPTS
AND CONSIDERATIONS

There are two preferred theoretical models utilized in group psychotherapy for patients with DID or other DDs: a systems model and a cognitive model.

The Systems Model

A systems framework functions as a structure for defining and maintaining boundaries. This framework puts boundaries (Agazarian, 1992) at the forefront of consideration and reflection in a group for patients with DID, where the number of alternate personalities (alters) is far greater than the actual number of physical bodies present in the group session. In group psychotherapy for patients with DID or other DDs, it is essential that the therapists be keenly aware of the nature of the boundaries of the individual patients, as well as the ways in which these function at a group level.

Boundaries differ in permeability and clarity. They may be rigid, enmeshed, diffuse, clear, or conflictual (Minuchin, 1974). Boundaries define who is in what system, the participation of each person within a system, the degree of differentiation within the system, and who and what are allowed inside and outside the system (Wilson & Kneisl, 1979). When boundaries are not appropriately managed, "the typical result is confusion, with rapid and unpredictable changes in topic, lack of continuity, limited follow-up, absence of a shared locus of attention, lack of closure and shifting levels of psychological discourse" (Klein & Kugel, 1981).

A system with "rigid" or "disengaged" boundaries is defined as one that is organized around rules prohibiting transactions and interactions with other systems. Little or no information is allowed to be exchanged between one system and another. For example, at an individual level, the amnestic boundaries of a patient with DID prevent the transmission of information between alters, as well as interactions between the patient's internal and external worlds. Rigid or disengaged boundaries can be seen in a group setting when individual group members do not respond to one another and maintain lengthy periods of silence.

At the other extreme, a system with "enmeshed" or "diffuse" boundaries is one that lacks differentiation and autonomy, with a consequent blurring of boundaries and decrease in distance among individual members of the system. The components of such a system have difficulty individuating from one another and from other systems. At the individual level, a patient with DID who is discussing feelings of suicidality may experience a blurring of the boundaries between personalities who function to contain feelings. Since the permeability of the boundaries between personalities is variable, it is fairly common for one personality who is more typically dysthymic than actually depressed to be "approached" by a very depressed personality whose only purpose is to think of ways to commit suicide. When this occurs, the dysthymic personality—seemingly "out of the blue," but actually through passive influence consequent to permeable amnestic boundaries—will become involved in formulating a complex suicide plan. The impetus for the suicide plan may be secondary to an external event (a disappointment in the patient's life, job stress, etc.) or may arise through a conflict between the personalities. At the group level, the consequences of blurred boundaries may be twofold: (1) One group member's suicidality because of lack of internal containment (blurred individual boundaries) may (2) trigger, through other group members' identification with the suicidal member, a domino effect (contagion effect) as the other members echo similar feelings of suicidality with full-blown affect (blurred group boundaries). Again, the role of the group therapists is to provide a model for maintaining clear boundaries and to function as boundary makers for both each individual and the group as a whole until the group can learn this function on its own. Therefore, the group therapists serve as selfobjects by facilitating and regulating transactions across boundaries, in terms of both systems and self-psychological models.

In groups for patients with DID or other DDs, the concept of boundaries is multidimensional and intertwined. The multiple categories of boundaries within each group member are the final vectors of varied boundaries between and among the alters/ego states. For example, a single group member can have an internal world composed of multiple configurations of alters/ego states with various types of boundaries. The group member may be amnestic for a configuration of alters/ego states with rigid boundaries that could be useful at a particular moment in time, and may be negatively influenced by a configuration of alters/ego states that symbolically represent the external abusers, which may have enmeshed boundaries. Alter/ego state configurations that are unable to differentiate between "here and now" and "there and then," or between "inside world" and "outside world," may have conflictual boundaries (e.g., child alters in relation to internalized abuser alters). Therefore the boundaries within each group member are complex and shifting, and changes in these will have an impact on the group boundaries as a whole. These group boundaries themselves can configure as in a parallel process according to the dynamics of one "stronger" member, or can unfold in ways similar to the forces that intrude on other individuals and be rigid, clear, conflictual, or enmeshed.

In regard to issues of boundaries, the therapists function in a dual capacity: they are both group members and overseers. In their role as group members, therapists need to acknowledge and deal with their own complex and perhaps fluctuating boundaries. If the therapists' boundaries are too rigid, the patients will feel as if they are attending a military school drill; however, if the therapists' boundaries are overly permeable, the patients will not feel safe and contained. The therapists are therefore models for imitation and internalization, as well as supportive selfobjects, and are consequently responsible for maintaining a group climate that will facilitate the work of the individual members within the group (Roback & Smith, 1987). In their role as overseers, the therapists must monitor, clarify, confront, and/or explore the patients' boundaries, and therefore must also maintain an appropriate and skilled observing ego on behalf of the group so that the group is capable of work. It is reasonable for the patients in the group to expect the therapists to manage both functions in their role as teachers and as objects of identification and imitation, which is why two therapists are recommended for such groups (see the discussion of cotherapy below). Being consistently under the microscope and under scrutiny can be wearing and confusing for only one group therapist. Having two therapists allows for appropriate therapist self-examination and self-correction as well as for healthy and helpful group activity; it also wards off "therapist bashing," due to the patients' transient identification of the therapists with internalized abusers. What information is exchanged, and how the information is exchanged, are valuable to the therapists in identifying and analyzing the group process as well as in selecting interventions.

The Cognitive Model

In work with a homogeneous psychotherapy group for patients with DDs, the cognitive model is more pragmatic than the systems model. It derives its strength from the solid and rich foundation of individual cognitive therapy for DDs (Fine, 1988, 1990, 1991, 1992, 1993). The cognitive model in work with such clients is founded on the Socratic perspective. Applying this viewpoint to a group implies addressing the members' plethora of cognitive distortions—misleading beliefs and values about the self, the world, and the future that patients with DID or other DDs bring to their current reality because of past traumatic events. The group members are expected to question their own and others' expressed convictions; to hone in on the automatic thoughts that drive these beliefs; to figure out whether these thoughts are accurate in today's reality; to explore alternative explanations for these thoughts; and, on their own behalf, to attend internally to which personalities/ego states could be driving these perspectives. The group's efforts surround the participants' respective abilities to solve problems, as well as to help create cognitive dissonance across cognitive, affective, sensory, and behavioral dimensions within each group member.

Brabender and Fallon (1993) describe a cognitive model of group therapy that identifies faulty cognitions as both causes of and maintenance factors in psychopathology. The repetitious nature of the exploration of such cognitions, both in individual therapy and in a group format, is helpful for the personalities and/or group members to learn from one another. The on-going review of distortions and false beliefs in both individual and group therapy promotes the notion for the patients themselves, as well as for their respective personalities, that their *Weltanschauung* requires review and that a new understanding is in order. It also supports the notion that if one group member can learn from another, then one personality can learn from another, and vice versa. The group cognitive perspective clearly views this model as a teaching model (Brabender & Fallon, 1993).

Instructing individuals with DDs to develop alternative ways to deal with thinking and feeling is a direct attack on trauma-based schemata (Fine, 1996a) that have given rise to such notions as "For me, nothing can change," or "I have no impact on my own life," or "I am helpless," or "I am invisible (if not physically, at least psychologically)." The group process clearly demonstrates that one group member can be affected by and can learn from another, that one personality can learn from another, and that one personality can learn from another group member or from a personality of another group member.

> For example, a group member with DID who believed that she "oozed evil" commented, "The reason the group is hard today for all of you is because it is my birthday. I am contaminating you." The group members responded immediately that this was not why things were difficult; they could explain very clearly what was going on in their respective lives that made that particular group session strained. The group then encouraged the "birthday" member to explore a bit in the group setting (and, of course, in her individual psychotherapy) what made her birthday so destructive to her. Her individual psychotherapist later commented to the group therapists that a few personalities within this patient were relieved that they had not "ruined" the day for other group members, whereas more negative personalities were distraught that they had "lost their touch" in wrecking the life of others.

The psychoeducational strength of the cognitive model with dissociative populations lies in its reinforcing the notion that dissociation and its concomitant sequelae are things that patients have learned and can unlearn (Fine, 1988, 1990), rather than unalterable aspects of who they are. The group can help promote the important cost–benefit analyses that are an integral part of righting false but deeply felt perceptions, and can champion the replacement of such beliefs with testable alternative views.

Paradigm Shifts and the Need for Integration of Models in the Approach to Group Treatment

A study by Caul (1984) determined that in the individual psychotherapy of DDs, the disorders rather than therapists' preferred theoretical models dictated the interventions. Indeed, Caul videotaped therapists who defined themselves according to preferred schools of thought, only to find that most of the competent therapists employed the same interventions in response to identical patient behaviors or comments. Similarly, group therapists do not necessarily share a common understanding about the nature of psychopathology (Dies, 1995). However, "a common bond among group therapists is the faith that individual patients . . . have the potential to contribute constructively in creating a powerful therapeutic environment for effecting meaningful clinical change" (Dies, 1995).

In our view, it is imprudent to adhere strictly to any one model of treatment in groups for patients with DDs. The group therapists must be fluent in several models of individual and group therapies and must straddle them appropriately—sometimes correcting misperceptions, sometimes commenting on family-of-origin structures being recreated in the group, at other times mentioning how transferential issues may be tainting the interpretations of behaviors, and so on. The art of group therapy for patients with DID or other DDs is for the therapists, through their interventions to be as flexible, supportive, and modeling as they would like the patients themselves to become.

CHARACTERISTICS OF OUTPATIENT GROUPS FOR TREATMENT OF DDs

As we have noted earlier, outpatient groups for the treatment of DDs are rarities rather than the norm; their inpatient counterparts are minimally useful in providing a model from which to work.

The Therapist(s)

Outpatient group therapists who are developing a group treatment module for crisis-prone patients with DDs will naturally revisit what has been learned from inpatient models; however, what is required of therapists in outpatient versus inpatient group therapies does differ. The use of single therapists versus cotherapists is also discussed here, as is the issue of confidentiality.

Differences between What Is Required of Therapists in Inpatient and Outpatient Group Therapies

Unlike inpatient group therapists, who may be assigned a fluctuating number of patients with DDs for an undetermined number of group sessions without having any training in or knowledge about DDs, outpatient group therapists must be knowledgeable about individual psychotherapy for DDs and must structure the group therapy encounters very predictably. Outpatient therapy groups need to be crisis-preemptive rather than crisis-reactive.

In any group psychotherapy (see Klein et al., 1986), errors will occur. An inpatient group therapist can afford to make a mistake, knowing that if a crisis occurs secondarily, the patient with a DD remains safe on the unit and there is a whole treatment team to take corrective measures. The inpatient unit functions as a safe holding environment (Klein, Orleans, & Soule, 1991; Klein et al., 1986). An outpatient group therapist for patients with DDs does not have such a luxury and is held to a higher standard of training and responsibility. An uncorrected error by an outpatient group therapist falls immediately back on a patient's individual psychotherapist, who is likely not to know the context for the problem and to be understandably leery of the patient's further group participation if such problems are to interfere regularly with the patient's progress in individual psychotherapy.

Another difference between the demands on therapists in inpatient and outpatient group therapies pertains to the determination of group size and other parameters. An inpatient group therapist is limited, with respect to the number of participating group members, to the number of patients present on the unit at one time; therefore, admission trends affect the size of the group, as does each patient's length of stay. In addition, the inpatient therapist defers group-related decisions to the unit director or some other administrative entity. By contrast, outpatient group therapists determine the size of the group, the length of each group session, and the number of sessions the group will meet, as part of a mutually acceptable and informed contractual agreement between the group therapists and the patients.

The Impact of Cotherapy on Group Therapy for DDs

Group psychotherapy for patients with DID or other DDs is led by two therapists, to assure that the majority of the exchanges in the group come under the scrutiny of two professionals trained in work with these patients; the two therapists monitor the various aspects of group process, and also oversee and regulate one another. There is a debriefing between the therapists after each group session, to revisit the main themes and dynamics of the group during the session and to hypothesize where to go next. Certain group dynamics are destructive to the group and to the individual members, and need to be anticipated and addressed in order for the group as a whole to take corrective measures.

Cotherapists are a necessity in outpatient groups for patients with DDs, in order to provide a sense of safety for the group as a whole. Two therapists are better able to negotiate the affect storms that arise in the group; the patients do not feel as if they have to protect or come to the defense of a lone therapist. If spontaneous abreactions do occur in the group context, two therapists can better arrest a chain reaction that could lead to behavioral dyscontrol.

Though abreactions are not encouraged in a group setting, abreactions do occur. Thus it is to the therapists' (and, of course, the patients') advantage to have an a priori action plan to negotiate such abreactions.

For example, a hand gesture as a nonverbal emphasis to a statement made by one of the therapists in one group was interpreted by a patient with DID as a threat. The gesture triggered the patient into a flashback, where an abreactive event became inevitable. The action plan was that the "nonoffending" therapist accompany the patient into another room, follow the abreaction, help the patient get regrounded, and return to the group. The group as a whole could then process the impact of this one patient's behavior; work on understanding the underlying concomitants; and come to appreciate that once an abreaction is over, life goes on.

It is essential that the cotherapists have respect for one another. They may or may not be members of the same discipline, but they must be able to get along with one another. The two therapists can compare notes, complement their respective interventions in the group, help maintain a group-level observing ego, and help diffuse intense and misguided transferences directed at one another. Because patients with DID or other DDs are by definition so highly hypnotizable (Spiegel, 1986), it is easy for the group *Zeitgeist* to function in altered states of consciousness as well. A possible consequence to the group of this natural progression is that a therapist and patient will shift into using trance logic (Orne, 1959) and therefore lose the useful problem-solving character of the group. With two therapists at work together, the group is less likely to get derailed in this manner; if there is a departure from anticipated cause-and-effect reasoning in the group, the presence of two therapists rather than one maximizes the chances of rapid redress. When such incidents happen, "mutual supervision" between the therapists can be used, as well as discussions with nongroup outpatient therapists. We ourselves have been unsuccessful in finding another experienced group therapist who has worked with DDs and who could provide either ongoing or as-needed supervision. In fact, other group therapists have told us, "Better you than me," when group discussions for supervisory purposes might have arisen. Being an outlier as a group therapist recapitulates, in a parallel-process way, many of the experiences of patients with DDs. This is another reason why cotherapy provides support for the helpers.

The Issue of Confidentiality

Patients with DDs are informed that it is primarily their responsibility to bring to their individual psychotherapists' attention the group themes and group issues that are relevant to them. However, the group therapists must request that confidentiality be waived between them and the individual psychotherapists, in order to further treatment cohesion and not to replicate dissociated and conflictual pools of knowledge and affect; of course, the reverse holds true as well. The role of the group therapists is a very direct one in instances where the rules and regulations of the group may differ somewhat from the practices promoted by individual therapists. These rules must be clarified by the group therapists a priori rather than post hoc. The referring individual therapists must be made aware of the group rules before the referral process is initiated.

Therefore, at the beginning of group treatment, patients with DDs know the dimensions of confidentiality. With this in place, the preferred type of communication at times of crisis is that the patients themselves report to their individual therapists. The severity of the emergency will dictate the responses of the group therapists, who need the freedom to act in the best interest of each individual patient as well as the group. In over a decade of group work with such patients, we have had two major crises calling for emergency action. In one case, we had to direct one group member to an emergency room for treatment of a potential overdose prior to coming to the group, because the patient's individual therapist was on vacation. In the other case, we had to call for an immediate psychiatric hospitalization when a patient did not control her rapid regression into a mute and primitive state (which persisted on the inpatient unit as well for several days).

The Group Format

The outpatient group format that we have developed and that satisfies all parties concerned (patients, group leaders, individual psychotherapists) is as follows.

The group itself is composed of six to eight patients with DDs and two group leaders. The group sessions have planned durations, and the boundaries of the time frame are maintained. Patients with greater ego strength are offered the option of participating in a 1½-hour group session once per week; patients with less ego strength seem to benefit more from a once-a-week group session that lasts only 1 hour (because it is less stimulating).

Though it is hoped that the group will be supportive in nature, it is understood that the group is a psychotherapy group. Therefore, there are no exchanges of phone numbers or last names, and no relationships are encouraged outside of the group. What happens in the group stays in the group; the issue of confidentiality is discussed at length in the group, just as it is when contractual agreements are drawn up between each group member, the group therapists, and the individual psychotherapist. This dictum promotes for the group members a budding understanding of the difference between secrecy and privacy. It also begins to clarify for the group members that they have an impact on one another (and therefore that they are important), and that they have responsibilities toward one another (and thus that separate connections can be hurtful if kept secret). In addition, contact outside of the group is discouraged because it can lead to dilution of the group process and can deprive the group of crucial data when issues are acted out in private. "Inappropriate" boundary crossings can lead a group member to ask another group member to manage a crisis, rather than turning to the individual or group therapists for help. Destructive alliances can be formed and remain undiscovered until a group member has a major crisis or until an outburst happens in a decontextualized manner in the group. Finally, contact outside of the group may jeopardize the day-to-day functioning of the various group members by unintentionally replaying traumatizing scenarios that are out of their respective awarenesses.

The group is a closed-ended group, with members expected to attend regularly each week. The group members contract for a 10- to 12-session series of groups; they are often offered an option to renew at the end of each group series. The rationale for these time-limited blocks of group sessions is that organizing the meetings in this fashion undermines the dissociative defenses of the patients while also preventing the recapitulation and reinforcement of the patients' pathological nondissociative defenses (e.g., avoidance, self-recrimination, self-blame, and self-shaming). These series of time-limited groups offer the group participants the options of continuing in a group if appropriate, of planning absences, or of arranging face-saving terminations. Opening up these options encourages deshaming and straight talk about needs, wishes, and fears. These groups frequently become the only place where patients with DDs can venture to speak up and be heard in a semipublic forum.

> For example, the termination from a group of a patient who was overly disruptive took the following pattern. The individual psychotherapist was contacted (see the discussion of confidentiality above), according to the contract between all the therapists and the patient; she was notified that regardless of the group therapists' persistent efforts, this patient consistently chose to get lost in trance states during group sessions and would then disown her behavior. In addition, this patient would compound her dyscontrol in the group by verbally attacking other group members, the group leaders, or her individual psychotherapist. The group therapists had tried to intervene with this patient by meeting with her individually on one occasion to process the problem outside of a group format, to no avail. Rather than confront-

ing her further in the group, the group therapists offered her the opportunity to take a leave of absence from the group at the natural termination of a group series. This "vacation from group" was a relief to the patient (and the group). It was promoted in an accurate, agreeable, and nonblaming way to the patient. The patient was able to address the group about her struggles in remaining grounded in the group psychotherapy; she stated that she intended to work more in individual therapy before returning to the group. The patient both told the truth and was not shamed in the process of group termination.

It is our belief as group leaders that many such difficult, embarrassing, and problematic confrontations can be handled in a gentle, straightforward manner if the group format fosters kindness, directness, and support.

In the same spirit of thoughtfulness, the sharing of graphic details of abuse is frankly discouraged. A therapy group for patients with DDs is not about "one-upmanship" on tales of horror and torture, as so many support groups have been. Giving the details of the abusive events is not as vital to the treatment goal as is sharing the feelings related to the events. Graphic details often lead other group members to dissociate frankly, going away into their own history; this retraumatizes them. In addition, the group member who is speaking is left "alone" again in the experience (another parallel to childhood). However, above all, it is essential for patients with DID or other DDs to figure out their own histories—or perhaps to realize that they may never really know what happened to them, and to mourn the loss of this knowledge. Encouraging the telling of graphic details in a group format creates an opportunity for the patients to dilute and/or distort what may have happened to them. In addition, accounts of detailed abuse may "contaminate" the experiences (memories) of other group members. If this happens, the group is no longer an agent of positive change for the patients, but an agent of quick rather than pondered solutions.

In the group psychotherapy structured as described, patients with DDs have an opportunity to observe and respond to peers with whom they have a common affective background. The initial pull in the group is actually parallel to the initial pulls in the individual psychotherapy for both patient and therapist. This pull is to come up rapidly with a solution, good or bad. Patients with DDs often believe that their perceived passivity in childhood in the face of overwhelming life experiences needs to be rectified in adulthood by an action-oriented stance. The initial group pressure is to engage in rapid problem solving to "fix" a member's feelings, behaviors, or thinking. The group therapists do well to question the immediacy of such responses, even though it will take time for the group to settle into a more affect-tolerant modality. It is an arena where the injunction to "make haste slowly" (Kluft, 1988) comes alive. In a similar vein, the group format will allow each patient to observe at first hand the active psychological resistances that accompany DDs, because it is always easier to recognize the errors in the ways of others then of oneself. The group members learn that making a cognitive decision is different from actualizing it in the world. In addition, and perhaps more importantly, the group format will help patients more rapidly discern the pervasiveness of the impact of abuse on people's lives, and will help them notice that "manifest" interpretations in the here and now may prove unhelpful in self-mastery. The impact of abuse is deep, and deep self-understanding is necessary; here there are no quick fixes.

Criteria for Group Membership

An essential criterion for group membership is that each patient be in individual psychotherapy for at least one session per week; in addition, it is expected that the individual psychotherapist will support the patient's participation in the group and will be openly communicative with the group therapists. Group therapy is not intended to compete with individual psychotherapy, but to complement it (see the section on confidentiality above). Though there should be a comfortable flow of information and concern between group and individual psychotherapists, the group therapists should in no way expect or encourage a breach of the precious confidentiality prerogative between group members and their individual psychotherapists.

Ensuring the individual psychotherapist's support is vital to exploring splitting and therapist bashing, if not actually preventing it.

For example, a patient with DID was angry with her individual psychotherapist and fired him without bringing this information to the group immediately. Eventually, one of her personalities guiltily confessed; the group therapists explored this new information in the group context, reminding her of the group rules. She spoke of her individual therapist in a malevolent way, accusing him of greed (like her father) when in reality she was very deeply in debt to the therapist financially. Other group members, rather than being able to help her notice the transferential quality of her accusations, rallied around her and joined her in bashing the individual therapist. Of course, when the group leaders did not support their attacks, the patients added them to the bashing for good measure. The issues of secrecy, transference, and anger emerged as group themes. In this particular instance, there was an additional opportunity for the group leaders to discuss countertransference openly—in other words, how it feels to be tarred and feathered for another person's false interpretation. The group leaders contributed by cautiously sharing their feelings in this instance; this became an additional opportunity for the group members to recognize a common dynamic (see the section on process below) in their respective families, where they (the patients, as children) were often the target of false accusations. They also learned how this time, through their identification with their abusers, they chose to slight and blame someone rather than examine the incoming data further. This allowed the group therapists to inquire, along with the group members, whether a path of investigation other than identification with victims or identification with abusers was possible. Confronting this all-or-none dynamic in the group continued to challenge the affect-driven cognitive limitations of these patients.

A second criterion for group membership is that each patient must be willing to submit to a screening interview with one or both of the group psychotherapists. In this initial interview, both the therapist(s) and the patient can question whether the patient can work within the group rules as these are presented and reviewed. A history of uncontrollable behaviors, violence, suicidality, or active substance abuse is not necessarily a criterion for exclusion from the group, but it will give pause to the group leaders, who understandably will want to know the status of those behaviors today. Such behaviors often indicate that the client continues to be in an abusive relationship, either with a member of the family of origin or with a harsh significant other. For patients with DID or other DDs, another common reason for ongoing self-abusive acting out is that the patients are refusing to acknowledge and deal with an internalized abuser alter/ego state that is forever attempting to take executive control over their behavior. This avoidance of inner dynamics may come to the forefront of any number of group sessions. Hence the initial screening process (as well as discussion with the individual psychotherapist) is vital to assessing whether a client has the capacity to manage these chronic self-destructive behaviors within the group context.

> For example, eating disorders are commonly comorbid with a diagnosis of a DD. A group member who had been restricting food and overexercising, and who had divulged in earlier groups that her doctor thought that she was anorectic, was willing to talk about her struggles with food once another group member inquired about her health. Though the anorectic behaviors did not immediately cease, the patient felt that she could ask for help in monitoring and redressing her food-restricting behaviors. She also began to explore, with the help of the group, which of her personalities were actively promoting her anorexia.

The initial screening interview, as stated earlier, also serves the purpose of familiarizing potential new group members with the group rules and giving them an opportunity to opt out of joining the group. Voluntary participation is essential. Possible new group members are reminded that different personalities/ego states may be differentially motivated to join and belong to the group, and that they need to "check inwardly with all parts of the mind" before signing on. Once they enroll, they are committed for one group series (10 or 12 sessions) no matter what. In a small but predictable way, commitment to the group represents a pledge to participation in the current world—today's reality. Patients who chose to belong to such a psychotherapy group must have true courage, because they will be revisiting the past and living life in the present as well.

Too many patients with DID or other DDs see themselves so much as victims that they revictimize themselves by living angrily in a past where they were helpless and rejecting the present, where "no one understands" or "no one cuts me a break." They isolate themselves from society, and in doing so commit themselves not to understanding and surpassing the past, but rather to continuing to live in it (in some derivative form). Not uncommonly, this pronounced yet denied fact drags the patients into perceptions that they are entitled to irresponsibility because they are "owed." Belonging to a homogeneous group for patients with DDs diminishes this sense of entitlement, lessens the cult of "woundology" (Myss, 1997), and assists the patients in adopting a compensatory model of responsibility (Fine, 1996b) that will further their functioning as active and participating members of society. This compensatory model of responsibility promotes the notion that though people may not have been responsible for their past problems, they are responsible for current solutions. This structured group psychotherapy bolsters this perspective for these patients.

In addition, the structure imposed by the group rules serves as a container for the patients (Klein & Kugel, 1981). Patients with DID or other DDs operate better in a setting where predictability, organization, and consistency reign. These characteristics of the group favor the emergence of traumatic material; this carries with it the components of posttraumatic stress disorder, which the group through this format can hold. Patients find this group structure a safe harbor to bring up questions and concerns that they have shamefully secreted away.

The third major criterion for group participation and maintenance is an expectation of respect for self and for other group members, regardless of what is discussed. An abuse survivor with a DD frequently reports feeling evil, bad, ugly, stupid, and worthless; there is no room in such a group to ignore these foundational beliefs about the self and let them go unchallenged. Silences, glances, or statements that even allude to the depreciation of others/self in a destructive context are challenged immediately—initially by the group therapists, and eventually by the group members themselves. The fact that *any* issue can be brought up in the group, as well as the fact that group members will be heard with compassion, sympathy, empathy, and respect, serves as an additional holding environment for traumatized patients with DDs. This containment field within the overall group structure is buttressed by a proposed structure within each group session proper.

This structure is "group-defined" (Yalom, 1983), but in the initial sessions the definition is modeled by the group therapists, who request from the group members that topics of concern be put forward and that the group as a whole agree to pursue the most pressing issue at hand. The group leaders always revisit by the end of the group session, and sometimes formally summarize, what was covered in the session and what was learned. Unfinished themes are revisited at the next group session.

Themes and Process

Though it is clear that no one will alone pick (1) the theme to be discussed, (2) what will be addressed within each theme, or (3) what is acceptable to say or not to say, each group session begins with a member's proposing a theme that may be relevant in his or her individual psychotherapy or in his or her life today, and asking whether other group members wish to make this theme one of the topics for the group on that occasion. This respectful process of agreeing on a topic continues the message delivered by the group therapists that anything can be discussed in the group in a productive and safe way. As the group themes unfold and one topic begets another, careful attention must be paid to the group's readiness for the current theme.

Though themes can emerge naturally from the group process, there are occurrences, especially in the initial group therapy sessions, when patients with DDs are totally silent—as a defense against the wish to flee the group situation, as part of an derivative enactment, or both. The patients will often question whether group has "begun yet," then lapse into silence. If the silence continues, the group therapists may intervene; the possible interventions differ, depending on the maturity of the group. If the group is relatively new, the therapists may choose to promote self-sufficiency and engage in problem solving with the patients by taking a piece of paper and beginning to list potential group topics. The list lengthens as therapists and patients brainstorm together. This list becomes a resource for the group, though it is seldom needed once it is available. If an established group is silent, the obvious intervention is to inquire directly about the nature of the silence and the feelings behind it. Commonly, silences reflect leftover unprocessed topics or unaddressed issues from the previous group session; if so, these must be revisited, clarified, and resolved.

Typically, process issues are connected to the multiple reality problems (Loewenstein, 1991) with which these patients grapple. Patients with DID or other DDs live in multiple, simultaneous, and sometimes mutually exclusive realities, which are confusing to sort out. In addition, problem solving in one reality does not imply problem solving in another; this holds true for both content and process concerns. Therefore, leaps into premature generalizations or quick "solutions" can be frustrating and pointless for these patients. The support from the group, the witnessing of parallel struggles in other patients, and the reaping of rewarding solutions once traumatic mechanisms are abandoned all contribute to the dissolution of amnestic barriers between the various ego states or personalities, and therefore to the integration of each person as a whole.

Early in the group process, the patients struggle to distinguish between the following constructs: "here and now" versus "there and then" "inside world" versus "external world," and "either–or" versus "both–and." Themes such as trust, loss, and control are often operationalized within these constructs. For example, a group member who as a life stance takes on the role of "making friends with the enemy" by being overly pleasant with everyone may have adopted a preemptive control strategy in the "here and now" that is probably an adaptation to not making waves in the "there and then" of his or her childhood environment.

As with any group of mentally ill clients, trust is an ongoing issue for each of the group members in each and every session. The traumata that underlie the dissociative pathology of these patients, and that were frequently experienced at the hands of caretakers, can contribute greatly to an atmosphere of mistrust.

> For example, a recent change in group leaders brought to the forefront a member's mistrust of the remaining therapist (though both therapists were, and are, equally knowledgeable in the treatment of DID and other DDs). The patient was reenacting a false belief, which she projected onto the therapists, that "if both Mom and Dad are present, nothing bad will happen." Clarification of this dynamic for the patient allowed her to say goodbye to the departing therapist, resettle with the remaining therapist, and return to her individual therapist with a clearer picture of her projections onto significant people in her current life.

Polarized presentations of issues such as trust versus mistrust are ongoing concerns in groups of patients with DID or other DDs; these reflect the all-or-none nature of their interpretations about the world today. And these represent only a small fraction of all the possible distortions and misinterpretations that can be addressed productively in these homogeneous groups.

CONCLUSION

In conclusion, we have been conducting groups for affectively labile patients with DID and other DDs for over 10 years. We are both recognized individual psychotherapists for the treatment of these disorders, and have learned to use our understanding of dissociative pathology to create a safe, predictable structure within which patients can increase their understanding of their issues and begin to take risks in a more "public" forum. Therapists' ability to shift paradigms rapidly within a predesignated structure contributes to the success of these groups. Close attention to the rules and regulations of group functioning, and an ability to justify each decision to therapists and group members alike, are also important. It must be kept in mind that patients with DID or other DDs have been on the receiving end of out-of-control and arbitrary behaviors by authority figures throughout their childhoods; they have also rarely been included in redressing circumstances gone awry. Therefore, a thoughtful and explainable group structure that can be reviewed and revised as necessary is the sine qua non of successful group management. It will support the patients' individual psychotherapy and will be a respectful environment within which to take risks and renew their connections with a nonabusive world.

NOTE

1. Here is a clarification of two terms from the medicohistorical literature on DDs: "Magnetic somnambulism" is a term commonly used in the 18th and 19th centuries to describe a state of hypnosis; "mental desegregation" is a term coined by Janet and Charcot to describe what would now be called "dissociation."

REFERENCES

Agazarian, Y. (1992). Contemporary theories of group psychotherapy: A systems approach to the group as a whole. *International Journal of Group Psychotherapy, 42,* 177–203.

American Psychiatric Association. (1980). *Diagnostic and statistical manual of mental disorders* (3rd ed.). Washington, DC: Author.

Baum, E. Z. (1993). Dance/movement group therapy with multiple personality disorder patients. In E. S. Kluft (Ed.), *Expressive and functional therapies in the treatment of multiple personality disorder* (pp. 125–141). Springfield, IL: Thomas.

Brabender, V., & Fallon, A. (1993). *Models of inpatient group psychotherapy.* Washington, DC: American Psychological Association.

Buchele, B. (1994). Group psychotherapy for persons with multiple personality disorder and dissociative disorders. *Bulletin of the Menninger Clinic, 57,* 362–370.

Caul, D. (1984). Group and videotape techniques for multiple personality disorder. *Psychiatric Annals, 14,* 43–50.

Despine, A. (1840). *De l'emploi du magnétisme animal et des eaux minérales dans le traitement des maladies nerveuses, suivi d'une observation très curieuse de guérison de névropathie.* Paris: Baillière.

Dies, R. R. (1995). Group psychotherapies. In A. Gurman & S. B. Messer (Eds.), *Essential psychotherapies: Theories and practice* (pp. 448–522). New York: Guilford Press.

Figley, C. R. (1995). Compassion fatigue: Towards a new understanding of the costs of caring. In B. H. Stamm (Ed.), *Secondary traumatic stress: Self-care issues for clinicians, researchers and educators* (pp. 3–28). Lutherville, MD: Sidran Press.

Fine, C. G. (1988). Thoughts on the cognitive–perceptual substrates of multiple personality disorder. *Dissociation*, 1(4), 5–10.

Fine, C. G. (1990). The cognitive sequelae of incest. In R. P. Kluft (Ed.), *Incest-related syndromes of adult psychopathology* (pp. 161–182). Washington, DC: American Psychiatric Press.

Fine, C. G. (1991). Treatment stabilization and crisis prevention: Pacing the therapy of multiple personality disorder patients. *Psychiatric Clinics of North America*, 14, 661–675.

Fine, C. G. (1992). Multiple personality disorder. In A. Freeman & F. M. Dattilio (Eds.), *Comprehensive casebook of cognitive therapy* (pp. 347- 360). New York: Plenum Press.

Fine, C. G. (1993). A tactical integrationalist perspective on multiple personality disorder. In R. P. Kluft & C. G. Fine (Eds.), *Clinical perspectives on multiple personality disorder* (pp. 135–153). Washington, DC: American Psychiatric Press.

Fine, C. G. (1996a). A cognitively-based treatment model for DSM-IV dissociative identity disorder. In L. K. Michelson & W. J. Ray (Eds.), *Handbook of dissociation: Theoretical, empirical and clinical perspectives* (pp. 401–411). New York: Plenum Press.

Fine, C. G. (1996b). Models of helping: The role of responsibility. In J. L. Spira (Ed.), *Treating dissociative identity disorder* (pp. 81–98). San Francisco, CA: Jossey-Bass.

Jacobson, M. (1993). Group art therapy with multiple personality disorder patients: A viable alternative to isolation. In E. S. Kluft (Ed.), *Expressive and functional therapies in the treatment of multiple personality disorder* (pp. 101–123). Springfield, IL: Thomas.

Janet, P. (1886). Les actes inconscients et le dédoublement de la personnalite pendant le somnambulisme provoqué. *Revue Philosophique*, 22(2), 577–792.

Klein, R. H., Hunter, D. E. K., & Brown, S. L. (1986). Long-term inpatient group psychotherapy: The ward group. *International Journal of Group Psychotherapy*, 36(3), 361–380.

Klein, R. H., & Kugel, B. (1981). Inpatient group psychotherapy from a systems perspective: Reflections through a glass darkly. *International Journal of Group Psychotherapy*, 31(3), 311–328.

Klein, R. H., Orleans, J., & Soule, C. (1991). The axis II group. *International Journal of Group Psychotherapy*, 41, 97–116.

Kluft, R. P. (1984). Aspects of treatment of multiple personality disorder. *Psychiatric Annals*, 14, 51–55.

Kluft, R. P. (1985). Childhood multiple personality disorder: Predictors, clinical findings and treatment results. In R. P. Kluft (Ed.), *Childhood antecedents of multiple personality disorder* (pp. 167–196). Washington, DC: American Psychiatric Press.

Kluft, R. P. (1988). On treating the older patient with multiple personality disorder: "Race against time" or "Make haste slowly." *American Journal of Clinical Hypnosis, 30,* 257–266.

Kluft, R. P. (1990). Incest and subsequent revictimization: The case of therapist–patient sexual exploitation, with a description of the sitting duck syndrome. In R. P. Kluft (Ed.), *Incest-related syndromes of adult psychopathology* (pp. 263–287). Washington, DC: American Psychiatric Press.

Kluft, R. P. (1999). Current issues in dissociative identity disorder. *Journal of Practical Psychiatry and Behavioral Health, 5,* 3–19.

Lego, S. (1984). Group therapy. In S. Lego (Ed.), *The American handbook of psychiatric nursing* (pp. 206–217). Philadelphia: Lippincott.

Loewenstein, R. J. (1991). An office mental status examination for chronic complex dissociative symptoms and multiple personality disorder. *Psychiatric Clinics of North America, 14,* 567–604.

Madden, N. E., & Fine, C. G. (1990). Issues in outpatient group psychotherapy in multiple personality disorder patients. In B. G. Braun & E. B. Carlson (Eds.), *Proceedings of the Seventh International Conference on Multiple Personality and Dissociative States: Altered states of consciousness* (p. 59). Chicago: Rush University Dissociative Disorders Program.

Minuchin, S. (1974). *Families and family therapy.* Cambridge, MA: Harvard University Press.

Myss, C. (1997). *Why people don't heal and how they can.* New York: Three Rivers Press.

Orne, M. T. (1959). The nature of hypnosis: Artifact and essence. *Journal of Abnormal and Social Psychology, 58,* 277–299.

Petetin, J.-H.-D. (1775). *Mémoire sur la découverte des phénomènes que présentent la catalepsie et le somnambulisme, symptômes de l'affection hystérique essentielle.* Lyon.

Prince, M. (1919). The psychogenesis of multiple personality. *Journal of Abnormal Psychology, 14,* 225–280.

Putnam, F. W. (1989). *Diagnosis and treatment of multiple personality disorder.* New York: Guilford Press.

Roback, H., & Smith, M. (1987). Patient attrition in dynamically oriented treatment groups. *American Journal of Psychiatry, 144,* 426–431.

Rossel, R. D. (1998). Multiplicity: The challenge of finding "place" in experience. *Journal of Constructivist Psychology, 3,* 221–240.

Schultz, R., Braun, B. G., & Kluft, R. P. (1989). Multiple personality disorder: Phenomenology of selected variables in comparison to major depression. *Dissociation, 2,* 48–51.

Spiegel, D. (1986). Multiple personality as a post-traumatic stress disorder. *Psychiatric Clinics of North America, 9,* 101–110.

Thigpen, C. H., & Cleckley, H. (1957). *The three faces of Eve.* New York: McGraw-Hill.

van der Kolk, B. A. (1987). The role of the group in the origin and resolution of the trauma response. In B. A. van der Kolk (Ed.), *Psychological trauma* (pp. 153–171). Washington, DC: American Psychiatric Press.

Watkins, J. G., & Watkins, H. H. (1997). *Ego states: Theory and therapy*. New York: Norton.

Wilbur, C. B. (1984). Multiple personality disorder and child abuse: An overview. *Psychiatric Clinics of North America, 7*, 3–7.

Wilson, H., & Kneisl, C. (1979). *Psychiatric nursing*. Menlo Park, CA: Addison-Wesley.

Yalom, I. (1983). *Inpatient group psychotherapy*. New York: Basic Books.

13

◄◦►

Group Treatment of Severe Clinical Disorders, Personality Disorders, and Substance Use Problems

RICHARD E. GALLAGHER
HOWARD D. KIBEL

The disorders discussed in this chapter refer to those individuals who carry a DSM-IV diagnosis of a major psychotic disorder, a serious mood disorder, or a severe personality disorder, and to those who have a long-standing alcohol or other substance use problem. Individuals in these treatment groups generally represent the most common, and are often seen as the most difficult, patients encountered in psychiatric hospitals, rehabilitation centers, and ambulatory care clinics. As a whole, these patients constitute a considerable public health problem. As individuals (though extremely varied, of course), they commonly undergo enormous personal suffering and present with very high levels of impairment.

Because of the prevalence and massive needs of these classes of patients, group psychotherapies are particularly attractive and economically sensible modalities to consider when feasible. Their effectiveness has been described for the chronically mentally ill (Kibel, 1991; Stone, 1996). Because many of these patients have been traumatized, therapy should optimally address in some way this aspect of their backgrounds. Beyond these points, however, it is extremely rash to generalize, since treatment must always be individualized; it must be geared to the person, not the disorder.

Two hallmarks of the nature, understanding, and treatment of these patients are precisely their complexity and heterogeneity. Optimal treatment is therefore often a matter of particularizing, practicality, and flexibility. Many of these patients have been traumatized, but many have not. In addressing issues of abuse and other forms of trauma, group clinicians must be sensitive to a host of issues: the highly complex and varied therapeutic needs of these patients, the timing of any trauma-centered interventions, the choice of patients appropriate to such a focus, and the imperative neither to underemphasize nor to overemphasize the relevance of the history of trauma. The last of these is most important. Clinicians run the risks of either neglecting the effects of trauma or prematurely focusing on it before the patients can tolerate exposure and exploration. It doesn't help that truly skilled and motivated group practitioners for these disorders are frequently lacking and underfunded.

There are major problems in discussing disorders in which there is a history of trauma. Three are highlighted here. First, many disorders are complex in themselves. The multiple diagnostic axes that were introduced in DSM-III (American Psychiatric Association [APA], 1980) alerted us to this phenomenon. Descriptive clinicians speak of "comorbidity," such as the existence of two or more personality disorders on Axis II, and the DSM system allows for multiple diagnoses of clinical disorders on Axis I. Our current nosology, which is necessary for scientific investigation and communication, arbitrarily compartmentalizes a person and his or her ailments. These allegedly separate entities, however, are often part of a unitary disorder that constitutes the psychopathology we treat. Second, many clinical investigators do not differentiate the treatment of the disorders considered here from one another; nor is this done in the literature on the group psychotherapy of trauma. So as not to run too far afield in the present discussion, however, this chapter treats each of these disorders separately. Third, posttraumatic stress disorder (PTSD) is not discussed; yet when PTSD occurs, there may be comorbidity and hence complexity. PTSD has been discussed separately, as a large subject in itself, in another chapter of this volume (see Johnson & Lubin, Chapter 6). Originally, PTSD was defined as psychological sequelae attendant upon experience "that is generally outside the range of usual human experience" (American Psychiatric Association, 1980, p. 236). However, over the years the definition has been broadened to include all sorts of trauma. Thus much of the material to follow can also be applied to PTSD.

In the context of the emphases in this book, two critical issues arise with respect to patients with clinical, personality, or substance use disorders:

1. How prevalent are traumatic backgrounds in these patients, and of what relevance are they to the presenting disorders?

2. Of what value and risks are attempts to address traumatic backgrounds with such patients, and what might be the optimal role of groups in this regard?

Unfortunately, the answers to these questions are not simple and are subject to a fair amount of controversy. Rather than trying to present simple cookbook recommendations about dealing with traumatized individuals, we attempt to sketch out some working guidelines about treating each group of such patients, emphasizing the maximal use of group modalities when practical with an appropriate clinical sensitivity to traumatic issues, as relevant. Clinical examples illustrate the therapeutic recommendations. It is indispensable first, however, to place this whole subject of the treatment of abused and other traumatized individuals in the context of its convoluted history.

ORIENTING PERSPECTIVE
AND BRIEF HISTORICAL OVERVIEW

It is important to put the subject of trauma with respect to serious psychopathology in proper historical perspective, both to attempt to clear up lingering confusions and prejudices in our field, and to orient the clinician working with more severely mentally impaired individuals. Current disagreements and controversies often reflect entrenched ideological and tendentious positions, rather than the humble and measured judgments that truly scientific discussion of this issue warrants.

It is important to keep in mind that among the major theoretical advances in the psychiatric literature during the past 20 years has indeed been the recognition of the frequency and importance of abuse and other forms of trauma trauma in the backgrounds of so many psychiatric patients. However, there is still little consensus as to the therapeutic relevance of these findings. In fact, it is fair to say that the topic of the relevance and prevalence of trauma in the backgrounds of seriously ill patients has been a confusing and heated one for at least a century now.

Contrary to what is often believed, Freud's findings in this area were by no means simplistic or categorical. Misconceptions of his views still abound. The traditional opinion is that Freud during the early 1890s, in energetically searching for a *caput Nili* (a "source of the Nile"—i.e., a central etiological factor) in the causation of the often severely neurotic (and probably at times near-psychotic) disorders of his practice, at first believed the spontaneous reports of his patients that they had been sexually abused. In time, however, Freud became convinced that his patients' psyches created these stories, and that such tales were more properly accounted for by deeply determined early fantasies, long repressed and now uncovered by his psychoanalytic methods. Standard, sympathetic biographies of Freud, such as those by Ernest Jones (1961) and Peter Gay (1988), proffer this view. Gay (1988), for instance, writes that Freud "for a time continued to accept as true his patients' lurid recitals . . . [but eventually recognized them as] . . . a collection of fairy tales his patients had . . . told him" (pp. 94, 96).

This historiographic view was often cited to support the emphasis given in early psychoanalytic treatment to the uncovering of repressed intrapsychic drive determinants at the expense of the impact of real events. Such a reading of Freud also buttressed the opinions of the psychoanalytic community for many years (even as etiological claims for neuroses became considerably more pluralistic). The general feeling among therapists trained both within and without the analytic community seemed to be that abuse and other forms of trauma in the histories of patients were probably rare; one text in the 1970s cited the rate of incest as one in a million children. In any case, it was assumed that the psychological processing of such experiences, rather than the traumatic impact of the events per se, was of most clinical relevance.

The inevitable backlash to this mindset occurred in the late 1970s and 1980s, when the full extent of patients' traumatic histories became clearer, and more recently, when a more sophisticated appreciation of the biological impact of such experiences came under investigation (van der Kolk & Saporta, 1991). In not a few cases, however, the pendulum swung too far in the opposite direction. In some therapeutic circles (and especially among the less sophisticated even to this day), uncovering and "healing" the "traumatized" self became the main and sometimes the only real focus of treatment. As the focus on trauma reached inordinate proportions, some practitioners were subtly (or not so subtly) pressuring their patients to retrieve remembrances that did not in fact reflect real events. This risk is especially prominent in dealing with the very impaired and chronic groups of patients under discussion here, whose dependency on their therapists makes them prone to subtle influencing.

> For example, a very disturbed young male allegedly recalled seeing the murder of a 5-year-old child by a local minister. It transpired that the therapist himself had actually witnessed the gruesome slaughter of a 5-year-old while on tour in Vietnam. When evidence was presented to suggest that the patient's memory was false, the therapist acknowledged that he must have unwittingly contributed to the formation of a bizarre and untrue recollection in his patient.

Although a scenario as dramatic as this case is probably fairly uncommon, some therapists can, and undoubtedly still do, become overly invested in seeking out trauma as a too exclusive pathogenic element. With the identification of "false-memory syndrome" has come recognition of the risks of trying to elicit memories under subtle pressure. While the prevalence of trauma is better known, the danger of making its resolution the sole focus of treatment is also slowly becoming clearer to most clinicians.

Ironically, a more careful reading of Freud than the standard one noted above might actually have anticipated the need for corrective balance and obviated polarized controversy. It appears that Freud himself unwittingly engaged for a brief time in the very same type of behavior that later became so suspect among our overenthusiastic "traumatists." An unbiased and close reading of the 1890s papers makes this argument nearly inescapable. For instance, in "The Aetiology of Hysteria," the published version of his famous, poorly received lecture in Vienna, Freud wrote that before they come for analysis the patients "know nothing about these scenes. They were indignant as a rule if he warned them that such scenes were going to emerge. Only the strongest compulsion of the treatment could induce them to embark on a reproduction of them" (Freud, 1896/1962, p. 204). His patients asserted that they have "no feeling of remembering the scene" and spoke to him "emphatically of their unbelief" (p. 204). In *Studies on Hysteria*, after having stated at a point that he had "laboriously forced some piece of knowledge" upon his patients, Freud wrote (with his colleague Breuer) that even as they accepted this point, they still insisted that they "can't remember having thought it" (Breuer & Freud, 1893–1895/1955, pp. 299–300).

Freud's efforts to dredge up false memories emanated from the very logic of his early methodology; after all, by his own schema, he was supposed to be working with memories that lay at an unconscious level, were subject to strong resistance, and therefore were *not* spontaneously generated. It is well known that Freud came to realize the power of the unconscious to create fantasy and to elicit narratives based more on unconscious need than on reality. Yet he never truly dismissed the importance of real-life trauma. Much of his theoretical system and many of his later adherents, however, appeared to minimize it.

In work with patients who have been traumatized, the first principle therefore must be to recognize how easily subject to distortion, confusion, and misplaced emphasis this whole subject matter can be. The second principle is no less significant and may serve to underscore the more specific points made in the rest of this chapter: Abuse and other forms of trauma, though easily subject to over- or underemphasis, are nevertheless very real phenomena in the backgrounds (and, of course, sometimes the present reality) of many of the sickest patients, and cannot be ignored conceptually or therapeutically.

BASIC PRINCIPLES

At the risk of a somewhat simplified schematization, the rest of this chapter focuses upon three categories of patient groups and proposes some general guidelines for use of group psychotherapies in addressing traumatic aspects of their respective histories. The three groups to be surveyed here are as follows:

1. Those patients with Axis I diagnoses of schizophrenia, schizo-affective disorder, or severe mood disorders.
2. Those patients with severe Axis II disorders, especially borderline and antisocial personality disorders (as paradigmatic of entrenched character pathology).
3. Those patients suffering from long-standing problems with alcohol or other substance use.

The precise theoretical understanding of the role of trauma in the backgrounds of most of these patients is still only poorly understood, even for the personality-disordered. Arguments for the etiological impact of such events are particularly controversial. Almost all these conditions emanate from a genetic predisposition to varying degrees. Yet they are all most fruitfully conceptualized as highly multifactorial and heterogeneous in origin. It should be obvious that treatment planning for such patients will thus encompass a broad mix of various psychosocial treatments and at times medications or other biological treatments, rather than any specific trauma-focused modality alone. At the same time, the issue of abuse or other traumatization is too pressing to ignore. With some of these conditions, traumatic histories may indeed have contributed in some fairly direct way to the disorder; for instance, many students of borderline and antisocial personality disorders do believe that a history of trauma is frequently highly determinative of the pathology (Gunderson & Chu, 1993; Silk, Lee, Hill, & Lohr, 1995). Nevertheless, even in these conditions there remains little consensus as to the exact degree of influence. Moreover, trauma has a widely divergent impact on phenomenology even within the same diagnostic groupings, especially since patients within each diagnostic group vary among themselves. Group psychotherapy for these patients cannot ignore the relevance of trauma, but must use the treatment in a way that is individualized to the specific needs of each patient.

After attention to such basic principles as relevant to the disorders discussed in this chapter, next will follow more specific guidelines with regard to each of these categories.

PSYCHOTIC AND SEVERE MOOD DISORDERS

For those with Axis I diagnoses of schizophrenia, schizoaffective disorder, and severe mood disorders, the role of trauma as an etiological factor to any degree is highly disputed and in some quarters even resented. The backgrounds of such patients are so enormously varied, and biological antecedents (especially genetic influences) are so powerful, that any generalization as to the specificity of the environmental damage involved—let alone "trauma"—is bound to be precariously grounded. Yet in careful surveys, to a surprising extent, it does appear that a fair amount of such individuals have been abused or otherwise traumatized. For some time, it has been known that general psychiatric populations have high rates of abusive backgrounds (e.g., Bryer, Nelson, Miller, & Krol, 1987; Carmen, Ricker, & Mills, 1984; Herman, 1986; Jacobson & Herald, 1990). Less well recognized is that more specialized studies of patients with psychotic disorders have more specifically shown that many such individuals have indeed suffered trauma in their families of origin. For instance, Stone (1990) found that 26.4% of his sample of patients with schizoaffective disorder reported intrafamilial sexual abuse. Beck and van der Kolk (1987) reported on a series of 12 state hospital patients diagnosed with schizophrenia, who had been severely abused. Our own detailed survey of hospitalized inpatients diagnosed with schizophrenia has found surprisingly high rates of physical, verbal, and sexual abuse alike (Gallagher, Flye, & Hurt, 2000).

In subsets of these diagnostic groups, do such events play a role as one of a multitude of influences in a multifactorial model of etiology? Undoubtedly so, although given how poorly understood the pathophysiology and pathogenesis of these states are, one is loath to claim definitude, especially with any particular case. It may be that many individuals who are genetically prone to severe clinical disorders become easy prey for abuse or other trauma subsequent to its development or earlier in life—that is, during premorbid ages. A small group of patients have become delusional about the whole subject; however, this population (which psychotically believes it was traumatized and probably was not) is, in our clinical experience, quite small. What is clear, at any rate, is that many of these individuals do in fact struggle with the effect of abuse or other trauma in their backgrounds; such histories and their consequences cannot be dismissed clinically.

The more severe and fulminant patients' clinical disorders are, the more problematic this aspect of their backgrounds is for the working group clinician. When these patients are acutely psychotic and/or grossly manic, most psychotherapies, whether individual or group-oriented, are not feasible and are even contraindicated. Bringing up the subject of trauma to acutely decompensated patients is generally disorganizing. Medications and the use of a structured milieu are called for to ameliorate the active symptoms, whether they be hallucinations, delusions, thought disorder, mania, or severe depression.

Once the patients' condition had been properly stabilized, consideration should then be given to discussion of traumatic material. But, in practice, this is rarely done. Much of the current literature discourages use of dynamically oriented groups for patients with major Axis I disorders.

This recommendation is not new. In fact, for many years there was controversy in the literature about the value of group psychotherapy at all for patients with psychotic disorders (Kibel, 1981). Early workers found that treatment caused such patients' condition to deteriorate. This finding was largely based on a misapplication of analytic, expressive models, without the parameters necessary to contain these patients' anxiety and regressive potentials. In short, an emphasis on insight into psychogenic conflict proved inappropriate and often harmful. As work with the severely mentally ill became more refined, the results proved better. Kanas (1986), in a meta-analysis of multiple studies on group psychotherapy with schizophrenic patients, showed that the treatments contributed significantly to positive outcome. However, most studies use criteria for success that are too narrowly defined, such as reduction in the rates of relapse and of positive symptoms. In other words, adaptation is valued over exploration, development of the self, and progress in the more comprehensive aspects of quality of life (Skolnick, 1999).

Kanas (1996) developed a group method for treating schizophrenic patients that has been repeatedly tested through clinical research. It is said to be an integrative approach, in that it combines a focus on symptoms with efforts to improve interpersonal relationships. However, some aspects of the method underline Skolnick's view. According to Kanas, the first goal is to help psychotic patients learn to cope with their symptoms. This means helping them learn to test reality and to deal with hallucinations and delusions. Only then does the therapist use the interactions between members to focus on interpersonal learning. Since this work is done in a context in which the control of symptoms is a priority, adaptation inevitably supersedes exploration.

In recent years, psychoeducational groups have become popular in the treatment of patients with major clinical disorders. Beginning with the work of Julian Leff (Leff, Kuipers, Berkowitz, & Sturgeon, 1985), who tried to assess the nature of interactions between families and patients, the work has evolved into formalized, sometimes manualized training programs in which patients and significant others are provided with information about specific illnesses and symptoms. There can be an assumption in these groups that the illnesses are completely biological, and so adaptation again becomes the chief goal of treatment. Paralleling this trend has been the use of social skills training (Dobson, McDougall, Busheikin, & Aldous, 1995; Douglas & Mueser, 1990), which is often administered in a group. This is usually part of a comprehensive rehabilitation program that includes counseling and groups helping patients to function more effectively in the community (Kanas, 1996).

In contrast, the reports of the effectiveness of cognitive-behavioral therapy (CBT) approaches have been less encouraging. Although patients seem to improve while they are in treatment, there remains insufficient evidence that the benefit carries over outside the treatment setting. This may be due, for the most impaired, to negative symptoms and persistent internal preoccupations that interfere with the kind of learning emphasized by standard CBT methods (Kanas, 1999). One positive report of group treatment using a psychoeducational and CBT model is worth noting (Gallagher & Nazarian, 1995). Selection criteria encompassed voluntary patients with a history of one or more psychotic episodes; the majority of those involved turned out to carry diagnoses of schizophrenia. This study included not a few patients with a history of trauma. It was somewhat unusual in two ways. First, the treatment did not eschew the use of dynamic insights, nor did it avoid highly sensitive topics—components especially appreciated by the more intelligent patients. Second, it was one part of a comprehensive inpatient milieu that provided support for the work done in the group and helped to contain psychotic anxiety. Since abuse and other trauma were frequently part of these patients' past, explicit attention was paid to including this subject matter as a routine topic in that setting. The case of a paranoid woman treated in that program is described in the third example provided below.

The vast majority of current group treatments for patients with major Axis I disorders stress adaptation and social adjustment over more substantive change in the personality. Consequently, they are not designed to work with histories of trauma. For the most part, they are not mutative treatments. They have limited goals and offer impersonal mirroring rather than transformation (Skolnick, 1999). They are not ineffective; they diminish emotional suffering and can restore a patient to the community and/or the family. They also reduce deviant behavior, thereby facilitating functioning in society. They are invariably short-term and less labor-intensive. There is a tradeoff, in a sense, in which stability is possible as long as the more disruptive aspects of personality (i.e., the psychotic core) are encapsulated (Skolnick, 1999).

It is then left to longer-term treatments to go further. Although many will argue that encapsulation and adaptation make longer-term treatment difficult, a different notion is expressed by some who have worked for years with such patients (Kibel, 1991; Chazan, 1993; Stone, 1996). They contend that the sense of safety that develops in a long-term group—that is, the sense of bonding and holding that occurs under the aegis of a protective leader—allows patients to gradually reveal the psychotic core of their personalities and to risk exploration. This sequence can be applied to the exposure and discussion of traumatic events. However, for that to occur, the group must be quite cohesive, stable, and functioning well. This can be the case even if all the members are quite impaired. There are times when a group can function in a way that seems to surpass the level of integration of its individual members. Kibel (1992) has noted that "a supportive, cohesive group of patients with severe psychopathology can help members contain their fragmented egos and enhance their adaptive functioning when they are . . . in session" (p. 152).

Granted, exploration and working through of trauma may be limited in many of these groups. But even the limited support that the group provides can be enormously therapeutic. It can pave the way for a patient to put experience into a conceptual framework, understand its relation to difficulties in later life, and thereby foster mastery of that experience. At times this is not possible to do entirely in the group, depending on its history, its ability to sustain the so-called "holding" function, and the occurrence of untoward intercurrent events; supplementary individual sessions are then required to help a patient achieve those goals. In any case, when conducted by experienced clinicians, psychodynamically informed groups have helped patients with major psychiatric disorders improve their quality of life. When such groups are conducted by less seasoned practitioners or trainees, supervision is mandatory. The supervision obviously guides the therapists and notably fosters confidence in the modality (Gallagher, 1994). Although psychodynamically informed group psychotherapy can be particularly effective with these patients, they are exceedingly difficult to conduct. A therapist must work hard to promote sufficient cohesion so that patients feel connected to one another. Yet, at the same time, the therapist needs to respect these patients' fear of merger. The therapist must modulate the level of anxiety in the group and be attuned to each member's ability to tolerate the intensity of the process. There is always a danger that some patients will be overwhelmed during periods of concentrated interaction and will flee or decompensate. For this reason, such groups require highly skilled leadership or leaders who are receiving capable supervision.

Much depends upon the proper mix of patients and the skill of the group's leadership. Too many overly paranoid or aggressive Axis I patients in any group can preclude constructive discussion of any highly sensitive subject, let alone abuse or other trauma. Similarly, group leaders who are uncomfortable or inexperienced may find that this subject matter and/or these patients' psychotic responses outweigh their ability to contain the patients' anxiety. Too often, such leaders react prematurely by using confrontation to suppress verbalization.

Three case examples will illustrate more precisely how the recommendations above work in practice.

The first example involved a 30-year-old male patient with schizoaffective disorder, originally misdiagnosed as primarily a mixed personality disorder. He was placed in a psychodynamically oriented group, but one in which peers were encouraged to confront one another's acting out. In this group, patients were not shy about challenging each other. Although not grossly delusional, this new patient (unbeknownst to the relatively inexperienced group leader, who was a resident in supervision) turned out to be more paranoid than originally thought.

Unexpectedly, the subject of his first session was, it turned out, the trauma many members had undergone as children. The patient in question, who had quickly alienated some of his peers by his rather entitled and angry stance from the outset, had in fact been physically abused himself and started to recount his own painful experiences. The group seemed to view this as an effort to justify his evident attitude toward them. The members quickly turned on him, whereupon the patient decompensated and became psychotic. He accused his peers of being worse than his sadistic father, became quite delusional about what he saw as "accusations," and stormed out of the session.

This example illustrates the danger of including such open-ended discussion of abuse and other trauma with poorly compensated patients who have such severe psychopathology. Their psychotic projections are likely to be quickly transferred onto any object that appears even mildly unsympathetic toward their concerns. This patient's inclusion in this type of group was a mistake and was quickly corrected. The notion seems warranted that for such patients, processing of their traumatic histories must be delayed until they are fully integrated into the group and until the other members have learned how to tolerate their level of pathology. Should that not happen, then any discussion of trauma may have to be avoided altogether.

The second example demonstrates a more satisfactory resolution of a similar case involving a paranoid patient. This time the mixed-diagnosis, psychodynamically oriented group was run more expertly. A gifted trainee, who had been very carefully supervised, conducted this stable group. This group seemed able to contain the patient's projections. The group leader was fully aware that the subject of sexual mistreatment might be a difficult one for the members to hear, but believed that a properly guided recounting of severe abuse by this relatively depressed and mildly paranoid young woman could be constructively handled. The patient, a woman in her 30s with a long-standing diagnosis of bipolar disorder, had been gang-raped as a teenager and had always been extremely sensitive and secretive about the subject. The leader had known from previous treatment that she was intensely mortified by others' knowing of her rape, and that she could get quite paranoid, falsely believing that people were talking about her and calling her "a slut." This point was especially poignant, since she had a subsequent history of promiscuity.

The patients in this cohesive group, whose members liked and valued her and who indeed felt protective toward her, proved quite adept in helping her discuss the effects of this trauma. She recounted how shameful she and her enmeshed family had found the painful incident, and how for years it was never mentioned at all in the family home. She wondered whether the group participants also felt that she was "a bad girl." She stammered as she said that she had begun to think people at her residence were continually staring at her body. The group leader complimented her on having the courage to bring up these disturbing memories, and asked the other members of the group (who had initially been silent) to comment.

The group members proved able to allay her concerns by pointing out how unlikely it was that people would spontaneously stare at her so many years after the incident. They added that they knew she was in fact not "bad," but a very kind-hearted and honorable person. It was clear that the patient benefited greatly from the acknowledgment of her value, and she eventually commented that, based on her experience in the group, she realized it seemed absurd to think that others around her would be as preoccupied with her sexual history as she had been.

The final example of a group-oriented treatment for severe Axis I mental illness that addressed trauma involved a patient in one of the CBT/psychoeducational groups discussed previously. This woman, also in her 30s, had a long history of untreated schizophrenia. She had recently been hospitalized for a psychotic episode in which she experienced ideas of reference and delusional grandiosity. She made it quite clear that she was not interested in any "therapy"; she had found no use for doctors, who, she stated, merely wanted to "pick my brain."

This patient did agree, however, to attend a "class," the instructional group format that was recommended for patients who expressed an interest in such an option. As noted, one of the many topics discussed in the didactic section was that of abuse and other trauma. After hearing the lecture, the patient spontaneously stated that for the first time, she had felt understood. She now realized that her mother was in fact an emotionally abusive person who had made her life miserable. The patient felt positive enough about this session that she remained an involved member throughout the subsequent lectures/discussions over the ensuing weeks prior to discharge. Shortly thereafter, this patient agreed to try one of the newer antipsychotic medications and to attend a more traditional group psychotherapy—both first time ventures for her.

These examples underscore the point that patients with psychotic and severe mood disorders have considerable problems discussing abuse and other forms of trauma. On the other hand, the more stable the group and the more motivated the patients (even if they retain psychotic potential), the more helpful group psychotherapeutic discussions of abuse and other trauma can be. Of course, in any truly long-standing group treatment effort, eventually the emotionally charged issue of trauma is bound to surface. It is important for clinicians to have neither utopian nor nihilistic attitudes toward fostering such discussions, especially with the very impaired patients considered here.

SEVERE PERSONALITY DISORDERS

Moving the focus from psychotic and serious mood disorders to severe personality disorders places the discussion on firmer ground. There seems to be less doubt of the relevance of abuse and other trauma to patients with the more severe and flamboyant personality disorders, especially those upon whom this section concentrates. The focus here is primarily upon borderline and antisocial personality disorders, prototypes of the complex and extreme character pathology under consideration. Both conditions have proven to be associated with high degrees of abuse and trauma in the patients' histories. They have been the most extensively studied of the personality disorders. Yet the findings in these conditions may apply to others as well.

Rates of various forms of abuse have been shown to be especially high in the history of patients who go on to develop borderline personality disorder. Two small studies in the early to mid-1980s alerted the field to this (Herman, 1986; Stone, Kahn, & Flye, 1981). A more recent one that used advanced research methodology (Gallagher, Flye, Hurt, Stone, & Hull, 1992) found at least some level of both sexual and physical abuse in an astounding 73% of a hospitalized sample. Numerous other researchers have similarly found high rates of abuse (compared to those in control groups) in the backgrounds of both adult and adolescent "borderline" populations (e.g., Westen, Ludolph, Misle, Ruffins, & Block, 1990), as well as high rates of what Ogata and colleagues have defined as "multiple abuse" (Ogata et al., 1990).

Abuse or other trauma as the primary pathogenic element should not be accepted as a given. With personality disorders in general, one is again undoubtedly dealing with heterogeneous conditions and multiple etiologies. Yet making trauma more of a focus of treatment for these patients is worth consideration, given such impressive frequencies.

When a patient has a severe personality disorder, a clinician ought to take a careful history. The clinician should be receptive to the history of trauma, but should be careful not to suggest it merely to reconfirm a preexisting expectation. When a history of trauma is found, it needs to be evaluated as to its more specific possible etiological role in the pathology. For example, the effect of a chaotic childhood is undoubtedly different from that of frank childhood sexual abuse. Likewise, the nature of childhood sexual abuse varies. At what age did the event(s) occur? Who was the perpetrator? What was the duration? What was the social context of the abuse? Silk and colleagues (1995) examined the relationship of specific symptoms of borderline personality disorder to dimensions of severity of sexual abuse. They found that most predictive of the severity of the personality disorder were three factors in abuse—namely, the perpetrator, the duration, and the type. Specifically, severity was more likely if the perpetrator was a parent rather than another relative or a nonrelative, if the sexual abuse was ongoing, and if it involved penetration. Ongoing sexual abuse was associated with parasuicidal behavior. The most prominent predictor of severity was the duration of abuse.

Even the significance of these compelling findings needs to be elucidated from a psychodynamic perspective if their clinical implications are to be fully appreciated. It has been part of contemporary clinical wisdom to conceptualize the effects of trauma on a continuum, depending on the age of the victim, the frequency and duration of the trauma, the extent of injury, and the degree of support the person received when the trauma occurred (Scharff & Scharff, 1994). Nicholas and Forrester (1999) correctly note that the "variables determining the psychological consequences of traumatic abuse include the closeness of the relationship between the abuser and abused before the trauma and the degree of betrayal felt by the abused, as well as the extent to which the trauma was acknowledged by others in the victim's family and social networks" (p. 324). They go on to note that recognition of the social nature of trauma—that is, its context—goes back to the work of Pierre Janet and is reflected in the work of today's contemporary leaders in the field.

Of the dimensions of trauma described above, the key elements appear to be those related to the impact on personality development—specifically, the sense of personal identity. A child who has been sexually abused by a parent over a period of time comes to feel betrayed by the family (but not always by the perpetrator); has been deprived of the social support that is ordinarily afforded to children; suffers damage to a wide network of relations; experiences relations as inherently duplicitous; has difficulty trusting others; and yet continues to maintain a complicated, often unconsciously eroticized, and clearly disturbed attachment to the abusing parent. This pathological connection, in turn, impairs separation–individuation and later inhibits the development of intimacy in adulthood (Ganzarain & Buchele, 1989).

Evaluation of the nature of trauma and its effects is a complicated process, and the full implications may only emerge during the course of treatment. Ganzarain and Buchele (1989) were so impressed by the intricacies of the relationship between perpetrators and abused individuals that they were reluctant merely to consider these patients to be victims in the usual sense of the word, and preferred to call them "individuals with a history of incest."

A focus on the history of trauma should not blind the clinician to the essence of the personality disorder. Severe psychopathology can occur in the presence of trauma and may have occurred regardless of what happened. A sobering finding is that survivors of sexual abuse who entered group psychotherapy were less likely to complete treatment if they had a previous history of psychiatric hospitalization (Hazard, Roger, & Angert, 1993). In other words, the severity of the condition is an intrinsic predictor of treatment response. So is the presence of antisocial aspects in the personality (Clarkin, Hull, Yeomans, Kakuma, & Cantor, 1994). Some patients (and unfortunately some clinicians) too readily accept patients' statements of verbal abuse as if it were as pathogenic as other trauma. In these instances, the patients may be merely justifying a history of socially destructive behavior. Many times these patients have a variant of borderline pathology that is infused with narcissistic and antisocial elements, which Kernberg (1984) has dubbed "malignant narcissism." Treating this as if it were as clinically significant as overt trauma runs the risk of reinforcing the patients' pathology.

Even when frank abuse is not evident, neglect and/or pathogenic family environments have been shown to occur commonly in these patients' backgrounds. As with major psychotic disorders, the need for caution in treatment and a regard for the complexity inherent to disorders in which there is a history of trauma must be emphasized. Not only is it true that not all those with severe character pathology have been traumatized; it is also neither always useful nor even desirable to focus on the traumatic history early on in treatment.

> One such case involved a patient with borderline personality disorder in her mid-30s who, despite a considerable and chronic level of distress, was actually quite functional by that time in her life. Appropriately, she sought psychotherapy for the first time and happened to land in the hands of a therapist who believed emphatically in working immediately with traumatic material. In short order this woman was, in her own words, a "basket case"; her long-standing job came into jeopardy, and her few solid relationships quickly dissipated. This patient simply could not deal with the level of anxiety, rage, and pain associated with the "trauma work" that was vigorously pursued by her well-meaning if overzealous therapist. It would have been better to defer detailed exploration until much later in the treatment, after the therapeutic alliance had solidified, so that the transference could help the patient better tolerate the work with such painful memories.

No single approach in general to borderline pathology is likely to dominate in today's climate, with its plethora of treatments. Individual and group psychotherapies each have their place; the orienting perspectives have become more pluralistic and commonly range at present between CBT and, with suitable modifications, psychodynamic approaches. In this context it is interesting to note the commentary of two of the most prolific clinical theoreticians of the treatment of borderline pathology. Neither Linehan (Linehan, Armstrong, Suarez, Allman, & Heard, 1991), who employs a CBT approach, nor Kernberg (1984), who uses a psychoanalytic one, discounts the role of trauma. In general, Linehan emphasizes its pathogenic potential more than Kernberg does. However, in their long-standing clinical and research experience with borderline personality disorder, neither views therapeutic work on abuse or other trauma as the first priority. Their positions reinforce the notion that working through traumatic experience ought to be part of the ongoing work with the basic pathology and should not be seen as distinct.

None of this is to suggest that the subject of trauma should be avoided. In fact, avoidance can have untoward effects, such as reinforcing a patient's feeling of shame and stigma. The issue for the clinician is when and how to bring up the subject. Gunderson and Chu (1993) have correctly noted that acknowledgment of the patient's victimization and empathy for the effects of early trauma on the person's life can serve to strengthen the therapeutic alliance. Reframing the patient's current problems as a consequence, in part, of childhood trauma can afford the individual much relief and pave the way for development of a sense of mastery. However, it is important to note that these constitute supportive maneuvers, not exploratory ones. They are usually done individually. The effect in a group is different, since the other members' reactions cannot be controlled and always contain some element of exploration (be that questioning, doubting, or merely underreacting).

One of us has observed a supportive, educational group used effectively early in treatment on an inpatient unit. These "trauma groups" for personality-disordered patients provided circumscribed instruction about trauma, yet discouraged the expression of high-intensity affect. The method was successful, particularly because it was conducted in a supportive and contained milieu.

Once patients with borderline personality disorder are stable and can tolerate long-term psychotherapy, group psychotherapy appears to offer certain advantages. Because of the social nature of trauma and its effect on interpersonal relationships, particularly impairing the development of intimacy in adulthood, group psychotherapy is suited to the task (Allen & Bloom, 1994; Nicholas & Forrester, 1999). Telling, understanding, and even achieving some mastery of the effects of trauma are not mutative in themselves. What is needed is exploration of the vicissitudes of attendant pathological relationships. A psychotherapy group is ideally suited to working on unconscious reenactments of the effects of trauma on relationships, as these are recapitulated in the transferences to the other members and the therapist (Ganzarain & Buchele, 1989; Tyson & Goodman, 1996). The therapist must be patient and let these patterns evolve over time in the course of treatment. They should never be forced. It takes time, and therapeutic benefit cannot be expected in a few months; it often takes a year or more before some progress is seen (Tyson & Goodman, 1996).

A more extended case example than those provided earlier illustrates some of the points already made and clearly demonstrates the unique value of group psychotherapy. The group session took place in a day hospital milieu program. Therefore, it was not the kind advocated for exploration and working out the intrapsychic manifestations of a personality disorder that has been affected by trauma. Yet it quite clearly shows how the social medium of the group is an ideal one for reenacting borderline pathology. In this case, the patient's use of self-justification and the degree of manipulation shown suggests the presence of antisocial features (Kernberg, 1984). The facts that the perpetrator was not a parent, that the abuse was short-lived, and that it did not include penetration suggest that the trauma was not as severe as the patient made it seem (Silk et al., 1995). Ironically, there was a second patient in the group who also had a history of incest, but hers occurred with a stepfather over some period of time. Even though that abuse was more severe, the second patient took a subordinate role in the session and supported the first. The dominance of the first patient again speaks to her facile, manipulative behavior.

The example demonstrates a particular aspect of the interpersonal relations of many patients with a history of sexual abuse. Having been "favorites," of a sort, of those family members with whom the incest occurred (Ganzarain & Buchele, 1989), in adulthood they seek the attention of parent surrogates and fantasize about gratifying them. In treatment, these efforts are directed toward therapists. In contrast, they may have rivalries with peers, who unconsciously represent siblings who could vie for that "favored" position. The family dynamics mesh with those of small groups as outlined by Freud (1921/1955) and were apparent in the session to be described here.

The focus of this example is on a 28-year-old, single woman, Miss Sandra Lee Child. She was referred to the day program after a brief hospitalization for suicidality; she had taken a minor overdose of medication in the presence of her roommate. Miss Child had borderline personality disorder with a long history of psychiatric treatment that included several hospitalizations. She had also had a series of psychotherapists. Her most recent therapist had elicited a history that her grandfather fondled her when she was 7 years old. This allegation of sexual abuse was confirmed by the parents, who admitted that they had often left her in his care and learned only years later that he had behaved inappropriately with several of his grandchildren. In retrospect, it was clear that at the time of the fondling, the grandfather had been showing early signs of cerebral vascular dementia. When this had occurred, the parents' marriage was in turmoil. The father had been having an extramarital affair; in response, the mother had threatened divorce. The accusations against the grandfather served to divert the family's attention away from the marital strife. In fact, the father subsequently gave up the affair, and the marriage was reconstituted.

The patient's previous psychotherapist was intrigued by the history of sexual abuse. She asked the patient whether she had ever had states of altered consciousness associated with uncharacteristic behavior. The patient responded positively to the therapist's suggestion and reported the presence of episodic, childlike patterns of behavior. The therapist, further fascinated by the patient's response, asked whether she thought that this state had a name. In compliance, the patient said, "Her name is Sarah." The therapist was thus convinced that the patient had multiple personality disorder (now known as dissociative identity disorder). At the time of the session to be described, the diagnosis was still in question for the staff members at the day hospital. They were still captivated, so to speak, by the patient's dramatic presentations on the unit. Only later, when the patient allegedly developed many more "personalities," did it become clear that these symptoms were part of a histrionic pattern of manipulative behavior. In retrospect, it seemed that the eagerness of the previous therapist had induced dissociative phenomena.

The psychotherapy group at the day hospital was conducted by two psychiatric residents, one of whom was on vacation for the week. At the morning community meeting, the unit chief announced that the psychiatric residents would be leaving the service in 4 weeks. These circumstances accentuated the feelings of emotional deprivation that patients already had by virtue of their psychopathology. In addition, the day before this session, Miss Child had had an episode of childlike, hysterical crying that became a focus of concern and absorbed much of the staff's attention, thereby depriving others.

There were seven patients in the group. Two others of note are now briefly described. Mr. Coke was a 36-year-old single man from an impoverished neighborhood in which there was a high crime rate and where substance misuse was prevalent. He had a schizophrenic-spectrum disorder, which was complicated by cocaine abuse. Mrs. Fragile was a 32-year-old married woman with mixed dependent and histrionic personality disorder, or what used to be called infantile personality disorder. She too had reported a history of incestuous abuse: She had described being sexually involved with her stepfather during her early teens. As an adult, she had had chaotic relations with men who abused her. She had been married for the last 2 years to a very kind, conscientious man from whom she demanded inordinate attention. While in the day hospital, she telephoned him several times each day. One day prior to the group session, he had appeared on the unit with some flowers for her. When he tried to leave, she began to cry in an uncontrolled manner. He had been unable to leave until a staff member restrained her.

At the outset of the group session, Miss Child expressed concern about the rotation (i.e., the pending change of therapists). She had no thought about the departing therapists, but rather was concerned about who her new therapist would be. Concurrently, she denied that she had given the matter much thought, because she had been upset about other (unspecified) matters. The therapist then asked the other group members how they felt about the change in therapists, noting that some patients would be changing individual therapists, that all would have new group therapists, and that her cotherapist would return from vacation on Monday.

Mrs. Fragile reported that she was pleased that the cotherapist (who was also her individual therapist) would be returning soon; the covering therapist had not had sufficient time for her. Another patient said that she did not mind that her therapist was away, especially since she would be discharged on Tuesday. The therapist noted that others would be discharged soon, and inquired how members might feel with fewer patients in the day hospital. Miss Child thereupon dismissed the inquiry by minimizing the effect that the discharges would have.

Mrs. Fragile began to complain about her medication. She reported that it was overly sedating and said that her doctor (the vacationing group leader) had prescribed medication that she did not need. Miss Child responded to her in a comforting manner, noting that the medication controlled her (Mrs. Fragile's) mood swings. Mrs. Fragile persisted with her complaint, and so Miss Child proceeded to document the ways in which her moodiness was at times excessive. She noted how unreasonable Mrs. Fragile had been when her husband visited and brought her flowers. Other group members joined Miss Child in confronting Mrs. Fragile. The latter persisted in her denial and began to cry. She stated that she was too upset to discuss the incident further and wanted to leave the session. She got up to leave, but was soothed by the intervention of the therapist, who noted that the members cared about her and were trying to help.

The group leader then turned to Mr. Coke, noting that this was to be his last session, as he would be discharged early the next day. She invited him to address the group members. Mr. Coke said that he appreciated the help he had received at the program, and spoke of being much improved. Yet, as he spoke, he clearly indicated that he was anxious about the future. He was unsure how he would spend his day without a full-time program. The group members encouraged him to be active and gave suggestions. Yet Mr. Coke remained anxious. He then began to talk in a somewhat stilted but quasi-philosophical way about the day hospital. He spoke of its mix of patients and compared it to the ethnically diverse neighborhood in which he lived. (It should be noted that the group leader was born in Eastern Europe and that the vacationing therapist was Asian American.) He said that he had once felt isolated in his neighborhood, and then segued to complaining about the adolescents on the unit. The therapist, recognizing the transference implications of what Mr. Coke had said, tried to encourage further discussion by group members. She asked how they felt about the age differences and the ethnic differences among patients on the unit. However, the group members were unable to respond in a meaningful way. Several said that it was not a problem for them. One spoke about the benefits he received from his medication. Anxiety in the group appeared to spread. Mr. Coke began to talk about his fears of relapse and asked, in a pleading manner, whom he should call if he should again develop symptoms.

Just then Mrs. Fragile began to laugh. The therapist inquired what seemed funny at that moment. She said that "Sandra Lee" (Miss Child) was smiling in a way that was amusing. At this point, everyone turned to Miss Child. (This appeared to organize the group and dissipated the transference anxiety.) One patient asked her, "Are you Sandra Lee or Sarah?," referring to the alter ego. Miss Child responded, "Sarah!" The therapist, evoking a treatment care plan, said, "You [Sarah] promised to stay in the foyer and not come into group meetings." Miss Child nodded, fluttered her eyelashes, and appeared to discard the childlike manner that she had just assumed. With this, the tension in the group seemed to subside.

The therapist asked Miss Child to explain what had just happened to her, noting that it would be confusing to those who were unfamiliar with her situation. Miss Child proceeded to tell the members about her alter ego, Sarah, who was 7 years old (the age at which Miss Child's grandfather had sexually abused her). She used this to explain her demanding, childlike behavior at the day hospital, and furthermore to claim that she should not be held accountable for her disruptive actions on the unit. There was a lengthy discussion of her "split personality" by the therapist and some of the group members. However, one member, who did not join in the discussion, repeatedly stated that the air in the room was stifling and that he could not breathe well. Another became restless; she stood up, paced, and left the room for a few moments, ostensibly to get a drink of water. Mrs. Fragile was the most empathic and said that she understood Miss Child because she too had been sexually abused as a youngster. She claimed that this was why she was anxious when she was not with her husband, and why she had cried when he left after delivering the flowers.

The man who complained of difficulty breathing asked the two women whether they felt hatred toward those who abused them. Miss Child reported that she felt that way toward her mother for allegedly not protecting her from the grandfather. She also felt hatred toward her 20-month-old niece (i.e., her mother's only grandchild). In fact, there were times when she felt an urge to abuse the niece as she had been abused. That, she believed, would serve as retaliation against her mother. Miss Child reported that guilt over such feelings accounted for her suicidality.

It was near the end of the session, so the therapist asked group members whether they had other reactions that they wished to share. Mrs. Fragile said that she felt better as a result of the session. She said, "If we don't talk and only keep it inside, we might become violent." The therapist, noting that earlier Mrs. Fragile had almost left the session, told her that it was of benefit that she had stayed and that the session had been productive for all. With this, the session ended.

The process in this session, to a large degree, was dominated by the transference. The announcement of the change of therapists undoubtedly triggered transference reactions in the patients. The absence of the cotherapist augmented these feelings. For much of the time, the patients struggled with attendant feelings of abandonment. These were expressed through displays of neediness and through discussion about discharges. The issues in the session were manifested around themes of inclusion and flight. When Mr. Coke reflected on his stay at the day hospital, the feelings of loss and abandonment were accentuated. There was a chance that these would emerge in expressions of a negative transference. That was too frightening for the patients; instead, Miss Child absorbed the projections, so to speak, and became the focus of attention. This served to diffuse the tension in the transference and gratified her need for attention. This dynamic of absorbing conflicts within the group (as she had done in her family of origin) and deflecting attention from a transference figure (analogous to her father, in a narrow sense, and her parents in general) reflected a reenactment of an unconscious object relations pattern from childhood. Dynamically, she once again became the fantasized "favorite" in the group; she got attention from everyone, which she craved, and rescued the therapist from attack.

This example demonstrates the vicissitudes of borderline dynamics associated with a history of abuse. These were complicated by the presence of manipulative behavior on the part of Miss Child. Of course, patients with borderline personality disorder pose many of the same special problems for group therapists as they do for individual ones. The risks include such displays of manipulativeness, as well as tendencies to acting out and self-destructiveness—traits that may be stimulated by the intensity of any expressive therapy for these patients. Levels of emotional intensity are sometimes less capable of being titrated in a group than in individual therapy, but in our experience, skilled direction by group leaders and supervisors make such risks much less problematic.

When manipulative conduct reflects outright antisocial tendencies, the prognosis is worse. When frank antisocial personality disorder is present, a less optimistic scenario can generally be predicted for group psychotherapeutic treatment. Although it was previously assumed that rates of traumatic backgrounds in patients with antisocial personality disorder were somewhat lower than in patients with borderline personality disorder, numerous studies over the years have proven that the former patients have often been emotionally, sexually, and especially physically abused (e.g., Herman, Perry, & van der Kolk, 1989; Zanarini, Gunderson, Marino, Schwartz, & Frankenburg, 1989).

In general, patients with antisocial personality disorder do not tolerate being made to feel too vulnerable, so that constructive discussion of their traumatic histories among peers is often difficult. Characterologically, they often skirt the issue and their painful affects in group settings, if indeed they agree to any treatment at all. Their characteristic dishonesty and manipulativeness often make them poor group members in general. Moreover, these patients frequently attempt to turn the group against the leader or try to control and deflect the discussion in an attempt to gratify their narcissistic needs. For this reason, most clinicians have had to exclude patients with antisocial personality disorder from psychotherapeutic groups.

In order for any depth treatment to work, patients with antisocial personality disorder generally need a firm "container," such as a therapeutic community or some ideal prison settings. Those groups are better organized along peer confrontational lines. This is similar to what is advocated for individuals with chronic substance addictions, as we note below. If such groups are properly conducted, it is sometimes surprisingly poignant how well the discussions of a sensitive subject such as abuse or other trauma can proceed.

Less has been said here about patients with other types of personality disorders, because they usually present fewer problems in group psychotherapy and because their rates of abuse and other trauma, though not trivial, appear to be lower. Those with histrionic and narcissistic personality disorders are among the best group candidates for exploration of traumatic histories. The entitlement and grandiosity of the former and the emotional displays of the latter stand in bold relief in a psychotherapy group, making these characteristics ripe for exploration. Although this is admittedly a generalization, patients with schizotypal, paranoid, and schizoid personality disorders seem less well suited to group sessions focused on trauma, given how tenuous and fragile their relationships to fellow group members usually are. With such patients, like those with major psychotic disorders, individualized treatment plans and flexibility in discussing histories of abuse or other trauma seem warranted.

ALCOHOL AND OTHER
SUBSTANCE USE DISORDERS

The final group of abused or otherwise traumatized individuals to be discussed consists of those with alcohol and other substance use problems. There are literally millions of individuals in these diagnostic categories, as in the first two groupings discussed in this chapter. By recent estimates, there are probably about 30 million individuals in the United States who seriously misuse alcohol or other drugs; excluding alcohol, 14 million people over the age of 12 use nonprescribed mood-altering substances at least once a week (National Institute on Drug Abuse, 1991; Substance Abuse and Mental Health Services Administration, 1995).

There is, of course, much overlap between this class of patients and both of the first two groups we have described. Such "dual diagnoses" are quite common and, it is fair to surmise, may be especially prevalent among substance users with abuse or other trauma in their backgrounds. The principles already enunciated for treating psychotic, severe mood, and personality disorders obviously apply to these conditions as well.

Since patients with substance use problems are such a heterogeneous group, once again it is treacherous to generalize. Nevertheless, some basic guidelines—first, with respect to stabilization—seem pertinent. Obviously, a proper psychiatric assessment and medical stabilization are the first priorities. Treatable medical or psychiatric symptoms, including withdrawal risks, must be vigorously addressed. Only when a patient is stabilized and sober can more sophisticated group treatment begin and the issues of abuse or other trauma be addressed. As further insurance, the majority of these patients will benefit from traditional Twelve-Step group programs (where trauma is usually not addressed). The group support and pressures—including confrontation by peers, as well as the host of other therapeutic factors intrinsic to these groups—play a critical role in allowing patients to remain sober so that they can proceed with psychological growth in traditional psychotherapies. In fact, because of their experience in Twelve-Step groups, many of these individuals are often more comfortable in a psychotherapy group than other patients and more willing to reveal personal details of their histories to peers.

It is only well after sobriety is achieved that addressing abuse or other trauma becomes feasible. Once stabilized, a majority of such patients can benefit from group psychotherapy. Yet, as noted earlier, those substance-misusing patients with very paranoid and/or sociopathic orientations will be unsuitable for outpatient group psychotherapy.

As in any well-functioning group, discussion of trauma is inevitable for those so afflicted, but can be of benefit to the other members too. Although there may be a role for circumscribed and time-limited "trauma groups" early in treatment, such an approach seems to have limited applicability with this population. The commonality of substance use problems seems more compelling for these patients and becomes the single factor that facilitates group bonding. The history of trauma takes a secondary position and only emerges later, during more advanced phases of group development.

The following clinical example came from a psychodynamically oriented psychotherapeutic group—one somewhat unusual in nature, in that (1) it consisted exclusively of alcoholics and (2) it had a stable population of about 10 members for 8 years. All these patients had been initially treated on an inpatient detoxification unit and then agreed to join the group; all were simultaneously in Alcoholics Anonymous (AA).

Issues of abuse and other trauma, though never a prolonged focus of the group, nevertheless surfaced frequently. Six of the members had histories of moderate to severe abuse, predominantly verbal and physical, and in two cases sexual as well. Generally, as expected, the abuse came at the hands of alcoholic or drug-addicted parents. Validation by sharing and comparing their respective experiences seemed therapeutic in itself. Recognizing the commonality of having turned to drink to deal with (at least in part) the rage and disappointment engendered by such mistreatment seemed to create an intense bond between the members, even for those who were not abused. Airing the issue seemed to facilitate other members' ability to talk of disappointing and more mildly "traumatic" events in their own backgrounds.

The patients continually struggled with the tension between the effects of abusive experiences and the perceived personal responsibility for their alcoholism. This struggle mirrored that often experienced by abused patients with borderline personality disorder as they attempt to explain their pathology to themselves. Perhaps because of the emphasis in AA on not allowing one's historical burdens to serve as "excuses," the group under discussion here seemed to be able to separate the actual abuse experience from any self-justification more readily than most patients with borderline personality disorder seem to do. One particularly intense session illustrates this dynamic. The following exchange occurred after the newest patient in the group, Adam, had temporarily relapsed over the previous week. Feeling embarrassed and upset, for the first time he shared his history of physical mistreatment at the hands of a sadistic stepfather:

BOB: Don't use that as no b.s. excuse.

ADAM: You know they always tell you in the program [i.e., AA] not to let your past make you feel sorry for yourself . . . but I think I've never allowed myself to feel the pain at all. I get confused.

CARL: Welcome to the club. Both things are true. You gotta feel it, you gotta deal with it . . . we go over in our heads this stuff all the time, believe me. (*To Bob*) You know we're not in the program here. You gotta see both sides. I don't mind you telling him like it is, but don't be afraid to show some humanity, man.

BOB: AA teaches humanity too. I just think we can't let him think this is a group for mama's boys.

A productive dialogue ensued about whether the present group and the members' respective AA groups would have any differences in philosophy about acknowledging abuse. The general consensus emerged that there are no real contradictions, just differences of emphasis. In the process, the leader pointed out how the use of splitting mechanisms—idealizing one of the groups at the expense of the other—was a frequent theme in recent sessions. The following dialogue then ensued:

DAVE: Let's face it. None of us like to talk of this stuff [i.e., abuse]. It makes us all feel weak, like babies ... maybe I would have said "mama's boys," like Bob, but that makes me *really* uncomfortable.

CARL: Look, it's the $64,000 question: Why are we here? Yeah, we gotta be able to share the pain—to talk of this stuff without feeling we're wimps or weak sisters. That's what I gotta say to you. Adam, let's hear your story ... believe me, we've *all* got one.

This example illustrates how problematic the discussion of abuse can be, especially for men, but also how conducive a truly supportive group atmosphere can be to facilitating its exposure. Males tend to perceive histories of abuse as castrating and shameful. For these members, the group seemed of enormous help in fostering the atmosphere of mutual revelation so critical to the success of effective psychotherapy. Certainly, their long-standing commitment to one another played an important part in assuring them that exposure would be safe.

The recommendation to consider dynamically oriented psychotherapy groups for patients with serious substance addictions must be qualified in one sense. The main caveat is to guard against inclusion of individuals with frank antisocial personality disorder. This risk is a rare one, however, because a truly antisocial individual rarely accepts dynamically oriented treatment. Many of those patients can and should be treated via peer confrontation, in the restricted types of group treatment environments recommended earlier.

CONCLUDING REMARKS

Abused and other traumatized individuals with the disorders discussed throughout this chapter represent an enormous and undertreated group of patients. We hope that this chapter has brought some order to a vastly heterogeneous field. Presented here are guidelines, albeit rough ones, for addressing these populations. Abuse and other forms of trauma are therapeutic foci that always require both special sensitivity and caution on the part of clinicians, especially in dealing with individuals early in treatment.

Attention to the therapeutic setting of the group is critical. Select inpatient units (especially longer-term ones) and day hospitals can sometimes allow clinicians to start encouraging exploration of traumatic issues with a level of safety and supervision that is less possible in outpatient treatments. Conversely, hospital units often contain decompensated patients who are unsuitable for such a focus until they are stabilized and truly settled into a clinic. In today's health care environment, clinicians engaged with such patients must be very cognizant of the complexities involved. They must be comfortable actively working and communicating with the various mental health professionals on a multimodality team. They must also carefully titrate the level of intensity devoted to the exploration of abuse or other trauma—remaining well aware, for instance, of such factors as phase of the treatment, individualized selection criteria, availability of backup resources, and knowledge of the level of skill and experience of other team members.

There are both risks and rewards in working with traumatized individuals with clinical, personality, or substance use disorders. The harvest is great, but skilled laborers are too few.

REFERENCES

Allen, S. N., & Bloom, S. L. (1994). Group and family treatment of post-traumatic stress disorder. *Psychiatric Clinics of North America, 17,* 425–437.

American Psychiatric Association (APA). (1980). *Diagnostic and statistical manual of mental disorders* (3rd ed.). Washington, DC: Author.

Beck, J. C., & van der Kolk. B. (1987). Reports of childhood incest and current behavior of chronically hospitalized psychotic women. *American Journal of Psychiatry, 144,* 1474–1476.

Breuer, J., & Freud, S. (1955). Studies on hysteria. In J. Strachey (Ed. and Trans.), *The standard edition of the complete psychological works of Sigmund Freud* (Vol. 2, pp. 1–305). London: Hogarth Press. (Original work published 1893–1895)

Bryer, J. B., Nelson, B. A., Miller, J. B., & Krol, P. A. (1987). Childhood sexual and physical abuse as factors in adult psychiatric illness. *American Journal of Psychiatry, 144,* 1426–1430.

Carmen, E., Ricker, P., & Mills, T. (1984). Victims of violence and psychiatric illness. *American Journal of Psychiatry, 141,* 378–383.

Chazan, R. (1993). Group analytic therapy with schizophrenic outpatients. *Group, 17,* 164–178.

Clarkin, J. F., Hull, J., Yeomans, F., Kakuma, T., & Cantor, J. (1994). Antisocial traits as modifiers of treatment response in borderline patients. *Journal of Psychotherapy Research and Practice, 3,* 307–312.

Dobson, D. J. G., McDougall, G., Busheikin, J., & Aldous, J. (1995). Effects of social skills training and social milieu treatment on symptoms of schizophrenia. *Psychiatric Services, 46,* 376–380.

Douglas, M. S., & Mueser, K. T. (1990). Teaching conflict resolution skills to the chronically ill. *Behavior Modification, 14,* 519–547.

Freud, S. (1955). Group psychology and the analysis of the ego. In J. Strachey (Ed. and Trans.), *The standard edition of the complete psychological works of Sigmund Freud* (Vol. 18, pp. 65–144). London: Hogarth Press. (Original work published 1921)

Freud, S. (1962). The aetiology of hysteria. In J. Strachey (Ed. and Trans.), *The standard edition of the complete psychological works of Sigmund Freud* (Vol. 3, pp. 189–221). London: Hogarth Press. (Original work published 1896)

Gallagher, R. (1994). Stages of group psychotherapy supervision: A model for supervising beginning trainees of dynamic group therapy. *International Journal of Group Psychotherapy, 44*(2), 171–185.

Gallagher, R., Flye, B., & Hurt, S. (1999). *Severity of abuse and trauma in the backgrounds of psychiatric patients.* Manuscript in preparation.

Gallagher, R., Flye, B., Hurt, S., Stone, M., & Hull, J. (1992). Retrospective Assessment of Traumatic Experiences (RATE). *Journal of Personality Disorders, 6*(2), 99–108.

Gallagher, R., & Nazarian, J. (1995). A comprehensive cognitive-behavioral/educational program for schizophrenic patients. *Bulletin of the Menninger Clinic, 59*(3), 357–371.

Ganzarain, R., & Buchele, B. J. (1989). *Fugitives of incest.* Madison, CT: International Universities Press.

Gay, P. (1988). *Freud: A life for our times.* New York: Norton.

Gunderson, J. G., & Chu, J. A. (1993). Treatment implications of past trauma in borderline personality disorder. *Harvard Review of Psychiatry, 1,* 75–81.

Hazard, A., Roger, J. H., & Angert, L. (1993). Factors affecting group therapy outcome for adult sexual abuse survivors. *International Journal of Group Psychotherapy, 43,* 453–466.

Herman, J. L. (1986). History of violence in an outpatient population. *American Journal of Orthopsychiatry, 56,* 137–141.

Herman, J. L., Perry, J. C., & van der Kolk, B. (1989). Childhood trauma in borderline personality disorder. *American Journal of Psychiatry, 146,* 490–495.

Jacobson, A., & Herald, C. (1990). The relevance of childhood sexual abuse to adult psychiatric inpatient care. *Hospital and Community Psychiatry, 41,* 154–156.

Jones, E. (1961). *The life and work of Sigmund Freud.* New York: Basic Books.

Kanas, N. (1986). Group psychotherapy with schizophrenics: Controlled studies. *International Journal of Group Psychotherapy, 36,* 339–351.

Kanas, N. (1996). *Group therapy for schizophrenic patients.* Washington, DC: American Psychiatric Press.

Kanas, N. (1999). Research reviews: Group therapy for patients with chronic psychotic disorders. *International Journal of Group Psychotherapy, 49,* 413–416.

Kernberg, O. (1984). *Severe personality disorders: Psychotherapeutic strategies.* New Haven, CT: Yale University Press.

Kibel, H. D. (1981). A conceptual model for short-term inpatient group psychotherapy. *American Journal of Psychiatry, 138,* 74–80.

Kibel, H. D. (1991). The therapeutic use of splitting: The role of the mother-group in therapeutic differentiation and practicing. In S. Tuttman (Ed.), *Psychoanalytic group theory and therapy: Essays in honor of Saul Scheidlinger* (pp. 113–132). Madison, CT: International Universities Press.

Kibel, H. D. (1992). The clinical application of object relations theory. In H. Bernard, R. Klein, & D. Singer (Eds.), *Handbook of contemporary group psychotherapy: Contributions from object relations, self psychology, and social systems theories* (pp. 144–176). Madison, CT: International Universities Press.

Leff, J., Kuipers, L., Berkowitz, R., & Sturgeon, D. (1985). A controlled trial of social intervention in the families of schizophrenic patients: Two-year follow-up. *British Journal of Psychiatry, 146,* 594–600.

Linehan, M., Armstrong, H., Suarez, A., Allman, D., & Heard, H. (1991). Cognitive-behavioral treatment of chronically parasuicidal borderline patients. *Archives of General Psychiatry, 48,* 1060–1064.

National Institute on Drug Abuse. (1991). *National Household Survey on Drug Abuse: Highlights.* Washington, DC: U.S. Government Printing Office.

Nicholas, M., & Forrester, A. (1999). Advantages of heterogeneous therapy groups in the psychotherapy of the traumatically abused: Treating the problem as well as the person. *International Journal of Group Psychotherapy, 49,* 323–342.

Ogata, S. N., Silk, K. R., Goodrich, S., Lohr, N. E., Westen, D., & Hill, E. M. (1990). Childhood sexual and physical abuse in adult patients with borderline personality disorder. *American Journal of Psychiatry, 147,* 1008–1012.

Scharff, J., & Scharff, D. (1994). *Object relations therapy of physical and sexual trauma.* Northvale, NJ: Aronson.

Silk, K. R., Lee, S., Hill, E. M., & Lohr, N. E. (1995). Borderline personality disorder symptoms and severity of sexual abuse. *American Journal of Psychiatry, 152,* 1059–1064.

Skolnick, M. R. (1999). Psychosis from a group perspective. In V. L. Schermer & M. Pines (Eds.), *Group psychotherapy of the psychoses: Concepts, interventions and contexts* (pp. 43–82). London: Kingsley.

Stone, M. H. (1990). *The fate of borderline patients: Successful outcome and psychiatric practice.* New York: Guilford Press.

Stone, M. H., Kahn, E., & Flye, B. (1981). Psychiatrically ill relatives of borderline patients: A family study. *Psychiatric Quarterly, 53,* 71–84.

Stone, W. N. (1996). *Group psychotherapy for people with chronic mental illness.* New York: Guilford Press.

Substance Abuse and Mental Health Services Administration, Office of Applied Studies. (1995). *Preliminary estimates from the 1995 National Household Survey on Drug Abuse.* Washington, DC: U.S. Government Printing Office.

Tyson, A. A., & Goodman, M. (1996). Group treatment for adult women who experienced childhood sexual trauma: Is telling the story enough? *International Journal of Group Psychotherapy, 46,* 535–542.

van der Kolk, B., & Saporta, J. (1991). The biological response to psychic trauma:

Mechanisms and treatment of intrusion and numbing. *Anxiety Research, 4,* 199–212.

Westen, D., Ludolph, P., Misle, B., Ruffins, S., & Block, J. (1990). Physical and sexual abuse in adolescent girls with borderline personality disorder. *American Journal of Orthopsychiatry, 60,* 55–66.

Zanarini, M. C., Gunderson, J. G., Marino, M. F., Schwartz, E. O., & Frankenburg, F. R. (1989). Childhood experiences of borderline patients. *Comprehensive Psychiatry, 30,* 18–25.

Index